Handbook of Intensive Care

Handbook of Intensive Care

Edited by Camilia Brooks

hayle medical

New York

Hayle Medical,
750 Third Avenue, 9th Floor,
New York, NY 10017, USA

Visit us on the World Wide Web at:
www.haylemedical.com

This book contains information obtained from authentic and highly regarded sources. Copyright for all individual chapters remain with the respective authors as indicated. All chapters are published with permission under the Creative Commons Attribution License or equivalent. A wide variety of references are listed. Permission and sources are indicated; for detailed attributions, please refer to the permissions page and list of contributors. Reasonable efforts have been made to publish reliable data and information, but the authors, editors and publisher cannot assume any responsibility for the validity of all materials or the consequences of their use.

ISBN: 978-1-63241-829-6

Trademark Notice: Registered trademark of products or corporate names are used only for explanation and identification without intent to infringe.

Cataloging-in-Publication Data

Handbook of intensive care / edited by Camilia Brooks.
p. cm.
Includes bibliographical references and index.
ISBN 978-1-63241-829-6
1. Critical care medicine. 2. Emergency medicine. 3. Intensive care units. I. Brooks, Camilia.
RC86.7 .H36 2020
616.028--dc23

Table of Contents

Preface

The diagnosis and management of various life-threatening conditions require sophisticated care and life support, as well as intensive monitoring. Such care is under the scope of intensive care medicine. Lethal cardiac arrhythmias, acute renal failure, multiple organ failure, cardiovascular instability and airway or respiratory compromise are some of the conditions that require intensive care. Serious infections such as severe pneumonia or sepsis, lethal short-term conditions like a heart attack or stroke, and major accidents also qualify for intensive care. Various equipment may be used in an intensive care unit or facility, such as a ventilator, monitoring equipment for assessing blood pressure, heart rate and oxygen levels in blood, feeding tubes, etc. This book aims to shed light on some of the unexplored aspects of intensive care and the recent researches in this field. Most of the topics introduced herein cover new techniques and the applications of intensive care medicine and support. For all those who are interested in this field, this book can prove to be an essential guide.

The information shared in this book is based on empirical researches made by veterans in this field of study. The elaborative information provided in this book will help the readers further their scope of knowledge leading to advancements in this field.

Finally, I would like to thank my fellow researchers who gave constructive feedback and my family members who supported me at every step of my research.

Editor

The association between FABP7 serum levels with survival and neurological complications in acetaminophen-induced acute liver failure

Constantine J. Karvellas[1]* ⓘ, Jaime L. Speiser[2], Mélanie Tremblay[3], William M. Lee[4], Christopher F. Rose[3] and For the US Acute Liver Failure Study Group

Abstract

Background: Acetaminophen (APAP)-induced acute liver failure (ALF) is associated with significant mortality due to intracranial hypertension (ICH), a result of cerebral edema (CE) and astrocyte swelling. Brain-type fatty acid-binding protein (FABP7) is a small (15 kDa) cytoplasmic protein abundantly expressed in astrocytes. The aim of this study was to determine whether serum FABP7 levels early (day 1) or late (days 3–5) level were associated with 21-day mortality and/or the presence of ICH/CE in APAP-ALF patients.

Methods: Serum samples from 198 APAP-ALF patients (nested case–control study with 99 survivors and 99 non-survivors) were analyzed by ELISA methods and assessed with clinical data from the US Acute Liver Failure Study Group (ALFSG) Registry (1998–2014).

Results: APAP-ALF survivors had significantly lower serum FABP7 levels on admission (147.9 vs. 316.5 ng/ml, $p = 0.0002$) and late (87.3 vs. 286.2 ng/ml, $p < 0.0001$) compared with non-survivors. However, a significant association between 21-day mortality and increased serum FABP7 early [log FABP7 odds ratio (OR) 1.16, $p = 0.32$] and late (log FABP7 ~ OR 1.34, $p = 0.21$) was not detected after adjusting for significant covariates (MELD, vasopressor use). Areas under the receiver-operating curve for early and late multivariable models were 0.760 and 0.892, respectively. In a second analysis, patients were grouped based on the presence ($n = 46$) or absence ($n = 104$) of ICH/CE. A significant difference in FABP7 levels between patients with or without ICH/CE at early (259.7 vs. 228.2 ng/ml, $p = 0.61$) and late (223.8 vs. 192.0 ng/ml, $p = 0.19$) time points was not identified.

Conclusion: Serum FABP7 levels were significantly elevated at early and late time points in APAP-ALF non-survivors compared to survivors. However, significant differences in FABP7 levels by 21-day mortality were not ascertained after adjusting for significant covariates (reflecting severity of illness). Our study suggests that FABP7 may not discriminate between patients with or without intracranial complications.

Keywords: Liver-type fatty acid-binding protein, Multiorgan failure, Prognosis, ALFSG index

Background

Acute liver failure (ALF) is defined by the occurrence of hepatic encephalopathy (HE) and hepatic synthetic dysfunction within 26 weeks of the first symptoms of liver disease [1]. Severe coagulopathy, encephalopathy and hemodynamic instability contribute to a picture of multiorgan failure. Currently, the most common cause of ALF in North America is acetaminophen (APAP) [2]. Particularly in APAP-induced ALF, cerebral edema (CE) and intracranial hypertension (ICH) are major causes of morbidity and mortality [3]. The pathogenesis for ICH

*Correspondence: dean.karvellas@ualberta.ca
[1] Division of Gastroenterology (Liver Unit), Department of Critical Care Medicine, University of Alberta, 1-40 Zeidler Ledcor Building, Edmonton, AB T6G-2X8, Canada

and CE in ALF is not fully understood, but astrocyte swelling causing cellular dysfunction as well as increased cerebral blood flow is believed to be implicated [4]. The degree of hyperammonemia has been demonstrated to be associated with ICH [5]. Ammonia, as a gas (NH_3) and ion (NH_4^+), freely crosses the blood–brain barrier and is primarily removed by glutamine synthetase, an enzyme solely found in astrocytes within the brain [6]. Glutamine synthetase catalyzes the amidation of glutamate to glutamine that subsequently leads to hyperosmotic changes and astrocyte swelling. However, studies have shown that hyperammonemia alone does not predict ICH [7].

Given the challenges presented in managing critically ill ALF patients with potential CE/ICH including the consideration for liver transplant (LT), the development of a noninvasive biomarker with the potential to predict ICH would be of great value, especially given the significant bleeding risks of invasive intracranial pressure monitoring in these coagulopathic patients [8].

Fatty acid-binding proteins (FABP) are small (15 kDa) cytoplasmic proteins that are abundantly expressed in tissues with active fatty acid metabolism, such as brain and liver. The primary function of FABPs is the intracellular transport of long-chain fatty acids [9]. The cellular expression of FABPs is responsive to changes in lipid metabolism, which can be induced during pathophysiological conditions, such as ischemia/inflammation or pharmacological stimuli [10]. Brain-type FABP (FABP7) is solely expressed in brain, exclusively in astrocytes [11]. Previous investigations have shown serum levels of FABP7 to be elevated in patients with various neurological diseases including stroke [12] and dementia [13]. While our group recently demonstrated the prognostic value of serum levels of liver-type FABP (FABP1) in ALF, to date FABP7 as a biomarker for the risk of ICH in ALF has not been investigated [14].

This nested case–control study of randomly selected samples from prospectively enrolled patients from the US Acute Liver Failure Study Group (ALFSG) registry aimed to examine levels of FABP7 in APAP-ALF patients. Specifically, our primary objectives were to test the following hypotheses

(a) Higher FABP7 serum levels are significantly associated with 21-day transplant-free mortality (in the absence of transplant) after adjusting for other significant covariates (Analysis 1).

(b) Elevated serum levels of FABP7 in APAP-ALF are significantly associated with ICH/CE after adjusting for other significant covariates (Analysis 2).

Methods

This study is a nested case–control study of prospectively collected data and biosamples of 198 patients enrolled in the US ALFSG registry/biorepository and is outlined in detail in Additional file 1: Figure S1. Between January 1998 and December 2014, 1027 APAP-ALF patients were enrolled in the registry from which 704 patients were alive at day 21 in the absence of LT. We identified 124 survivors with early and late serum samples from which 99 were randomly selected for analysis. Of 224 patients who died in the absence of LT, 87 patients with early and late samples were also included in this analysis. A further 12 patients with exclusively an early sample (of a possible 92) were randomly selected for inclusion in this analysis. Personnel not involved in the analysis of the samples or statistical analysis for the paper performed random selection of patients. All enrolling centers were tertiary academic centers, and all but one were LT centers. The authors' Institutional Review Board (IRB)/Health research ethics boards of all enrolling US ALFSG sites have approved all research, and all clinical investigation has been conducted according to the principles expressed in the 1975 Declaration of Helsinki. Given patients were unable to provide written consent (critical illness, HE), written assent was obtained from the next of kin from each patient. Each center implemented monitoring and therapeutic interventions according to institutional standards of care. Reporting of the analysis of this study followed the STROBE Guidelines for reporting case–control studies [15]. Consistent with ALFSG studies [16], the primary outcome (Analysis 1) was 21-day LT-free survival (no patients included in the analysis received LT). Secondary outcome (Analysis 2) was the development of ICH/CE.

Participants

Inclusion criteria were: (1) evidence of ALF according to the enrollment criteria for the ALFSG (see operational definitions); (2) age ≥ 18 years; (3) HE during the first seven days of study admission (West Haven Criteria) [17]; and (4) patients within the ALFSG registry with primary diagnoses of APAP determined by the site investigator. *Exclusion criteria* were: (1) cirrhosis/acute-on chronic liver failure; (2) patients without a primary diagnosis of APAP; and (3) patients who received a LT. Serum samples were analyzed on study admission (early; day 1) and late (either day 3, 4 or 5) where available. Patients who received a LT *were excluded from our study* because listing for transplant is a clinical decision, which is not standardized among ALFSG sites. A further 51 healthy controls were analyzed (University of Alberta) for FABP7 only.

Operational definitions

For the purposes of this study, ALF was defined as INR ≥ 1.5 and HE within the first 26 weeks of liver disease in a patient with an acute hepatic insult [18]. HE coma grade was defined by the West Haven Criteria (simplified) as follows: grade 1 ~ any alteration in mentation, grade 2 being somnolent or obtunded but easily rousable or presence of asterixis, grade 3 being rousable with difficulty, and grade 4 being unresponsive to deep pain [17]. In this study, we defined 'low coma grade' as grade 1 or 2 and 'high coma grade' as grade 3 or 4. The KCC [19] predicts poor outcome (death/transplant) if: (a) pH is less than 7.3 or (b) if INR is greater than 6.5, creatinine is greater than 3.4 mg/dl, and coma grade is high (3 or 4). The model for end-stage liver disease (MELD) is defined as $10*(0.957*\log(4) + 0.378*\log(\text{bilirubin}) + 1.12*\log(\text{INR}))$ for dialyzed patients and $10*(0.957*\log(\text{creatinine}) + 0.378*\log(\text{bilirubin}) + 1.12*\log(\text{INR}))$ for patients not dialyzed [20].

Laboratory Assays of FABP7

FABP7 was measured in serum samples with a solid-phase enzyme-linked immunosorbent assay (ELISA) following manufacturer's instructions (Biomatik, USA). Briefly, samples were incubated 2 h on a monoclonal anti-FABP7 pre-coated plate. A specific FABP7 biotin-conjugated polyclonal antibody solution was added for 2 h. After washing plates, avidin conjugated to horseradish peroxidase was added for 30 min. Finally, substrate tetramethylbenzidine was added for 15 min. Reactions were stopped by addition of sulfuric acid, and absorbance was read at 450 nm. Standard curve ranges from 0.47 to 30 ng/ml. Samples were performed in duplicate and accepted valid with a variation coefficient less than 25%.

Statistical methods aim one: FABP7 and 21-day survival in APAP-ALF

For differences between outcome groups (APAP-ALF survivors, $n = 99$, APAP-ALF non-survivors, $n = 99$), categorical variables were compared using the Chi-squared test or Fisher's exact test (if $n < 10$ in any cell of the two-by-two table). FABP7 was treated as a continuous variable. Continuous variables were reported as medians with interquartile range (IQR) and compared using the Wilcoxon rank-sum test. Survival was defined as the dichotomous outcome, alive or dead at 21 days after enrollment into the registry (no patients received a LT in this analysis). A two-sided p value of < 0.05 was considered statistically significant for all comparisons (Additional file 2).

In order to control for variables that may confound the effect of FABP7 on 21-day mortality, logistic regression analysis was performed [21]. Aside from FABP7, covariates considered in multivariable modeling included MELD, lactate, vasopressors use, RRT, MV and high coma grade. Separate multivariable (logistic) regression models were derived for FABP7 early (day 1) and late

(days 3–5) by including variables, which were significant on univariate analysis and performing backward elimination with a p value threshold of 0.05.

Statistical methods aim two: FABP7 and ICH in APAP-ALF

In this secondary analysis, the outcome of interest examined was intracranial hypertension (ICH) either based on (a) intracranial pressure monitoring with ICP > 25 mm Hg or based on (b) computed tomography (CT) imaging of the brain. CT evidence of cerebral edema was defined as a hypodense signal, effacement of the gray white matter junction, loss of differentiation of the lenticular nucleus and decreased visualization of the sulci, insula and cisterns [22]. Out of the 150 APAP-ALF patients where data were available to determine the presence or absence of ICH, 46 deceased patients had evidence of ICH based on these criteria. Statistical methods for this analysis will be similar to the first analysis except the primary outcome (ICH). Multivariable logistic regression analysis (as described above) was performed [21] to assess independent variables associated with ICH including FABP7. The pre-specified prognostic variables were based on previous publications [5] included at admission into the registry; age, lactate value, MELD [20] score (admission) and other variables with statistical significance on univariable analysis. Model performance for both Aim 1 and Aim 2 was assessed using area under the receiver-operating curve (AUROC) and the Hosmer–Lemeshow test for goodness of fit. SAS software version 9.3 was used for univariate comparisons and multivariable logistic regression modeling.

Results

Analysis one: comparative analysis of 198 APAP-ALF patients

Demographic and clinical outcomes stratified by mortality (alive at day 21, $n = 99$; deceased, $n = 99$) are listed in Table 1. No patients in this analysis received LT. Comparing APAP-ALF survivors and non-survivors at day 21, survivors required significantly less organ support during the 7 days of inpatient study (MV 65 vs. 93%; vasopressors 12 vs. 70%; RRT 27 vs. 45%; $p < 0.008$ for all). Survivors were less likely to achieve high (3 or 4) HE coma grade (62 vs. 93%, $p < 0.0001$) and less likely to receive mannitol for intracranial hypertension (22 vs. 46%, $p = 0.0003$). APAP-ALF survivors were less likely to have complications during the first 7 days of study including seizures (3 vs. 21%, $p < 0.0001$), arrhythmias (25 vs. 38%, $p = 0.047$) or gastrointestinal bleeding (8 vs. 19%, $p = 0.037$). On admission, 7% of APAP-ALF survivors and 16% of non-survivors met KCC ($p = 0.13$). Among the 99 APAP-ALF non-survivors, the most common causes of death reported were multiorgan failure (53%)

Table 1 Demographic, clinical and biochemical parameters in 198 APAP-ALF patients by outcome

	APAP alive day 21 ($n = 99$)		APAP dead day 21 ($n = 99$)		p value
	N	Number (%) or median (IQR)	N	Number (%) or median (IQR)	
Age	99	35 (28–43)	99	40 (30–48)	0.084
Sex (female)	99	75 (76%)	99	72 (73%)	0.63
Race					0.23
White	99	83 (84%)	99	79 (80%)	
African-American	99	8 (8%)	99	15 (15%)	
Other	99	8 (8%)	99	5 (5%)	
Organ support (days 1–7)					
Mechanical ventilation	99	64 (65%)	99	93 (93%)	< 0.0001
Vasopressors	99	12 (12%)	99	69 (70%)	< 0.0001
Renal replacement therapy	99	27 (27%)	99	45 (45%)	0.0078
KCC	87	7 (7%)	87	16 (16%)	0.13
Coma grade 3/4 (worst days 1–7)	99	61 (62%)	98	91 (93%)	< 0.0001
ICP-directed therapies (days 1–7)					
ICP monitor	99	12 (12%)	99	21 (21%)	0.086
Mannitol	99	22 (22%)	99	46 (46%)	0.0003
Hypertonic saline	99	11 (11%)	99	14 (14%)	0.52
Barbiturates	99	9 (9%)	99	20 (20%)	0.043
Hypothermia	99	17 (17%)	99	14 (14%)	0.56
Sedatives	99	70 (71%)	99	88 (89%)	0.0014
Blood products (days 1–7)					
Red blood cells	99	34 (34%)	99	50 (51%)	0.021
Fresh-frozen plasma	99	50 (51%)	99	76 (77%)	0.0001
Recombinant VIIA	99	3 (3%)	99	5 (5%)	0.72
Platelets	99	17 (17%)	99	36 (36%)	0.0023
ICU complications (days 1–7)					
Seizures	99	3 (3%)	99	21 (21%)	< 0.0001
Arrhythmias	99	25 (25%)	99	38 (38%)	0.047
GI bleeding	99	8 (8%)	99	19 (19%)	0.037
ARDS	99	0 (0%)	99	3 (3%)	0.25
CT (cerebral edema)	55	7 (13%)	72	32 (44%)	< 0.001
Abnormal CXR	99	88 (89%)	99	83 (84%)	0.30
Bacteremia/blood stream infection	99	7 (7%)	99	10 (10%)	0.61
Cause of death					
Multiorgan failure			99	52 (53%)	
Cerebral edema			99	38 (38%)	
Unknown			99	9 (9%)	

N frequency, *IQR* interquartile range, *ARDS* acute respiratory syndrome, *CT* computed tomography, *CXR* chest x-ray

and neurological complications (38%). Cause of death was unknown in 9% of cases.

Clinical parameters in 198 APAP-ALF patients: admission (early)

Comparisons of clinical parameters on study admission are listed in Table 2. APAP-ALF survivors demonstrated significantly lower MELD scores (23 vs. 29, $p < 0.0001$) than non-survivors on admission. Survivors were significantly less likely to be on organ support (MV 58 vs. 80%, $p = 0.0007$; vasopressors, 9 vs. 42%, $p < 0.0001$) or achieve high HE grade (57 vs. 71%, $p = 0.034$) on admission.

FABP7 levels at admission (early) are listed in Table 2 and graphically shown in Fig. 1. APAP-ALF survivors had significantly lower admission serum FABP7 levels (147.9 vs. 316.5 ng/ml) compared with non-survivors ($p = 0.0002$). In comparison, 52 healthy

Table 2 Demographic, clinical and biochemical parameters in 198 APAP-ALF patients by outcome (admission)

Early (admission)	APAP alive day 21 ($n = 99$)		APAP dead day 21 ($n = 99$)		p value
	N	Number (%) or median (IQR)	N	Number (%) or median (IQR)	
Biochemistry					
Hemoglobin (g/dl)	99	10.4 (9.2–12.5)	97	10.9 (9.5–12.2)	0.52
White blood count (10^9/l)	98	8.6 (6.4–11.2)	97	10.9 (7.3–17.5)	0.0008
Platelet count (10^9/l)	98	132.5 (90.0–195.0)	97	110.0 (67.0–160.0)	0.0045
INR	99	2.7 (1.8–4.1)	96	3.4 (2.3–4.8)	0.0023
ALT (IU/l)	98	3380 (1949–6576)	99	3235 (1483–5716)	0.37
Bilirubin (mg/dl)	98	4.1 (2.5–5.6)	99	5.0 (3.6–7.8)	< 0.0001
pH	88	7.4 (7.4–7.5)	88	7.4 (7.3–7.5)	0.22
Ammonia (venous) (µmol/l)	51	92 (73–140)	32	139 (72–205)	0.068
Creatinine (mg/dl)	98	1.4 (0.8–3.0)	98	2.6 (1.2–3.8)	0.0007
Lactate (mmol/l)	71	2.8 (1.7–5.5)	68	7.0 (4.8–11.8)	< 0.0001
Phosphate (mg/dl)	88	2.3 (1.7–3.4)	76	3.2 (2.1–4.5)	0.0061
MELD	98	23.4 (12.7–27.7)	96	29.1 (23.8–34.5)	< 0.0001
High coma grade (3 or 4)	99	56 (57%)	97	69 (71%)	0.034
Organ support					
Mechanical ventilation	99	57(58%)	99	79 (80%)	0.0007
Vasopressors	99	9 (9%)	99	42 (42%)	< 0.0001
Renal replacement therapy	99	19 (19%)	99	24 (24%)	0.39
FABP7 (ng/ml)	99	147.9 (66.6–296.2)	99	316.5 (119.8–562.2)	0.0002
Late ($n = 186$)	**APAP alive day 21 ($n = 99$)**		**APAP dead day 21 ($n = 87$)**		**p value**
Late (days 3–5)	N	Number (%) or median (IQR)	N	Number (%) or median (IQR)	
Biochemistry					
Hemoglobin (g/dl)	94	9.9 (9.0–11.1)	81	10.2 (9.2–10.9)	0.63
White blood count (10^9/L)	94	8.1 (5.9–11.6)	81	11.3 (7.1–15.0)	0.0029
Platelet count (10^9/L)	95	111.0 (68.0–153.0)	81	66.0 (47.0–100.0)	< 0.0001
INR	94	1.5 (1.3–1.8)	75	2.5 (1.8–4.4)	< 0.0001
ALT (IU/L)	94	1172 (612–2007)	78	938 (383–1995)	0.31
Bilirubin (mg/dl)	92	5.5 (2.7–8.2)	78	9.8 (6.7–13.7)	< 0.0001
pH	55	7.4 (7.4–7.5)	76	7.4 (7.3–7.5)	0.042
Ammonia (venous) (µmol/L)	25	62 (44–84)	17	119 (78–133)	0.0038
Creatinine (mg/dl)	94	1.2 (0.7–2.5)	82	2.4 (1.3–4.0)	< 0.0001
Lactate (mmol/L)	31	1.7 (1.0–2.2)	41	3.8 (2.6–6.7)	< 0.0001
Phosphate (mg/dl)	73	2.8 (2.3–3.6)	35	3.3 (2.5–4.5)	0.054
PO$_2$/FiO$_2$ ratio	48	3.3 (2.1–4.5)	71	2.5 (1.4–3.9)	0.0087
MELD	87	14.2 (5.4–24.6)	73	29.7 (23.5–35.4)	< 0.0001
High coma grade (3 or 4)[a]	59	35 (59%)	82	72 (88%)	< 0.0001
Organ support					
Mechanical ventilation	99	49 (49%)	88	74 (85%)	< 0.0001
Vasopressors	99	5 (5%)	88	45 (52%)	< 0.0001
Renal replacement therapy	99	10 (19%)	88	27 (31%)	0.062
FABP7 (ng/ml)	99	87.3 (48.0–261.5)	87	286.2 (146.7–536.9)	< 0.0001

N frequency, *IQR* interquartile range, *INR* international normalized ratio, *AST* aspartate aminotransferase, *ALT* alanine aminotransferase, *MELD* model for end-stage liver disease

[a] Hepatic encephalopathy grade according to West Haven criteria

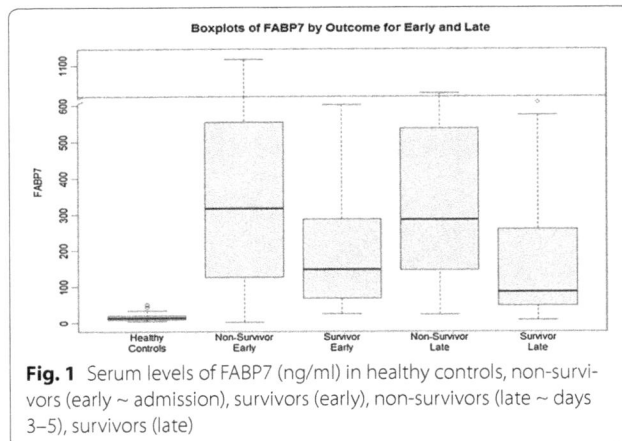

Fig. 1 Serum levels of FABP7 (ng/ml) in healthy controls, non-survivors (early ~ admission), survivors (early), non-survivors (late ~ days 3–5), survivors (late)

controls had median serum levels of 13.5 (8.7–20.2) ng/ml.

Clinical parameters in 186 APAP-ALF patients: days 3–5 (late)

Comparisons of clinical parameters on *days 3–5 (late)* are listed in Table 2. Of the 99 APAP-ALF non-survivors, samples of late time points were available in 87 patients as 12 died before days 3–5. APAP-ALF survivors ($n = 99$)

were significantly less likely to be on MV (49 vs. 85%, p < 0.0001) and vasopressors, (5 vs. 52%, p < 0.0001) or achieve high HE grade (59 vs. 88%, p < 0.0001) than non-survivors.

Late (days 3–5) FABP7 are listed in Table 2 and graphically shown in Fig. 1. APAP-ALF survivors had significantly lower late serum FABP7 levels (87.3 vs. 286.2 ng/ml) compared with non-survivors ($p < 0.0001$). FABP7 levels were significantly higher in all ALF patients (survivors and non-survivors) compared to healthy controls for both early and late time points ($p < 0.0001$).

Multivariable analysis: associations with 21-day mortality

In order to adjust for covariates, multivariable logistic regression for 198 APAP-ALF patients to determine associations (adjusted) with 21-day mortality was performed (Table 3). Two models were derived: one on admission (early) and one at days 3–5 (late). Values of serum FABP7 were transformed to their natural logarithm (log FABP1) to comply with the linearity assumption in logistic regression.

Early (admission) model

FABP7 was not associated with 21-day mortality [odds ratio OR 1.001 per increment, 95% CI (1.000, 1.001), $p = 0.18$] after adjusting for significant covariates

Table 3 Early (day 1) and late (days 3–5) predictors of 21-day mortality in 198 APAP-ALF patients

Early	Unadjusted				Multivariable model ($N = 194$), AUROC = 0.766			
	N	OR	95% OR CI	p value	Included in Model	OR	95% CI	p value
FABP7	198	1.001	(1.000, 1.002)	0.0078	Yes	1.001	(1.000, 1.001)	0.18
MELD	194	1.083	(1.047, 1.119)	< 0.0001	Yes	1.056	(1.020, 1.093)	0.0021
Lactate	132	1.205	(1.095, 1.327)	0.0001	No			
Vasopressors	198	7.368	(3.335, 16.287)	< 0.0001	Yes	4.138	(1.769, 9.677)	0.0011
Renal replacement therapy	198	1.347	(0.683, 2.658)	0.390	No			
Mechanical ventilation	198	2.910	(1.547, 5.475)	0.0009	No			
High coma grade (3 or 4)	196	1.892	(1.047, 3.421)	0.0348	No			
Late (days 3–5)	Unadjusted				Multivariable model ($N = 160$), AUROC = 0.891			
	N	OR	95% OR CI	p value	Included in model	OR	95% CI	p value
FABP7	186	1.003	(1.001, 1.004)	0.0001	Yes	1.001	(0.999, 1.003)	0.40
MELD	160	1.115	(1.075, 1.157)	< 0.0001	Yes	1.084	(1.038, 1.132)	0.0003
Lactate	71	6.908	(2.592, 18.406)	0.0001	No			
Vasopressors	186	20.143	(7.462, 54.370)	< 0.0001	Yes	20.419	(6.221, 67.021)	<0.0001
Renal replacement therapy	186	1.895	(0.964, 3.724)	0.0638	No			
Mechanical ventilation	186	5.808	(2.859, 11.802)	< 0.0001	No			
High coma grade (3 or 4)	141	4.936	(2.129, 11.446)	0.0002	No			

Early: lactate ($p = 0.52$), high coma grade ($p = 0.46$), and mechanical ventilator ($p = 0.084$) were not significant on multivariable analysis so not included in the final early model

Late: mechanical ventilation ($p = 0.69$) and high coma grade ($p = 0.53$) were not significant on multivariable analysis so not included in the final late model. Lactate was not included due to missing data

including MELD [OR 1.056 (1.020, 1.093) per increment, $p = 0.0021$] and requirement for vasopressors [OR 4.14 (1.77, 9.07), $p = 0.0011$]. This early model demonstrated AUROC of 0.766.

Late (days 3–5) model
FABP7 was not associated with 21-day mortality [OR 1.001 (0.999, 1.003) per increment, $p = 0.40$] after adjusting for significant covariates including MELD [OR 1.084 (1.038, 1.132) per increment, $p = 0.0003$] and requirement for vasopressors [OR 20.42 (6.22, 67.02), $p < 0.0001$]. This late model demonstrated AUROC of 0.891.

Analysis two: comparative analysis of 150 APAP-ALF patients
Demographic and clinical outcomes of 150 patients stratified by the presence ($n = 46$) and absence ($n = 104$) of ICH/CE based on review of subject data (ICP measurements, CT brain, cause of death) are shown in Additional file 3: Table S1. (In 48 patients, the presence or absence of ICH/CE could not be determined.) There were no significant differences in age (36 vs. 39, $p = 0.11$) or gender (female 74 vs. 69%, $p = 0.56$). During the 7 days of inpatient study, APAP-ALF patients with ICH/CE had higher requirements for ventilation (MV 100 vs. 75%, $p < 0.0001$) and were more likely to achieve high (3 or 4) HE coma grade (100 vs. 72%, $p < 0.0001$). APAP-ALF patients with evidence of ICH/CE were less likely to be alive at day 21 (17 vs. 41%, $p = 0.0049$) but were more likely to be listed for LT (33 vs. 13%, $p = 0.0062$).

Clinical parameters in 150 APAP-ALF patients: admission (early)
Comparisons of clinical parameters on study admission are shown in Additional file 4: Table S2. APAP-ALF patients with ICH/CE had significantly higher serum INR (3.6 vs. 2.9) compared to patients without ICH/CE ($p = 0.024$). On study admission, patients who went on to develop ICH/CE were significantly more likely to be on mechanical ventilation (MV 85 vs. 65%, $p = 0.019$) and achieve high HE grade (76 vs. 59%, $p = 0.043$). Admission (early) levels of FABP7 are listed in Additional file 4: Table S2 and graphically shown in Fig. 2. There were no significant differences in FABP7 levels on admission between APAP-ALF patients with or without ICH/CE (259.7 vs. 228.2 ng/ml, $p = 0.61$).

Clinical parameters in 186 APAP-ALF patients: days 3–5 (late)
Comparisons of clinical parameters on *days 3–5 (late)* are shown in Additional file 4: Table S2. Patients who developed ICH/CE were significantly more likely to be on mechanical ventilation (MV 95 vs. 63%, $p < 0.0001$) and

achieve higher grades of HE (100 vs. 75%, $p = 0.0004$). Days 3–5 (late) levels of FABP7 are shown in Additional file 4: Table S2 and graphically in Fig. 2. There were no significant differences in late FABP7 levels between APAP-ALF patients with or without ICH/CE (223.8 vs. 192.0 ng/ml, $p = 0.19$).

Multivariable analysis: associations with 21-day mortality
Multivariable logistic regression for 198 APAP-ALF to determine associations (adjusted) with the development of ICH/CE was performed (Table 4). Two models were derived; one on admission (early) and one at days 3–5 (late). Values of serum FABP7 were transformed to their natural logarithm (log FABP1) to comply with the linearity assumption in logistic regression.

Early (admission) model
FABP7 was not associated with the development of ICH/CE [OR 1.000 per increment, 95% CI (1.000, 1.001), $p = 0.65$] after adjusting for the only significant covariate, mechanical ventilation [OR 2.880 (1.166, 7.111), $p = 0.022$]. This early model demonstrated AUROC of 0.590.

Late (days 3–5) model
FABP7 was not associated with the development of ICH/CE [OR 1.000 per increment, 95% CI (0.999, 1.001), $p = 0.57$] after adjusting for the only significant covariate, high hepatic coma grade [OR 25.76 (1.40, 472.5), $p = 0.029$]. This late model demonstrated AUROC of 0.641.

Discussion
Key results
In this nested case–control study, we report the first published analysis of FABP7 in a large series of 198

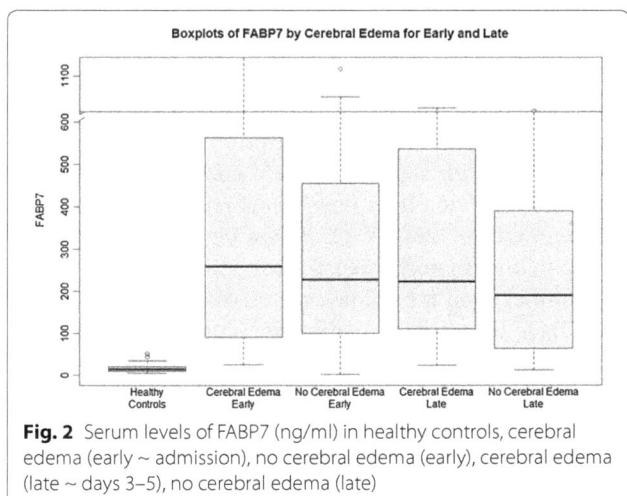

Fig. 2 Serum levels of FABP7 (ng/ml) in healthy controls, cerebral edema (early ~ admission), no cerebral edema (early), cerebral edema (late ~ days 3–5), no cerebral edema (late)

Table 4 Early (admission) and late (days 3–5) predictors of cerebral edema in 150 APAP-ALF patients

Early	Unadjusted				Multivariable model (N = 148), AUROC = 0.590			
	N	OR	95% OR CI	p value	Included in model	OR	95% CI	p value
FABP7	150	1.000	(1.000, 1.001)	0.58	Yes	1.000	(1.000, 1.001)	0.65
MELD	146	1.036	(0.997, 1.078)	0.072	No			
Lactate	100	1.000	(0.997, 1.002)	0.80	No			
Vasopressors	150	0.777	(0.363, 1.660)	0.51	No			
Renal replacement therapy	150	1.313	(0.598, 2.886)	0.50	No			
Mechanical ventilation	150	2.950	(1.199, 7.257)	0.019	Yes	2.880	(1.166, 7.111)	0.022
High coma grade (3 or 4)	148	2.227	(1.017, 4.878)	0.045	No			
Late (days 3–5)	**Unadjusted**				**Multivariable model (N = 113), AUROC = 0.641**			
	N	OR	95% OR CI	p value	Included in model	OR	95% CI	p value
FABP7	138	1.000	(0.999, 1.001)	0.96	Yes	1.000	(0.999, 1.001)	0.57
MELD	118	1.030	(0.994, 1.066)	0.10	No			
Lactate	53	1.031	(0.979, 1.086)	0.25	No			
Vasopressors	138	2.043	(0.947, 4.408)	0.069	No			
Renal replacement therapy	138	1.756	(0.789, 3.909)	0.17	No			
Mechanical ventilation	138	10.115	(2.300, 44.491)	0.0022	No			
High coma grade (3 or 4)*	113	24.324	(1.326, 446.243)	0.0316	Yes	25.759	(1.404, 472.46)	0.029

Early: high coma grade ($p = 0.69$) was not significant on multivariable analysis so not included in the final early model

Late: mechanical ventilation ($p = 0.65$) was not significant on multivariable analysis so not included in the final late model

*Statistically significant on multivariable analysis

well-characterized APAP-ALF patients. Compared with survivors, serum FABP7 levels were significantly higher at serial time points (early and late) in APAP-ALF non-survivors. However, significant differences in FABP7 levels by 21-day mortality were not ascertained after adjusting for significant covariates reflecting severity of illness (MELD, vasopressor dependence). No differences in the FABP7 levels were detected for APAP-ALF patients with and without evidence of ICH/CE.

Comparison with literature

In our study, ICH/CE was the cause of death in 39% of patients, similar to what has been previously reported [16]. ICH/CE arises due to astrocyte swelling, cerebral vasodilatation, dilated cerebral arterioles and altered cerebral blood flow [23, 24]. Furthermore, it has been shown that patients with signs of cerebral edema and ICH have increased cerebral blood flow compared to patients without brain edema [25, 26]. Given the bleeding risks associated with direct intracranial pressure monitoring [8], there is an unmet need for noninvasive markers of brain edema and ICH to help inform medical decisions. In the setting of ALF, astrocyte swelling/injury leads to astrocyte dysfunction and consequently impairs neuronal function leading to HE. However, in parallel, swollen astrocytes release small proteins, molecules and osmolytes in response to

astrocyte hypertonicity to reduce swelling. In the past 20 years, several biochemical biomarkers have been investigated for the detection of cerebral injury, including protein S100b [27], neuron-specific enolase (NSE) [27] and glial fibrillary protein (GFAP) [9]. Studies by Strauss et al. [27], as well as Vaquero et al. [28], which included 35 and 54 ALF patients, respectively, concluded that S-100b was not a useful marker of neurological outcome in ALF. Furthermore, despite a consistent increase of S-100b in serum, levels did not correlate with severity of HE, development of brain herniation or outcome. In the same patients, Strauss et al. found that serum levels of NSE were higher in ALF patients with ICH than those who survived without ICH [27]. However, this univariate comparison did not adjust for significant confounding factors/covariates, an important limitation to the study.

Major components of the brain are lipids with brain cells having a high cell membrane/cytoplasm ratio. Cell membranes are formed of lipid bilayers consisting of saturated and unsaturated fatty acids, which can also be oxidized for generating ATP. The primary function of FABPs is to facilitate the transport of intracellular long-chain fatty acids. In the brain, FABP7 and heart FABP (FABP3) are expressed with FABP7 primarily found in astrocytes [29] and FABP3 in neurons [30]. With astrocyte swelling being a neuropathological landmark of ALF along with a hyperdynamic circulation frequently occurring in ALF leading to an increased myocardial demand, FABP3 may be confounded with myocardial injury. Therefore, FABP7 is more specific to brain injury in ALF.

FABP7 has physiological properties that render this protein advantageous as a prognostic biomarker in ALF: (i) it is abundantly present in astrocytes (between approximately 0.8 and 3.1 µg/g of brain tissue), (ii) it has a lower molecular mass (14 kDa); it is smaller than S-100b (21 kDa), enolase (47 kDa) and GFAP (50 kDa) with a much shorter plasma half-life (11 min) [31–33]. Smaller proteins such as FABP7 diffuse more rapidly (via transcytosis) than larger proteins though the interstitial space and cross the blood–brain barrier (BBB).

The release of cerebrovascular proteins into blood plasma is dependent on the status (breakdown) of the BBB, which in ALF is dependent on the underlying mechanisms of cerebral edema, cytotoxic and vasogenic [34]. Astrocyte swelling plays a definitive role in the development of cytotoxic brain edema. In cytotoxic edema, the BBB is intact in the presence of intracellular swelling [35], whereas in vasogenic edema there is breakdown of the BBB and water and plasma constituents accumulate in the extracellular space [36]. Although a complete breakdown of the blood–brain barrier is not evident in ALF, increased permeation to water and other small molecules such as ammonia has been demonstrated resulting from subtle alterations in the protein composition of paracellular tight junctions [37].

Despite elevated levels in ALF patients (survivors and non-survivors) in this analysis, FABP7 did not discriminate between patients who went on to develop significant signs of ICH/CE either on imaging, ICP measurements or at death. One explanation is that variability in BBB permeability during ICH/CE could impact the diffusion rate of FABP7 into the peripheral circulation. In this study, we speculate that heterogeneity in the permeability of the BBB in ALF patients likely impacted the discriminatory ability of serum FABP7 measurements and important neurological outcomes in ALF. While FABP7 in cerebrospinal fluid may be more discriminatory between patients with and without astrocyte swelling/injury, this would not be feasible as a noninvasive biomarker as it would require an interventricular drain.

Limitations
The following limitations of this study warrant consideration. It is a nested case–control study, and as such the event rate of the primary outcome (21-day mortality) was 50%, higher than published in cohort series. Although patients were enrolled and samples were collected prospectively, analysis was performed

retrospectively and therefore can comment on association and discrimination (between survivors and non-survivors) and not on the absolute risks of death and intracranial complications according to serum FABP7 levels. To account for potential confounding in the study design, we performed multivariable analysis to adjust for other significant covariates reflecting severity of illness (MELD, vasopressors, mechanical ventilation, hepatic coma grade). To avoid confounding related to LT since transplant listing decisions for APAP-ALF and the organ availability were not consistent between study centers (Simmons et al., ALFSG unpublished data), samples from patients who received a LT were not evaluated in this study. The case–control design of the study may have introduced selection bias, as the primary outcome of survival is automatically unbalanced within the clinical profile of the groups. However, in an attempt to reduce observation bias, data were collected prospectively and within this specific study design, researchers measuring FABP7 were blinded to the clinical and outcome data of patients at the time of patient selection and sample analysis. Finally, we acknowledge that determinations of ICH were done retrospectively using available data from death summaries: cranial imaging and ICP measurements (if a monitor was used), and this may have introduced further bias. The decision to order computed tomography of the brain and the use of ICP monitors were individual decisions made by the practicing clinician, and these were not standardized across the ALFSG registry and may have varied between centers. While renal function may have impacted serum FABP7 levels, we attempted to adjust for this by including renal function (MELD) in multivariable analysis. Nonetheless despite these limitations, we believe these results are robust as they include APAP-ALF cases from across 16 tertiary liver transplant centers comprising the US ALFSG and are the first report of FABP7 in acute liver failure.

Conclusions
Brain FABP levels were elevated in APAP-ALF patients with significantly higher serum levels at early and late time points in APAP-ALF non-survivors. However, significant differences in FABP7 levels by 21-day mortality were not ascertained after adjusting for significant covariates reflecting severity of illness (MELD, vasopressor dependence). No differences in the FABP7 levels were detected for APAP-ALF patients with and without evidence of ICH/CE. FABP7 does not appear to discriminate between patients who did and did not have significant intracranial complications of APAP-ALF.

Abbreviations

ALF: acute liver failure; ALFSG: Acute Liver Failure Study Group; APAP: acetaminophen; FABP7: brain-type fatty acid-binding protein; HE: hepatic encephalopathy; ICU: intensive care unit; INR: international normalized ratio; IQR: interquartile range; KCC: King's College criteria; LT: liver transplantation; MELD: model for end-stage liver disease score; MV: mechanical ventilation; OR: odds ratio; RRT: renal replacement therapy.

Authors' contributions

CJK conceived the study concept and design, performed analysis and interpretation of the data, and drafted the final manuscript. JLS performed statistical analysis and interpretation of data and critically revised the final manuscript. MT performed laboratory analysis and revised the final manuscript. WML supervised the entire US Acute Liver Failure Study Group (U-01 Grant) and critically revised the manuscript for important intellectual content. CFR conceived the idea of the study, assisted in developing study design and interpretation of data and critically revised the final manuscript for important intellectual content. All authors read and approved the final manuscript.

Author details

[1] Division of Gastroenterology (Liver Unit), Department of Critical Care Medicine, University of Alberta, 1-40 Zeidler Ledcor Building, Edmonton, AB T6G-2X8, Canada. [2] Department of Public Health Sciences, Medical University of South Carolina, Charleston, SC, USA. [3] Hepato-Neuro Laboratory, CRCHUM, Université de Montréal, Montreal, Canada. [4] Division of Digestive and Liver Diseases, Department of Internal Medicine, University of Texas Southwestern Medical Center, Dallas, TX, USA.

Acknowledgements

 Current members and institutions participating in the Acute Liver Failure Study Group are as follows: W.M. Lee, M.D. (Principal Investigator); Anne M. Larson, M.D., Iris Liou, M.D., University of Washington, Seattle, WA; Michael Schilsky, M.D., Yale University, New Haven, CT; Daniel Ganger, M.D., Northwestern University, Chicago, IL; Robert Fontana, M.D., University of Michigan, Ann Arbor, MI; Brendan McGuire, M.D., University of Alabama, Birmingham, AL; David Koch MD, Medical University of South Carolina, Charleston, SC; R. Todd Stravitz, M.D., Virginia Commonwealth University, Richmond, VA; Constantine J. Karvellas MD, University of Alberta, Edmonton, AB; Jody Olson MD, University of Kansas, Kansas City, KA; Ram Subramanian MD, Emory, Atlanta, GA; James Hanje MD, Ohio State University, Columbus, OH; Bilal Hameed MD, University of California San Francisco, CA.

 The University of Texas Southwestern Administrative Group included Grace Samuel, Ezmina Lalani, Carla Pezzia, and Corron Sanders, Ph.D., Nahid Attar, Linda S. Hynan, Ph.D., and the Medical University of South Carolina Data Coordination Unit included Valerie Durkalski, Ph.D., Wenle Zhao, Ph.D., Jaime Speiser, Catherine Dillon, Holly Battenhouse and Michelle Gottfried.

Competing interests

The authors declare that they have no competing interests.

Format

This paper followed the STROBE guideline for reporting cohort studies (BMJ 2007): See Additional file 5.

Funding

The study was sponsored by NIH Grant U-01 58369 (from NIDDK) and a Grant from the University of Alberta Hospital Foundation (UHF).

References

1. O'Grady JG, Williams R. Classification of acute liver failure. Lancet. 1993;342(8873):743.
2. Larson AM, Polson J, Fontana RJ, Davern TJ, Lalani E, Hynan LS, et al. Acetaminophen-induced acute liver failure: results of a United States multicenter, prospective study. Hepatology. 2005;42(6):1364–72.
3. Bernal W, Wendon J. Acute liver failure; clinical features and management. Eur J Gastroenterol Hepatol. 1999;11(9):977–84.
4. Blei AT, Larsen FS. Pathophysiology of cerebral edema in fulminant hepatic failure. J Hepatol. 1999;31(4):771–6.
5. Bernal W, Hall C, Karvellas CJ, Auzinger G, Sizer E, Wendon J. Arterial ammonia and clinical risk factors for encephalopathy and intracranial hypertension in acute liver failure. Hepatology. 2007;46(6):1844–52.
6. Martinez-Hernandez A, Bell KP, Norenberg MD. Glutamine synthetase: glial localization in brain. Science. 1977;195(4284):1356–8.
7. Davern TJ. Predicting prognosis in acute liver failure: ammonia and the risk of cerebral edema. Hepatology. 2007;46(6):1679–81.
8. Karvellas CJ, Fix OK, Battenhouse H, Durkalski V, Sanders C, Lee WM, et al. Outcomes and complications of intracranial pressure monitoring in acute liver failure: a retrospective cohort study. Crit Care Med. 2014;42(5):1157–67.
9. Pelsers MM, Glatz JF. Detection of brain injury by fatty acid-binding proteins. Clin Chem Lab Med. 2005;43(8):802–9.
10. Bass NM, Barker ME, Manning JA, Jones AL, Ockner RK. Acinar heterogeneity of fatty acid binding protein expression in the livers of male, female and clofibrate-treated rats. Hepatology. 1989;9(1):12–21.
11. Glatz JF, van der Vusse GJ. Cellular fatty acid-binding proteins: their function and physiological significance. Prog Lipid Res. 1996;35(3):243–82.
12. Wunderlich MT, Hanhoff T, Goertler M, Spener F, Glatz JF, Wallesch CW, et al. Release of brain-type and heart-type fatty acid-binding proteins in serum after acute ischaemic stroke. J Neurol. 2005;252(6):718–24.
13. Teunissen CE, Veerhuis R, De Vente J, Verhey FR, Vreeling F, van Boxtel MP, et al. Brain-specific fatty acid-binding protein is elevated in serum of patients with dementia-related diseases. Eur J Neurol. 2011;18(6):865–71.
14. Karvellas CJ, Speiser JL, Tremblay M, Lee WM, Rose CF, Group USALFS. Elevated FABP1 serum levels are associated with poorer survival in acetaminophen-induced acute liver failure. Hepatology 2017;65(3):938–49.
15. von Elm E, Altman DG, Egger M, Pocock SJ, Gotzsche PC, Vandenbroucke JP. Strengthening the Reporting of Observational Studies in Epidemiology (STROBE) statement: guidelines for reporting observational studies. BMJ. 2007;335(7624):806–8.
16. Reuben A, Tillman H, Fontana RJ, Davern T, McGuire B, Stravitz RT, et al. Outcomes in adults with acute liver failure between 1998 and 2013: an observational cohort study. Ann Intern Med. 2016;164(11):724–32.
17. Conn HO, Lieberthal MM, editors. The hepatic coma syndromes and lactulose. Baltimore: Williams & Wilkins; 1979.
18. O'Grady JG, Schalm SW, Williams R. Acute liver failure: redefining the syndromes. Lancet. 1993;342(8866):273–5.
19. O'Grady JG, Alexander GJ, Hayllar KM, Williams R. Early indicators of prognosis in fulminant hepatic failure. Gastroenterology. 1989;97(2):439–45.
20. Kamath PS, Wiesner RH, Malinchoc M, Kremers W, Therneau TM, Kosberg CL, et al. A model to predict survival in patients with end-stage liver disease. Hepatology. 2001;33(2):464–70.
21. Li X, Song X, Gray RH. Comparison of the missing-indicator method and conditional logistic regression in 1:m matched case-control studies with missing exposure values. Am J Epidemiol. 2004;159(6):603–10.
22. Shawcross DL, Wendon JA. The neurological manifestations of acute liver failure. Neurochem Int. 2012;60(7):662–71.
23. Larsen FS, Ejlersen E, Hansen BA, Knudsen GM, Tygstrup N, Secher NH. Functional loss of cerebral blood flow autoregulation in patients with fulminant hepatic failure. J Hepatol. 1995;23(2):212–7.
24. Strauss G, Hansen BA, Kirkegaard P, Rasmussen A, Hjortrup A, Larsen FS. Liver function, cerebral blood flow autoregulation, and hepatic encephalopathy in fulminant hepatic failure. Hepatology. 1997;25(4):837–9.
25. Wendon JA, Harrison PM, Keays R, Williams R. Cerebral blood flow and metabolism in fulminant liver failure. Hepatology. 1994;19(6):1407–13.

26. Aggarwal S, Kramer D, Yonas H, Obrist W, Kang Y, Martin M, et al. Cerebral hemodynamic and metabolic changes in fulminant hepatic failure: a retrospective study. Hepatology. 1994;19(1):80–7.

27. Strauss GI, Christiansen M, Moller K, Clemmesen JO, Larsen FS, Knudsen GM. S-100b and neuron-specific enolase in patients with fulminant hepatic failure. Liver Transpl. 2001;7(11):964–70.

28. Vaquero J, Jordano Q, Lee WM, Blei AT. Group USALFS: serum protein S-100b in acute liver failure: results of the US Acute Liver Failure Study group. Liver Transpl. 2003;9(8):887–8.

29. Owada Y, Abdelwahab SA, Kitanaka N, Sakagami H, Takano H, Sugitani Y, et al. Altered emotional behavioral responses in mice lacking brain-type fatty acid-binding protein gene. Eur J Neurosci. 2006;24(1):175–87.

30. Myers-Payne SC, Hubbell T, Pu L, Schnutgen F, Borchers T, Wood WG, et al. Isolation and characterization of two fatty acid binding proteins from mouse brain. J Neurochem. 1996;66(4):1648–56.

31. Ghanem G, Loir B, Morandini R, Sales F, Lienard D, Eggermont A, et al. On the release and half-life of S100B protein in the peripheral blood of melanoma patients. Int J Cancer. 2001;94(4):586–90.

32. Mrozek S, Dumurgier J, Citerio G, Mebazaa A, Geeraerts T. Biomarkers and acute brain injuries: interest and limits. Crit Care. 2014;18(2):220.

33. Wunderlich MT, Ebert AD, Kratz T, Goertler M, Jost S, Herrmann M. Early neurobehavioral outcome after stroke is related to release of neurobiochemical markers of brain damage. Stroke. 1999;30(6):1190–5.

34. Scott TR, Kronsten VT, Hughes RD, Shawcross DL. Pathophysiology of cerebral oedema in acute liver failure. World J Gastroenterol. 2013;19(48):9240–55.

35. Traber PG, Dal Canto M, Ganger DR, Blei AT. Electron microscopic evaluation of brain edema in rabbits with galactosamine-induced fulminant hepatic failure: ultrastructure and integrity of the blood-brain barrier. Hepatology. 1987;7(6):1272–7.

36. Cui W, Sun CM, Liu P. Alterations of blood-brain barrier and associated factors in acute liver failure. Gastroenterol Res Pract. 2013;2013:841707.

37. Nguyen JH, Yamamoto S, Steers J, Sevlever D, Lin W, Shimojima N, et al. Matrix metalloproteinase-9 contributes to brain extravasation and edema in fulminant hepatic failure mice. J Hepatol. 2006;44(6):1105–14.

2

Predictors of response to fixed-dose vasopressin in adult patients with septic shock

Gretchen L. Sacha[1*], Simon W. Lam[1], Abhijit Duggal[2], Heather Torbic[1], Stephanie N. Bass[1], Sarah C. Welch[1], Robert S. Butler[3] and Seth R. Bauer[1]

Abstract

Background: Vasopressin is often utilized for hemodynamic support in patients with septic shock. However, the most appropriate patient to initiate therapy in is unknown. This study was conducted to determine factors associated with hemodynamic response to fixed-dose vasopressin in patients with septic shock.

Methods: Single-center, retrospective cohort of patients receiving fixed-dose vasopressin for septic shock for at least 6 h with concomitant catecholamines in the medical, surgical, or neurosciences intensive care unit (ICU) at a tertiary care center. Patients were classified as responders or non-responders to fixed-dose vasopressin. Response was defined as a decrease in catecholamine dose requirements and achievement of mean arterial pressure $\geq$ 65 mmHg at 6 h after initiation of vasopressin.

Results: A total of 938 patients were included: 426 responders (45%), 512 non-responders (55%). Responders had lower rates of in-hospital (57 vs. 72%; $P < 0.001$) and ICU mortality (50 vs. 68%; $P < 0.001$), and increased ICU-free days at day 14 and hospital-free days at day 28 (2.3 $\pm$ 3.8 vs. 1.6 $\pm$ 3.3; $P < 0.001$ and 4.2 $\pm$ 7.2 vs. 2.8 $\pm$ 6.0; $P < 0.001$, respectively). On multivariable analysis, non-medical ICU location was associated with increased response odds (OR 1.70; $P = 0.0049$) and lactate at vasopressin initiation was associated with decreased response odds (OR 0.93; $P = 0.0003$). Factors not associated with response included APACHE III score, SOFA score, corticosteroid use, and catecholamine dose.

Conclusion: In this evaluation, 45% responded to the addition of vasopressin with improved outcomes compared to non-responders. The only factors found to be associated with vasopressin response were ICU location and lactate concentration.

Keywords: Sepsis, Septic shock, Vasopressors, Vasopressin, Norepinephrine, Catecholamines

Background

Due to its vasoconstrictive properties, arginine vasopressin (AVP) is often utilized in practice for patients with shock requiring hemodynamic support. The Surviving Sepsis Campaign guidelines suggest AVP as an adjunct to norepinephrine (NE) at a fixed dosage of 0.03 units/min to achieve mean arterial pressure (MAP) goals or decrease NE requirements [1]. However, due to limited data these recommendations have a weak grading. In the landmark Vasopressin and Septic Shock Trial (VASST), patients were randomized to either AVP plus NE or NE monotherapy, with no mortality difference detected between treatment approaches [2]. However, further analyses have suggested that patients with less severe forms of septic shock may benefit from AVP [2, 3]. Despite limited data supporting the efficacy of this agent and weak guideline recommendations, clinicians commonly utilize AVP in practice.

The importance of targeting and maintaining goal MAP along with early initiation of vasoactive agents in patients with septic shock has been associated with reduced mortality rates [4, 5]. In fact, delays in vasoactive initiation were associated with increased mortality [5]. Conversely, the importance of limiting catecholamines (CA)

*Correspondence: sachag@ccf.org
[1] Department of Pharmacy, Cleveland Clinic, 9500 Euclid Avenue (Hb-105), Cleveland, OH 44195, USA

and utilizing non-CA vasoactive agents, such as AVP, is becoming more apparent and may ultimately improve patient outcomes [6–8]. Similarly, initiating AVP early in shock presentation may yield beneficial results [9, 10].

Unfortunately, there are still many unknowns regarding the most appropriate management strategy in patients with septic shock and the choice of vasoactive agent (especially second line) involves the weighing of a dynamic interplay of mechanisms and resultant responses of these agents. Specifically, one such agent is AVP and the ideal patient population to initiate AVP is unknown. There are limited data that may indicate a benefit in patients that are less severely ill [2, 3], have renal dysfunction [11, 12], or are receiving corticosteroids [13–15]. This study was designed to describe the impact of fixed-dose AVP on hemodynamic response and determine factors associated with response to AVP in a large cohort of adult patients with septic shock. The primary objective was to ascertain patient-specific factors at AVP initiation associated with a higher likelihood of response to AVP therapy. Secondary objectives included comparing clinical outcomes between responders and non-responders, and evaluating clinical characteristics over time, including MAP, lactate and CA dosage.

Methods

This was a retrospective, single-center evaluation of fixed-dose AVP at a large tertiary care academic medical center. Adults over the age of 18 with active orders for AVP between September 2011 and August 2015 were screened for inclusion. Patients with septic shock, receiving adjunctive, fixed-dose AVP for at least 6 h in the medical intensive care unit (ICU), surgical ICU, or neurosciences ICU were included. Patients must have received one or more CA agent for at least 1 h prior to AVP initiation and only the first course of AVP was included. Patients were excluded if they had incomplete electronic data or AVP was initiated in the operating room.

Patients were classified as responders to AVP if they achieved both a decrease in CA dosage and MAP $\geq$ 65 mmHg 6 h after AVP initiation. Six hours was chosen based on an evaluation showing MAP during the first 6 h was independently associated with mortality in patients with septic shock [16]. CA dosage was described in NE-equivalent dosage requirements from the following formula [NE (mcg/min)] + [Epinephrine (mcg/min)] + [Dopamine (mcg/kg/min)/2] + [Phenylephrine (mcg/min)/10] [2]. Septic shock was defined as meeting two or more systemic inflammatory response syndrome criteria with the presence of antibiotics and hypotension requiring CAs. The presence of acute kidney injury (AKI) was determined and patients were categorized into one of the risk, injury, failure, loss, and end-stage kidney disease

(RIFLE) categories based on serum creatinine increase at ICU admission and AVP initiation [11]. Total fluid bolus volume was calculated as crystalloid volume, with colloid equivalent doses [17, 18] and defined as total volume of fluids given 6 h prior to NE initiation until AVP initiation. Corticosteroid receipt was defined as receiving at least one dose of corticosteroids at AVP initiation up to 6 h after initiation.

Outcomes collected included in-hospital and ICU mortality, alive ICU-free days at day 14, alive hospital-free days at day 28, duration of mechanical ventilation, SOFA score change 48 h after AVP initiation, CA dosage change at 6 h after AVP initiation, need for continuous renal replacement therapy (CRRT) initiation, and CA duration. Cohorts of interest were defined a priori based on previous literature suggesting beneficial outcomes with AVP: NE-equivalent CA dose < 15 mcg/min at AVP initiation [2], lactate concentration $\leq$ 1.4 mmol/L at AVP initiation [2], receipt of corticosteroids [13, 15] obesity category [19, 20], the use of > 1 vasoactive agent at AVP initiation [2], and renal insufficiency per RIFLE category [11].

Data are presented as mean $\pm$ SD for continuous variables and n (%) for categorical variables. Univariate analyses between responders and non-responders were tested using either Chi-Square or Fisher's exact test, as appropriate, for categorical variables or ANOVA for continuous variables. Between-group differences in change in MAP, lactate concentration, CA dosage requirements, and central venous oxygen saturation (ScvO$_2$) were assessed at consecutive time intervals from AVP initiation to 72 h. A Bonferroni correction was applied to the pairwise comparisons. The effect of baseline variables on AVP response and ICU mortality were assessed using stepwise multivariable logistic regression. Statistically significant and variables with biologic plausibility for influencing the outcome were considered for the model and tested for colinearity using variance inflation factors and condition indices. If two variables were determined to be collinear [21], only one was included in the multivariable regression analysis. P values < 0.05 were considered to be statistically significant. All statistical analyses were performed with SAS 9.4 Software (SAS Institute Inc., Cary, NC) and StataIC 14 (StataCorp LLC, College Station, Tx). This study was approved by the Cleveland Clinic institutional review board (Study Number 15-2100).

Results

Of the 2555 screened, 938 (36.7%) met criteria for inclusion and of these, 426 (45.4%) were classified as responders to AVP and 512 (54.6%) as non-responders (Fig. 1). The average age was 62 $\pm$ 14 years, most patients were Caucasian (69.5%) and treated in the medical ICU (75.9%;

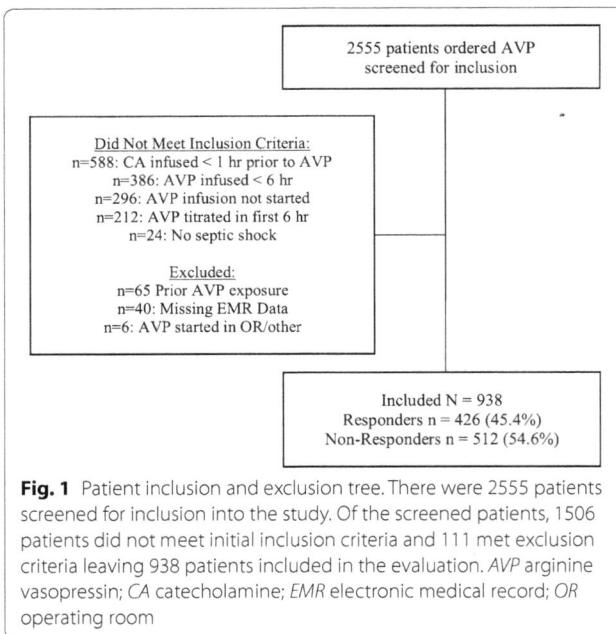

Fig. 1 Patient inclusion and exclusion tree. There were 2555 patients screened for inclusion into the study. Of the screened patients, 1506 patients did not meet initial inclusion criteria and 111 met exclusion criteria leaving 938 patients included in the evaluation. *AVP* arginine vasopressin; *CA* catecholamine; *EMR* electronic medical record; *OR* operating room

Table 1). When compared to responders, non-responders had higher rates of hepatic failure (19.3 vs. 14.3%; $P = 0.04$), lower MAP values (65 ± 12 vs. 69 ± 12 mmHg; $P < 0.001$) and higher lactate concentrations (5.4 ± 4.8 vs. 4.0 ± 3.6 mmol/L; $P < 0.001$) at AVP initiation. The average AVP initial dose was 0.03 units/min (range 0.01–0.08 units/min).

Responders had lower rates of in-hospital and ICU mortality (56.6 vs. 71.7%; $P < 0.001$ and 50.2 vs. 67.8%; $P < 0.001$, respectively), more ICU-free days at day 14 (2.3 ± 3.8 vs. 1.6 ± 3.3 days; $P < 0.001$), more hospital-free days at day 28 (4.2 ± 7.2 vs. 2.8 ± 6.0 days; $P < 0.001$) and less frequent need for CRRT within 72 h after AVP initiation (20.2 vs. 30%; $P = 0.002$) (Table 2). There was a significant difference between groups in the change in SOFA score from AVP initiation until 48 h (responders 0.30 ± 2.9 vs. non-responders 0.83 ± 2.9; $P = 0.02$) and CA dose change from AVP initiation until 6 h (responders -12.8 ± 9.6 mcg/min vs. non-responders $+13.8 \pm 51.2$ mcg/min; $P < 0.001$). Responders also had more CA-free and MV-free days on day 14 compared to non-responders (both $P < 0.001$). On multivariable logistic regression, treatment in the surgical or neurosciences ICU compared to the medical ICU and lower lactate concentrations was independently associated with higher odds of response to AVP ($P = 0.005$ and $P < 0.001$, respectively). Additionally, a positive hemodynamic response to AVP was independently associated with lower ICU mortality (Table 3).

In the predefined cohorts of interest, there was no association between the cohort designation and

hemodynamic response in patients whether classified on the receipt of corticosteroids, obesity category, number of vasopressors required at AVP initiation, or RIFLE-defined AKI. Patients with lactate concentrations ≤ 1.4 mmol/L had higher odds of response to AVP while patients with NE-equivalent CA doses < 15 had a decreased odds of response to AVP (Table 4).

There was a significant difference in CA dosage between responders and non-responders at every time point from AVP initiation through 48 h (Fig. 2a). There was also a significant difference in MAP change from AVP initiation in the responders compared to the non-responders at 3 and 24 h: $+5.4$ versus $+2.6$ mmHg ($P < 0.001$) and $+2.0$ versus -2.0 mmHg ($P < 0.001$) (Fig. 2b). Finally, lactate concentration differed significantly between responders and non-responders at every time point evaluated from AVP initiation through 48 h (Fig. 2c). There was no difference in ScvO$_2$ at any time point (Fig. 2d).

Discussion

This evaluation identified 938 patients in which 45% had a positive hemodynamic response to AVP which was associated with decreased mortality, increased ICU- and hospital-free days, and decreased CA dosage requirements. The improvement in outcomes in responders indicates the definition used for hemodynamic response may be an appropriate pharmacodynamic marker of response to AVP therapy and should be further evaluated in future studies. Furthermore, on multivariable analyses, non-medical ICU treatment and decreasing lactate concentrations were independently associated with a positive response to AVP and AVP response was independently associated with decreased ICU mortality. It is important to understand that the clinical utilization of AVP and its place in therapy relies on imperfect data, clinical experience, and weak guideline recommendations. Regardless of this, it is commonly used in clinical practice as an adjunct to NE in patients with refractory septic shock [22]. Its proposed mechanism of action is twofold, by causing V1 receptor-mediated vasoconstriction in some vascular smooth muscle beds [23], AVP can be utilized as a vasopressor similar to CAs. Additionally, in patients with septic shock, a relative endogenous vasopressin deficiency may exist and fixed, low dose exogenous AVP can be utilized as an endocrine supplement with resultant improvements in hemodynamics [12, 24–27]. Clinicians are often put in challenging situations in which they must determine if AVP should be initiated for an individual patient with few data available to inform the decision. The results of this study identify patient characteristics associated with response to AVP and can assist with decision-making regarding AVP initiation.

Table 1 Baseline characteristics

Characteristic	Total (N = 938)	Non-responders (N = 512)	Responders (N = 426)	P value
Characteristics at ICU admission				
Age, years	62 ± 14	61 ± 15	62 ± 14	0.17
Male, n (%)	493 (52.6)	272 (53.1)	221 (51.9)	0.70
Race, n (%)				0.10
Caucasian	652 (69.5)	357 (69.7)	295 (69.2)	
African American	241 (25.7)	124 (24.2)	117 (27.5)	
Other	45 (4.8)	31 (6.1)	14 (3.3)	
ICU type, n (%)				0.06
Medical	712 (75.9)	401 (78.3)	311 (73.0)	
Neurological	65 (6.9)	27 (5.3)	38 (8.9)	
Surgical	161 (17.2)	84 (16.4)	77 (18.1)	
Weight, kg	90.5 ± 34.0	92.0 ± 37.1	88.6 ± 29.9	0.13
BMI, kg/m^2	31.5 ± 11.7	31.9 ± 12.6	31.0 ± 10.4	0.22
ESRD, n (%)	119 (12.7)	58 (11.3)	61 (14.3)	0.17
APACHE III	106 ± 34	107 ± 36	104 ± 30	0.09
APS	90 ± 32	92 ± 35	88 ± 29	0.14
Comorbid conditions, n (%)				
Diabetes mellitus	286 (30.5)	152 (29.7)	134 (31.5)	0.56
Hepatic failure	160 (17.1)	99 (19.3)	61 (14.3)	0.04
Immune suppression	196 (20.9)	109 (21.3)	87 (20.4)	0.75
Leukemia/myeloma	65 (6.9)	38 (7.4)	27 (6.3)	0.52
Moderate COPD	13 (1.4)	9 (1.8)	4 (0.9)	0.45
Severe COPD	85 (9.1)	42 (8.2)	43 (10.1)	0.45
No chronic health issues, n (%)	232 (24.7)	118 (23.0)	114 (26.8)	0.19
Characteristics at time of AVP initiation				
Appropriate antibiotics, n (%)[a]	887 (94.6)	487 (95.1)	400 (93.9)	0.41
Fluids prior to AVP, mL/kg	30.7 ± 34.4	30.6 ± 35.1	30.8 ± 33.6	0.95
MAP, mmHg	67 ± 12	65 ± 12	69 ± 12	< 0.001
Lactate, mmol/L	4.8 ± 4.4	5.4 ± 4.8	4.0 ± 3.6	< 0.001
SOFA score	13 ± 4	12 ± 3	13 ± 4	0.49
Total CA dose				
mcg/min	28.2 ± 19.9	27.8 ± 21.9	28.6 ± 17.3	0.54
mcg/kg/min	0.34 ± 0.26	0.33 ± 0.27	0.35 ± 0.25	0.18
Catecholamine agent, n (%)				
Norepinephrine	937 (99.9)	511 (99.8)	426 (100.0)	0.99
Phenylephrine	66 (7.0)	31 (6.1)	35 (8.2)	0.20
Epinephrine	25 (2.7)	11 (2.1)	14 (3.3)	0.28
Dopamine	4 (0.4)	2 (0.4)	2 (0.5)	0.99
AVP dose				
Units/min	0.0314 ± 0.0063	0.0317 ± 0.0064	0.0312 ± 0.0062	0.24
Units/kg/h	0.0226 ± 0.0084	0.0224 ± 0.0084	0.0227 ± 0.0083	0.66
Corticosteroids, n (%)	571 (60.9)	320 (62.5)	251 (58.9)	0.26
AKI, n (%)				0.21
Risk	79 (8.4)	50 (9.8)	29 (6.8)	
Injury	32 (3.4)	21 (4.1)	11 (2.6)	
Failure	142 (15.1)	75 (14.6)	67 (15.7)	
Loss	0 (0)	0 (0)	0 (0)	
CRRT, n (%)	159 (17.0)	81 (15.8)	78 (18.3)	0.31

AKI acute kidney injury, *AVP* arginine vasopressin, *APS* acute physiology score, *BMI* body mass index, *CA* catecholamine, *COPD* chronic obstructive pulmonary disease, *CRRT* continuous renal replacement therapy, *ESRD* end-stage renal dysfunction, *MAP* mean arterial pressure, *SOFA* sequential organ failure assessment

[a] Antibiotics were considered to be appropriate if patients received antibiotics described in the Centers for Medicare & Medicaid Services sepsis measure or received an appropriately de-escalated antibiotic regimen for an isolated pathogen on the day of AVP initiation

Table 2 Patient outcomes

Outcome	Total (N = 938)	Non-responders (N = 512)	Responders (N = 426)	P value
In-hospital mortality, n (%)	608 (64.8)	367 (71.7)	241 (56.6)	< 0.001
ICU mortality, n (%)	561 (59.8)	347 (67.8)	214 (50.2)	< 0.001
ICU-free days at day 14	1.9 ± 3.6	1.6 ± 3.3	2.3 ± 3.8	< 0.001
Hospital-free days at day 28	3.4 ± 6.6	2.8 ± 6.0	4.2 ± 7.2	< 0.001
MV-free days at day 14	2.8 ± 4.9	2.2 ± 4.5	3.6 ± 5.3	< 0.001
SOFA score change[a]	0.6 ± 2.9	0.8 ± 2.9	0.3 ± 2.9	0.02
Respiration score change	2.3 ± 1.5	2.0 ± 1.5	2.5 ± 1.4	< 0.001
Coagulation score change	0.46 ± 1.0	0.5 ± 0.9	0.4 ± 1.0	0.19
Liver score change	0.1 ± 0.7	0.1 ± 0.8	0.7 ± 0.6	0.90
Neurological score change	− 0.1 ± 1.1	0.1 ± 1.1	− 0.2 ± 1.0	< 0.001
Cardiovascular score change	− 1.9 ± 1.7	− 1.6 ± 1.7	− 2.1 ± 1.7	< 0.001
CRRT initiation between AVP start and 72 h, n (%)[b]	190 (25.0)	112 (30.0)	78 (20.2)	0.002
CA dose change[c], mcg/min	+1.7 ± 40.6	+13.8 ± 51.2	− 12.8 ± 9.6	< 0.001
CA-free days at day 14	5.0 ± 5.8	3.9 ± 5.5	6.3 ± 6.0	< 0.001

CA catecholamine, CRRT continuous renal replacement therapy, MV mechanical ventilation, SOFA sequential organ failure assessment

[a] Evaluated at hour 48 after vasopressin initiation

[b] Evaluated only in patients who survived at least 24 h after vasopressin initiation

[c] Evaluated at hour 6 after vasopressin initiation

VASST is the largest trial of AVP in septic shock and randomized patients to either AVP plus NE or NE monotherapy [2]. While no mortality difference was detected between groups in the main analysis, several subsequent analyses have suggested benefit in specific subgroups of patients. In a priori-defined subgroup analyses, VASST showed improved 28- and 90-day outcomes in patients allocated to AVP with "less severe septic shock" (CA requirements < 15 mcg/min) and patients receiving one vasopressor at baseline (compared to two or more) [2], findings which were not corroborated in the current study. Furthermore, in contrast to VASST, the current study found patients with CA doses < 15 mcg/min had lower odds of response to AVP. The cutoff of 15 mcg/min was based on the results of VASST; however, it is unknown if an optimal CA dose threshold for achieving hemodynamic response with AVP exists and 15 mcg/min may not be the ideal threshold to evaluate. In fact, in a recent retrospective cohort study, increasing the AVP initiation threshold from a NE dose of 10 mcg/min to 50 mcg/min was not associated with increased mortality [28]. It should be noted that in clinical practice, AVP is frequently initiated in patients with NE dosage requirements exceed 15 mcg/min. In fact, the average NE dose at AVP initiation was 28 mcg/min in the current study which is similar to VASST (20 mcg/min) [2].

In an additional VASST post hoc subgroup analysis, patients receiving AVP with baseline lactate concentration ≤ 1.4 mmol/L had lower 28-day mortality rates than those receiving NE [2]. A subsequent re-analysis of VASST based on the updated definitions for septic shock also found improved survival in patients initiated on AVP with a lactate concentration ≤ 2 mmol/L [3]. The current study parallels these findings, with lower lactate concentrations independently associated with higher odds of hemodynamic response. Altogether, low lactate concentrations appear to be a useful biomarker for initiation of AVP. In comparison with VASST, which found no effect on renal replacement therapy, the current evaluation showed that fewer responders required a new initiation of CRRT compared to non-responders. These findings corroborate those from the Vasopressin versus Norepinephrine as Initial Therapy in Septic Shock (VANISH) trial which showed a decreased rate of renal replacement therapy initiation in patients who received vasopressin (when compared to NE) [29].

In addition, this study found no association with corticosteroid use and hemodynamic response; a combination previously thought to have a positive interaction [13]. The lack of an effect observed in this evaluation compared to previous studies could be due to differences of corticosteroid use. In the VASST analysis, the use of corticosteroids was regarded as receipt of at least one dose within the 28-day observation period, whereas the current study ensured corticosteroids were used concomitantly with AVP. However, it is important to note that patients could have received corticosteroids up to 6 h after AVP initiation, potentially affecting their ability to detect a response

Table 3 Results of multivariable analyses

Outcome	OR (95% CI)	P value
Multivariable analysis and association with response to vasopressin[a]		
Non-medical ICU	1.70 (1.18–2.46)	0.005
Lactate at AVP initiation, mmol/L	0.93 (0.89–0.97)	< 0.001
Multivariable analysis and association with ICU mortality		
Hemodynamic response to AVP	0.51 (0.35–0.76)	0.001
Catecholamine dose, mcg/kg/min	3.14 (1.36–7.28)	0.008
Lactate at AVP initiation, mmol/L	1.10 (1.04–1.18)	0.002
AKI presence		
Rifle versus no AKI	3.64 (1.77–7.49)	< 0.001
Injury versus no AKI	5.80 (1.13–29.60)	0.035
Failure versus no AKI	2.63 (1.38–5.01)	0.003
ESRD versus no AKI	2.37 (1.27–4.43)	0.007
APACHE III score	1.01 (1.01–1.02)	< 0.001
SOFA score	1.16 (1.08–1.25)	< 0.001
Medical ICU	1.58 (1.02–2.45)	0.040
Race (Caucasian)	1.72 (1.14–2.60)	0.010
Age	1.01 (1.00–1.03)	0.036
Hepatic failure	0.89 (0.48–1.62)	0.696

AKI acute kidney injury, AVP vasopressin, ESRD end-stage renal dysfunction, SOFA sequential organ failure assessment

[a] Variables entered into the model but without a statistically significant association with vasopressin response include RIFLE-defined AKI category, corticosteroid use, SOFA score, APACHE III score, hepatic failure, race, age, and catecholamine dosage (in mcg/kg/min)

to corticosteroids in the evaluated time frame. Furthermore, the lack of detected benefit with corticosteroids could be due to differences in the outcomes evaluated in the current study (hemodynamic response) versus historical studies (mortality) [2, 13–15]. However, the lack of association seen in the current evaluation corroborates the findings seen in VANISH which detected no interaction between AVP and corticosteroid use on 28-day mortality [29]. Additional studies are needed to determine the relationship between corticosteroid use and hemodynamic response to AVP in patients with septic shock.

An additional finding of the current study was the CA-sparing effect, in that CA dosages decreased in responders at every time point from AVP initiation until 48 h. In fact, because the MAP was > 65 mmHg when AVP was added, a CA-sparing effect was likely the intended goal of AVP initiation. Responders also had more CA-free days at day 14 compared to non-responders, further showing the CA-sparing effect observed in this group. The benefit of sparing CAs in patients with septic shock has recently become more apparent [6–8]. One analysis found that raising MAP values above 70 mmHg with increasing vasoactive doses resulted in increased organ failure events [6]. Additionally, excess CAs can have a negative effect on the immune system and can cause tachyarrhythmias, hyperglycemia, splanchnic hypoperfusion, and myocardial depression. This new perspective emphasizes

the importance of limiting CA doses while maintaining goal MAP, a method that can be achieved through AVP utilization.

Upon multivariable logistic regression, treatment in the medical ICU was associated with lower odds of response to AVP. Patients with sepsis secondary to medical (vs. surgical) conditions have higher mortality [30], which may influence AVP response. Additionally, these patient populations can present with a differing mix of comorbidities, which may alter patient outcomes differently [31], and medical patients may have lower frequencies of infectious source control (due to the prevalence of in-operable infections, i.e., pneumonia), which could decrease their response to treatment, including vasoactive therapies. It is also possible that there were residual confounders between medical ICU and non-medical ICU patients unable to be controlled for in the multivariable model. This finding of differing AVP response by treatment ICU and the potential mechanisms should be explored further.

This study has important implications for practice and future research. Regardless of the patients' CA dose, the association between low lactate concentration and hemodynamic response with AVP suggests that this marker of "less severe septic shock" is a useful indicator for AVP initiation. Furthermore, because of the improved outcomes in patients who had a positive hemodynamic response to

Table 4 Predefined cohorts of interest

Cohort of interest	Responders N (%)	Non-responders N (%)	P value	OR (95% CI) hemodynamic response	OR (95% CI) ICU mortality
Corticosteroids					
Yes	251 (58.9)	320 (62.5)	0.26	0.86 (0.66–1.12)	1.01 (0.77–1.32)
No[a]	175 (41.1)	192 (37.5)			
Lactate concentration					
> 1.4 mmol/L[a]	211 (78.4)	321 (88.7)	< 0.001	2.15 (1.39–3.32)^	0.39 (0.25–0.60)^
≤ 1.4 mmol/L	58 (21.6)	41 (11.3)			
BMI classification					
Underweight[a]	18 (4.2)	20 (3.9)	0.98		
Normal	94 (22.1)	106 (20.7)		0.99 (0.50–1.97)	1.09 (0.53–2.12)
Overweight	114 (26.8)	140 (27.3)		0.90 (0.46–1.79)	1.02 (0.51–2.05)
Obesity class I	81 (19.0)	101 (19.7)		0.89 (0.44–1.80)	0.91 (0.45–1.86)
Obesity class II	48 (11.3)	53 (10.4)		1.01 (0.48–2.12)	1.13 (0.52–2.43)
Obesity class III	71 (16.7)	92 (18.0)		0.86 (0.42–1.74)	0.77 (0.37–1.57)
CA equivalent dose					
≥ 15 mcg/min[a]	370 (86.9)	424 (82.8)	0.087	0.57 (0.36–0.92)^	0.62 (0.44–0.89)^
< 15 mcg/min	56 (13.1)	88 (17.2)			
Total vasopressor quantity					
1 Vasopressor[a]	370 (86.9)	463 (90.4)	0.084	1.43 (0.95–2.15)	1.98 (1.26–3.12)^
> 1 Vasopressor	56 (13.1)	49 (9.6)			
Renal insufficiency					
Yes	220 (51.6)	268 (52.3)	0.83	0.97 (0.75–1.26)	1.59 (1.23–2.07)^
No[a]	206 (48.4)	244 (47.7)			
AKI class					
No AKI presence[a]	258 (60.6)	308 (60.2)	0.21		
AKI-risk	29 (6.8)	50 (9.8)		0.69 (0.43–1.13)	2.40 (1.43–4.03)^
AKI-injury	11 (2.6)	21 (4.1)		0.63 (0.30–1.32)	3.30 (1.41–7.76)^
AKI-failure	67 (15.7)	75 (14.6)		1.07 (0.74–1.54)	3.06 (2.00–4.66)^
AKI-end stage	61 (14.3)	58 (11.3)		1.26 (0.85–1.87)	1.64 (1.09–2.46)^

AKI acute kidney injury, *BMI* body mass index, *CA* catecholamine

^ $P < 0.05$

[a] The reference group used for the odds ratio result

AVP at 6 h, monitoring for the achievement of hemodynamic stability can be an important early warning sign for the bedside clinician. Specifically, in patients who do not achieve hemodynamic stability within 6 h of starting AVP, alternative therapeutic interventions such as epinephrine [32], corticosteroids [33, 34], angiotensin II [35] (if available), or increasing AVP dose (especially when NE requirements exceed 0.6 mcg/kg/min) [36] should be considered. The use of this trigger and the next best step should be further investigated. Future trials should incorporate the observed factors associated with AVP response into their design, which may improve their likelihood of finding a target population for AVP use. Additionally, trials should evaluate when to initiate additional adjunctive agents and also compare efficacy between adjunctive agents.

Strengths of this evaluation include its a priori-defined cohorts for analysis, and evaluation of fixed-dose AVP (which removes the potential confounder of titrated doses on AVP response). Limitations of this evaluation include the fact that it was a single-center, retrospective study with no randomization and relied on medical record charting that may not instantaneously capture exact medication administration timing and hemodynamic change. Secondly, the definition of AVP response was not developed based on previous literature or able to be validated in this current study, but was created in an attempt to reflect hemodynamic response to this agent. However, based on the observed differences between responders and non-responders, it appears to accurately reflect a clinically meaningful response. Albeit, with this definition, patients who were already in the recovery

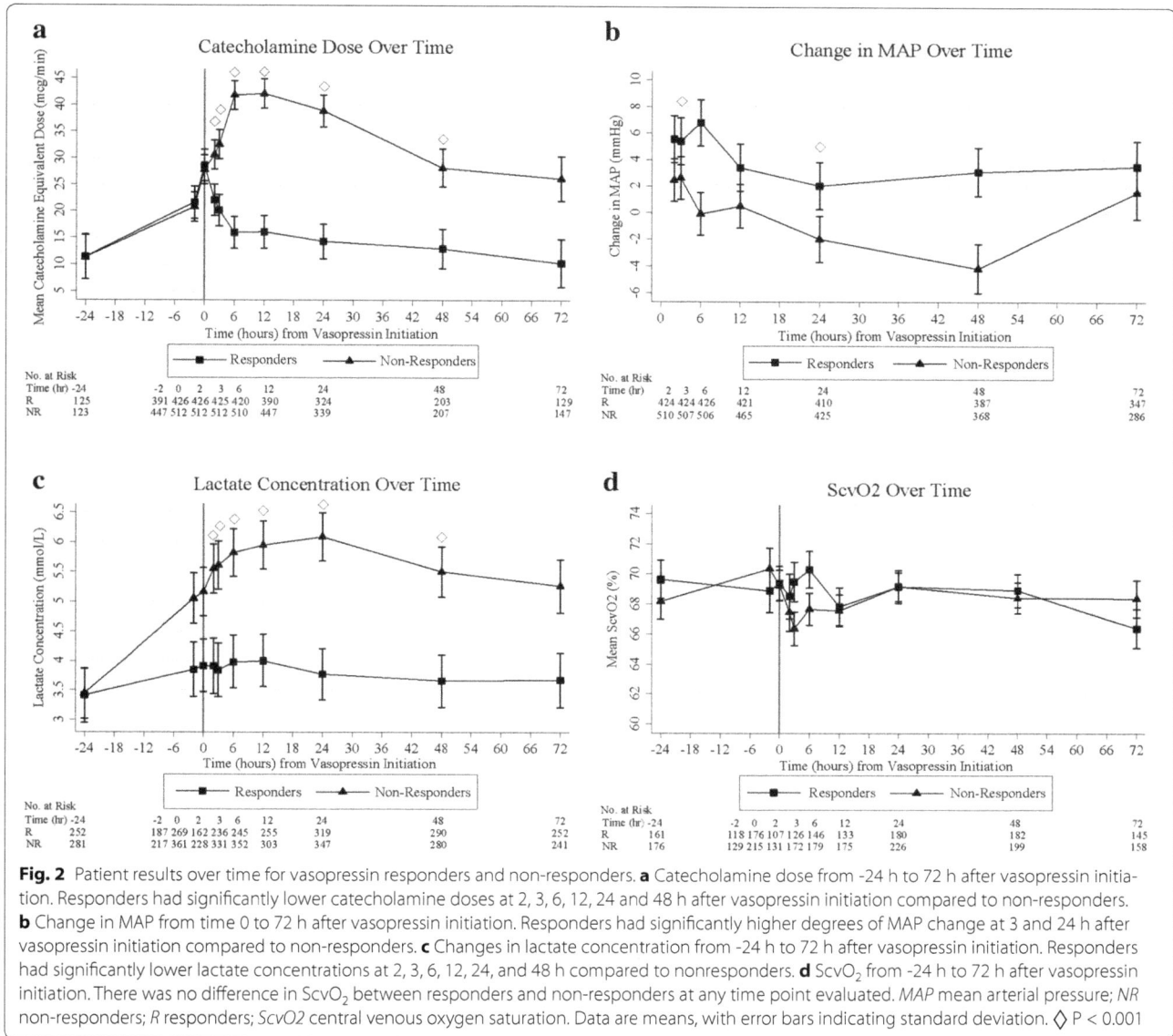

Fig. 2 Patient results over time for vasopressin responders and non-responders. **a** Catecholamine dose from -24 to 72 h after vasopressin initiation. Responders had significantly lower catecholamine doses at 2, 3, 6, 12, 24 and 48 h after vasopressin initiation compared to non-responders. **b** Change in MAP from time 0 to 72 h after vasopressin initiation. Responders had significantly higher degrees of MAP change at 3 and 24 h after vasopressin initiation compared to non-responders. **c** Changes in lactate concentration from -24 h to 72 h after vasopressin initiation. Responders had significantly lower lactate concentrations at 2, 3, 6, 12, 24, and 48 h compared to nonresponders. **d** ScvO$_2$ from -24 h to 72 h after vasopressin initiation. There was no difference in ScvO$_2$ between responders and non-responders at any time point evaluated. *MAP* mean arterial pressure; *NR* non-responders; *R* responders; *ScvO2* central venous oxygen saturation. Data are means, with error bars indicating standard deviation. ◊ P < 0.001

phase of septic shock with decreasing CA dosage at AVP initiation were regarded as "responders." Additionally, patients classified as "non-responders" may have had decreased overall CA exposure with AVP than if they were not started on AVP, which was not accounted for in our definition of response. This study was also unable to incorporate markers of tissue perfusion (e.g., lactate, urine output, pH) into the definition of hemodynamic response, because these parameters were not consistently or frequently monitored and documented for every included patient. The importance of markers of tissue perfusion should not be overlooked as patients could potentially be at goal MAP, with reductions in CA doses as a result, but still have tissue hypoperfusion. This study

also classified patients as having septic shock based on the previous definition and not the updated 2016 definition [1] which may result in more patients being included than those who had septic shock per the newest definition. Furthermore, cardiac output data were not available for most patients and therefore not collected. Although ScvO$_2$ values were elevated at baseline and not significantly different between responders and non-responders, we cannot adequately compare cardiac output between response groups. Additionally, the retrospective nature of this study makes identifying patients with true septic shock difficult, and as such, patients may have been included or excluded inadvertently. Finally, excluding patients who did not receive AVP for at least 6 h may have influenced the rates of response to therapy, as there may have been patients who responded earlier than 6 h and no longer needed vasoactive support with AVP (true responders) or patients who died within 6 h (true non-responders) and subsequently were excluded from the evaluation.

Conclusion

The current evaluation identified a large cohort of patients receiving fixed-dose AVP in which 45% responded to therapy. AVP response was associated with improved mortality and ICU and hospital-free days, indicating the definition used for hemodynamic response may be an appropriate pharmacodynamic marker of AVP therapy that can be used in future trials. In agreement with historical trials, patients with less severe forms of septic shock (lower lactate concentrations at baseline) appear to benefit more from AVP in comparison with patients with more severe forms. Future studies should incorporate the observed factors related to AVP response into their subsequent design to definitively identify the most appropriate patient population that would benefit from AVP.

Abbreviations

AKI: acute kidney injury; AVP: arginine vasopressin; CA: catecholamine; CRRT: continuous renal replacement therapy; ICU: intensive care unit; NE: norepinephrine; MAP: mean arterial pressure; RIFLE: risk, injury, failure, loss, end-stage kidney disease category; ScVO$_2$: central venous oxygen saturation; SOFA: sequential organ failure assessment; VASST: vasopressin and septic shock trial.

Authors' contributions

GLS contributed to study design, acquisition of data, analysis and interpretation of data, statistical analysis, drafting of the manuscript, critical revision of the manuscript for important intellectual content and provided final approval of the version to be published. SWL contributed to study conception and design, acquisition of data, analysis and interpretation of data, critical revision of the manuscript for important intellectual content and provided final approval of the version to be published. AD contributed to study conception, critical revision of the manuscript for important intellectual content and provided final approval of the version to be published. HT, SNB, and SCW contributed to study design, critical revision of the manuscript for important intellectual content and provided final approval of the version to be published. RSB contributed to statistical analysis and interpretation of data and provided intellectual input to the research and manuscript. SRB contributed to study conception and design, acquisition of data, analysis and interpretation of data, statistical analysis, drafting of the manuscript, critical revision of the manuscript for important intellectual content and provided final approval of the version to be published. All authors agree to be accountable for all aspects of work in ensuring that questions related to the accuracy or integrity of any part of the work are appropriately investigated and resolved. The authors would like to thank Eric Vogan for his assistance with this project. All authors read and approved the final manuscript.

Author details

^{1} Department of Pharmacy, Cleveland Clinic, 9500 Euclid Avenue (Hb-105), Cleveland, OH 44195, USA. ^{2} Respiratory Institute, Cleveland Clinic, Cleveland, OH, USA. ^{3} Department of Quantitative Health Sciences, Cleveland Clinic, Cleveland, OH, USA.

Acknowledgements

The results of this evaluation were presented in abstract form at the Society of Critical Care Medicine's 2017 Critical Care Congress on January 23rd, 2017 in Honolulu, Hawaii.

Competing interests

The authors declare that they have no competing interests.

Funding

No funding was received for this project.

References

1. Rhodes A, Evans LE, Alhazzani W, Levy MM, Antonelli M, Ferrer R, et al. Surviving sepsis campaign: international guidelines for management of sepsis and septic shock: 2016. Intensive Care Med. 2017;43(3):304–77.
2. Russell JA, Walley KR, Singer J, Gordon AC, Hebert PC, Cooper DJ, et al. Vasopressin versus norepinephrine infusion in patients with septic shock. N Engl J Med. 2008;358(9):877–87.
3. Russell JA, Lee T, Singer J, Boyd JH, Walley KR, Vasopressin, et al. The septic shock 3.0 definition and trials: a vasopressin and septic shock trial experience. Crit Care Med. 2017;45(6):940–8.
4. Beck V, Chateau D, Bryson GL, Pisipati A, Zanotti S, Parrillo JE, et al. Timing of vasopressor initiation and mortality in septic shock: a cohort study. Crit Care. 2014;18(3):R97.
5. Bai X, Yu W, Ji W, Lin Z, Tan S, Duan K, et al. Early versus delayed administration of norepinephrine in patients with septic shock. Crit Care. 2014;18(5):532.
6. Dunser MW, Ruokonen E, Pettila V, Ulmer H, Torgersen C, Schmittinger CA, et al. Association of arterial blood pressure and vasopressor load with septic shock mortality: a post hoc analysis of a multicenter trial. Crit Care. 2009;13(6):R181.
7. Rudiger A, Singer M. Decatecholaminisation during sepsis. Crit Care. 2016;20(1):309.
8. Andreis DT, Singer M. Catecholamines for inflammatory shock: a Jekyll-and-Hyde conundrum. Intensive Care Med. 2016;42(9):1387–97.
9. Hammond DA, Cullen J, Painter JT, McCain K, Clem OA, Brotherton AL, et al. Efficacy and safety of the early addition of vasopressin to norepinephrine in septic shock. J Intensive Care Med. 2017. https://doi.org/10.1177/0885066617725255.
10. Clem OPJ, Cullen J, McCain K, Kakkera K, Meena N, Hammond D. Norepinephrine and vasopressin vs norepinephrine alone for septic shock: randomized controlled trial [abstract]. Crit Care Med. 2016;44(12 Suppl 1):1350.
11. Gordon AC, Russell JA, Walley KR, Singer J, Ayers D, Storms MM, et al. The effects of vasopressin on acute kidney injury in septic shock. Intensive Care Med. 2010;36(1):83–91.
12. Holmes CL, Walley KR, Chittock DR, Lehman T, Russell JA. The effects of vasopressin on hemodynamics and renal function in severe septic shock: a case series. Intensive Care Med. 2001;27(8):1416–21.
13. Russell JA, Walley KR, Gordon AC, Cooper DJ, Hebert PC, Singer J, et al. Interaction of vasopressin infusion, corticosteroid treatment, and mortality of septic shock. Crit Care Med. 2009;37(3):811–8.
14. Bauer SR, Lam SW, Cha SS, Oyen LJ. Effect of corticosteroids on arginine vasopressin-containing vasopressor therapy for septic shock: a case control study. J Crit Care. 2008;23(4):500–6.
15. Torgersen C, Luckner G, Schroder DC, Schmittinger CA, Rex C, Ulmer H, et al. Concomitant arginine-vasopressin and hydrocortisone therapy in severe septic shock: association with mortality. Intensive Care Med. 2011;37(9):1432–7.
16. Varpula M, Tallgren M, Saukkonen K, Voipio-Pulkki LM, Pettila V. Hemodynamic variables related to outcome in septic shock. Intensive Care Med. 2005;31(8):1066–71.
17. Finfer S, Bellomo R, Boyce N, French J, Myburgh J, Norton R, et al. A comparison of albumin and saline for fluid resuscitation in the intensive care unit. N Engl J Med. 2004;350(22):2247–56.

18. Brunkhorst FM, Engel C, Bloos F, Meier-Hellmann A, Ragaller M, Weiler N, et al. Intensive insulin therapy and pentastarch resuscitation in severe sepsis. N Engl J Med. 2008;358(2):125–39.

19. Wacharasint P, Boyd JH, Russell JA, Walley KR. One size does not fit all in severe infection: obesity alters outcome, susceptibility, treatment, and inflammatory response. Crit Care. 2013;17(3):R122.

20. Miller JT, Welage LS, Kraft MD, Alaniz C. Does body weight impact the efficacy of vasopressin therapy in the management of septic shock? J Crit Care. 2012;27(3):289–93.

21. DA Belsley KE, Welsch RE. Regression diagnostics: identifying influential data and sources of collinearity. Hoboken: Wiley; 1980.

22. Vail EA, Gershengorn HB, Hua M, Walkey AJ, Wunsch H. Epidemiology of vasopressin use for adults with septic shock. Ann Am Thorac Soc. 2016;13(10):1760–7.

23. Russell JA. Bench-to-bedside review: vasopressin in the management of septic shock. Crit Care. 2011;15(4):226.

24. Landry DW, Levin HR, Gallant EM, Ashton RC Jr, Seo S, D'Alessandro D, et al. Vasopressin deficiency contributes to the vasodilation of septic shock. Circulation. 1997;95(5):1122–5.

25. Landry DW, Levin HR, Gallant EM, Seo S, D'Alessandro D, Oz MC, et al. Vasopressin pressor hypersensitivity in vasodilatory septic shock. Crit Care Med. 1997;25(8):1279–82.

26. Holmes CL. Vasopressin in septic shock: does dose matter? Crit Care Med. 2004;32(6):1423–4.

27. Holmes CL, Patel BM, Russell JA, Walley KR. Physiology of vasopressin relevant to management of septic shock. Chest. 2001;120(3):989–1002.

28. Wu JY, Stollings JL, Wheeler AP, Semler MW, Rice TW. Efficacy and out- comes after vasopressin guideline implementation in septic shock.

29. Gordon AC, Mason AJ, Thirunavukkarasu N, Perkins GD, Cecconi M, Cepkova M, et al. Effect of early vasopressin vs norepinephrine on kidney failure in patients with septic shock: the VANISH randomized clinical trial. JAMA. 2016;316(5):509–18.

30. Angus DC, Linde-Zwirble WT, Lidicker J, Clermont G, Carcillo J, Pinsky MR. Epidemiology of severe sepsis in the United States: analysis of incidence, outcome, and associated costs of care. Crit Care Med. 2001;29(7):1303–10.

31. Esper AM, Martin GS. The impact of comorbid [corrected] conditions on critical illness. Crit Care Med. 2011;39(12):2728–35.

32. Annane D, Vignon P, Renault A, Bollaert PE, Charpentier C, Martin C, et al. Norepinephrine plus dobutamine versus epinephrine alone for manage- ment of septic shock: a randomised trial. Lancet. 2007;370(9588):676–84.

33. Sligl WI, Milner DA Jr, Sundar S, Mphatswe W, Majumdar SR. Safety and efficacy of corticosteroids for the treatment of septic shock: a systematic review and meta-analysis. Clin Infect Dis. 2009;49(1):93–101.

34. Annane D, Sebille V, Charpentier C, Bollaert PE, Francois B, Korach JM, et al. Effect of treatment with low doses of hydrocortisone and fludrocortisone on mortality in patients with septic shock. JAMA. 2002;288(7):862–71.

35. Khanna A, English SW, Wang XS, Ham K, Tumlin J, Szerlip H, et al. Angiotensin II for the treatment of vasodilatory shock. N Engl J Med. 2017;377(5):419–30.

36. Torgersen C, Dunser MW, Wenzel V, Jochberger S, Mayr V, Schmit- tinger CA, et al. Comparing two different arginine vasopressin doses in advanced vasodilatory shock: a randomized, controlled, open-label trial. Intensive Care Med. 2010;36(1):57–65.

3

Procalcitonin-guided antibiotic therapy in intensive care unit patients

Hui-Bin Huang[1,2], Jin-Min Peng[1], Li Weng[1], Chun-Yao Wang[1], Wei Jiang[1] and Bin Du[1*]

Abstract

Background: Serum procalcitonin (PCT) concentration is used to guide antibiotic decisions in choice, timing, and duration of anti-infection therapy to avoid antibiotic overuse. Thus, we performed a systematic review and meta-analysis to seek evidence of different PCT-guided antimicrobial strategies for critically ill patients in terms of predefined clinical outcomes.

Methods: We searched for relevant studies in PubMed, Embase, Web of Knowledge, and the Cochrane Library up to 25 February 2017. Randomized controlled trials (RCTs) were included if they reported data on any of the predefined outcomes in adult ICU patients managed with a PCT-guided algorithm or according to standard care. Results were expressed as risk ratio (RR) or mean difference (MD) with accompanying 95% confidence interval (CI).

Data synthesis: We included 13 trials enrolling 5136 patients. These studies used PCT in three clinical strategies: initiation, discontinuation, or combination of antibiotic initiation and discontinuation strategies. Pooled analysis showed a PCT-guided antibiotic discontinuation strategy had fewer total days with antibiotics (MD − 1.66 days; 95% CI − 2.36 to − 0.96 days), longer antibiotic-free days (MD 2.26 days; 95% CI 1.40–3.12 days), and lower short-term mortality (RR 0.87; 95% CI 0.76–0.98), without adversely affecting other outcomes. Only few studies reported data on other PCT-guided strategies for antibiotic therapies, and the pooled results showed no benefit in the predefined outcomes.

Conclusions: Our meta-analysis produced evidence that among all the PCT-based strategies, only using PCT for antibiotic discontinuation can reduce both antibiotic exposure and short-term mortality in a critical care setting.

Keywords: Procalcitonin, Antibiotic strategies, Meta-analysis, Systematic review, Intensive care unit

Background

Timely diagnosis and appropriate antimicrobial treatment of infection remain a major challenge in critical care settings. Delay in diagnosis due to lack of specific clinical signs in the early stage of infection may withhold or delay antibiotic therapy. On the other hand, concern of not treating potentially life-threatening infection and the risk of recurrence frequently leads clinicians to antimicrobial overuse in intensive care unit (ICU) [1, 2]. Studies have demonstrated that up to 50% of antibiotics prescribed in hospital settings are either unnecessary or inappropriate [3]. Nowadays, long-term antimicrobial regimens applied to critically ill patients are common and often based on empiric rules [4, 5]. This may result in increased medical costs, emergence of resistant pathogens, prolonged length of stay (LOS), and risk of mortality [6, 7].

Recently, procalcitonin (PCT) has shown to be a promising biomarker for identification of bacterial infections and is correlated with the severity of infection [8–11]. The 2016 Surviving Sepsis Campaign (SSC) guidelines offered a weak recommendation (low quality of evidence), favouring that measurement of procalcitonin levels can be used to support shortening the duration of antimicrobial therapy in sepsis patients [12]. However,

---
*Correspondence: dubin98@gmail.com
[1] Medical ICU, Peking Union Medical College Hospital, Peking Union Medical College and Chinese Academy of Medical Sciences, 1 Shuai Fu Yuan, Beijing 100730, People's Republic of China

one recent large study failed to show any benefit of daily PCT measurement with regard to time to appropriate therapy or survival, but resulted in a longer antibiotic course and ICU stay [13]. To date, several meta-analyses have assessed the value of PCT to guide antibiotic stewardship in ICU patients [14–22]. Findings of these reports showed that utilizing PCT to guide antibiotic decisions could significantly reduce antibiotics use, but did not improve patient outcomes, such as mortality, hospital, or ICU LOS. However, one major limitation of these meta-analyses was unexplainable significant heterogeneity among included trials, possibly due to the fact that the different PCT guidance strategies (including antibiotic initiation, discontinuation, or combination of antibiotic initiation and discontinuation strategies) had been evaluated in these trials. Since the considerable differences in methodologies and research purposes associated with the different PCT-guided strategies, the previous meta-analyses might not accurately evaluate the effects of PCT-based algorithms (Additional file 1: Table S1). Recently, two large-scale randomized controlled trials (RCTs) of PCT-guided antibiotic strategy in ICU patients have been published, with inconsistent results [23, 24]. Of note, the study by de Jong et al., the largest PCT trial to date, demonstrated an unexpected and significant survival benefit, in addition to less antibiotic exposure.

Therefore, with the aid of increased power of meta-analytic techniques, we sought to expand the previous analyses by including studies published recently, stratifying different strategies to have a more accurate analysis of the influence of different PCT algorithms to guide antimicrobial decisions.

Methods
Search strategy and selection criteria
This systematic review and meta-analysis were conducted in accordance with the PRISMA guidance [25]. We searched RCTs in PubMed, Embase, Web of Science, and Cochrane Central Register of Controlled Trials from inception through 25 February 2017 to identify potentially relevant studies. Search included the following key words: ("Procalcitonin" OR "PCT") AND ("intensive care" OR "critically ill" OR "critical care"). No language restriction was imposed. Reference lists of relative articles were also reviewed.

Studies were included if they are enrolling adult ICU patients, with confirmed or suspected infection, assigned to either a PCT-guided therapeutic strategy group or a standard care group. Standard care referred to antimicrobial regimens based on clinical signs, laboratory results, and empiric rules or guidelines, without consideration of PCT level. We excluded studies enrolling children or patients without any evidence of infection and studies

without mentioning of PCT assay methods. Articles available only in abstract form or meeting reports were also excluded.

Data extraction and outcomes
Two reviewers independently extracted data from included studies on the first author, year of publication, country, sample size, study design, ICU type, compared protocols, methods of PCT assay, methodological quality, as well as all outcomes of interest.

We stratified different PCT-guided strategies according to medical decision with regards to antimicrobial therapy. In brief, strategy of antibiotic initiation referred to the decision to or not to start antibiotics, and decision of the intensified monitoring, diagnostic efforts, and interventions to explore uncontrolled sources of infection based on a predefined threshold of baseline PCT concentration, while strategy of antibiotic discontinuation meant making the decision to stop antibiotics according to a predefined threshold of PCT concentration, or the PCT level dropped by a certain proportion predefined compared with the previous value. The primary outcomes were the duration of antibiotic use and the short-term mortality, while the latter was defined as ICU or hospital or 28-day mortality [26, 27]. Secondary outcomes included ICU and hospital LOS.

Quality assessment
Two independent reviewers evaluated the quality of studies using the risk of bias tool recommended by the Cochrane Collaboration [28]. We assigned a value of high, unclear, or low to the following items: sequence generation; allocation concealment; blinding; incomplete outcome data; selective outcome reporting; and other sources of bias. Discrepancies were identified and resolved through discussion.

Statistical analysis
The results from all relevant studies were combined to estimate the pooled risk ratio (RR) and associated 95% confidence intervals (CIs) for dichotomous outcomes. As to the continuous outcomes, mean differences (MD) and 95% CI were estimated as the effect results. Heterogeneity was tested by using the I^2 statistic. An $I^2 < 50\%$ was considered to indicate insignificant heterogeneity, and a fixed-effect model was used, whereas a random-effect model was used in cases of significant heterogeneity ($I^2 > 50\%$). Before data analysis, we estimated mean from median and standard deviations (SD) from IQR using the methods described in previous studies [29]. Sensitivity analyses were performed by excluding trials that potentially biased the results of primary outcomes. Publication bias was evaluated by visually inspecting funnel plots. All

analyses were performed using Review Manager version 5.3.

Results

Study selection

The literature search yielded 881 records through database searching, and 13 RCTs fulfilled inclusion criteria were eligible for the final analysis [13, 23, 24, 30–39]. The overview of the study selection process is presented in Fig. 1. In the study by Jensen et al., some patients without infection were also included [13]; therefore, we only included patients with severe sepsis or septic shock that fulfilled our inclusion criteria from this study. The Cochrane risk of bias score for each citation varied across the studies (Additional file 2: Table S2).

Study characteristics

The main characteristics and predefined outcomes of the 13 included studies are shown in Table 1 and Additional file 3: Table S3. The degree of non-compliance with PCT algorithm recommendations for antibiotics varied among

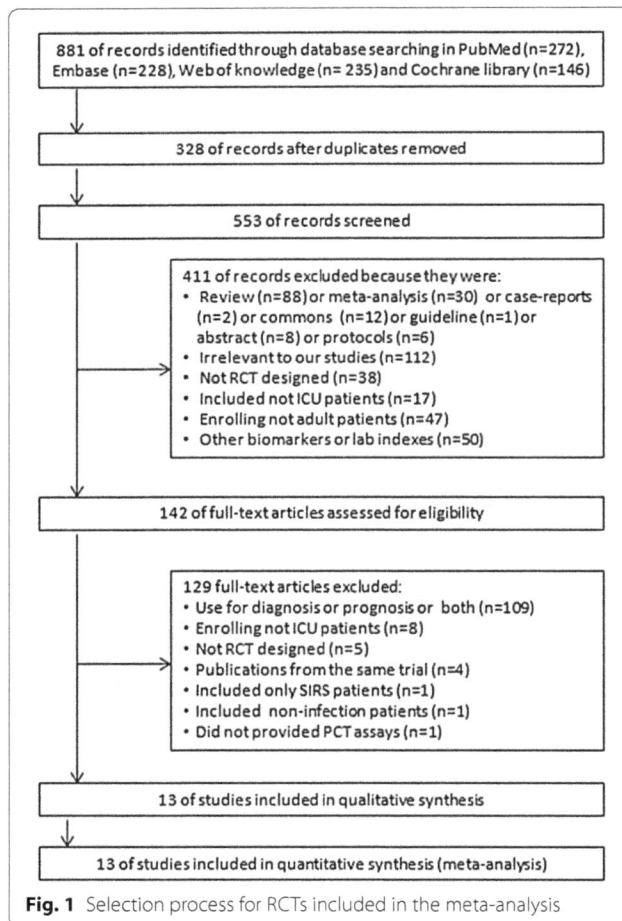

881 of records identified through database searching in PubMed (n=272), Embase (n=228), Web of knowledge (n= 235) and Cochrane library (n=146)

328 of records after duplicates removed

553 of records screened

411 of records excluded because they were:
• Review (n=88) or meta-analysis (n=30) or case-reports (n=2) or commons (n=12) or guideline (n=1) or abstract (n=8) or protocols (n=6)
• Irrelevant to our studies (n=112)
• Not RCT designed (n=38)
• Included not ICU patients (n=17)
• Enrolling not adult patients (n=47)
• Other biomarkers or lab indexes (n=50)

142 of full-text articles assessed for eligibility

129 full-text articles excluded:
• Use for diagnosis or prognosis or both (n=109)
• Enrolling not ICU patients (n=8)
• Not RCT designed (n=5)
• Publications from the same trial (n=4)
• Included only SIRS patients (n=1)
• Included non-infection patients (n=1)
• Did not provided PCT assays (n=1)

13 of studies included in qualitative synthesis

13 of studies included in quantitative synthesis (meta-analysis)

Fig. 1 Selection process for RCTs included in the meta-analysis

the included RCTs (Additional file 4: Table S4). Of these included studies, seven were multicenter studies. A total of 5136 patients comprised 2588 in the PCT-guided group and 2548 in the standard care group. These studies evaluated the effects of PCT-guided strategies in antibiotic discontinuation ($n = 8$) [23, 24, 31–34, 37, 39], antibiotic initiation ($n = 3$) [13, 30, 36], or the combination of the antibiotic initiation and discontinuation ($n = 2$) [35, 38]. Study population included surgical patients ($n = 3$) [30, 31, 33] and mixed medical–surgical patients ($n = 10$) [13, 23, 24, 32, 34–39]. PCT assays adopted varied across the included studies.

Data synthesis

Procalcitonin-guided discontinuation of antibiotics

The use of a PCT algorithm compared with standard care to guide antibiotic discontinuation in critically ill patients was evaluated in eight RCTs [23, 24, 31–34, 37, 39]. All eight studies reported outcomes including total days with antibiotics or antibiotic-free days. The aggregated data suggested that the duration of antibiotic treatment was 1.67 days shorter in PCT-guided group ($n = 3404$; MD − 1.66 days; 95% CI − 2.36 to − 0.96; $I^2 = 71\%$; $P < 0.00001$) [23, 24, 31–34, 37, 39] (Fig. 2), while antibiotic-free days were 2.26 days longer ($n = 2120$; MD 2.26 days; 95% CI 1.40–3.12; $I^2 = 0\%$; $P < 0.00001$) [23, 24, 32, 34] when compared with that of standard care group. Results showed patients in PCT-guided group had lower short-term mortality than standard care group ($n = 3414$; RR 0.86; 95% CI 0.76–0.98; $I^2 = 0\%$; $P = 0.02$) [23, 24, 31–34, 37, 39] (Fig. 3), while no differences were found in ICU LOS ($n = 3326$; MD − 0.00 days; 95% CI − 0.58 to 0.58; $I^2 = 0\%$; $P = 0.99$) [23, 24, 31–33, 37, 39] and hospital LOS ($n = 3290$; MD 0.43 days; 95% CI − 0.83 to 1.70; $I^2 = 30.4\%$; $P = 0.50$) [23, 24, 32, 34, 37, 39]. There was significant heterogeneity in the outcome of duration of antibiotic treatment between the pooled studies. Therefore, we conducted sensitivity analyses to explore potential sources of heterogeneity. Exclusion of the trial by Bloos and colleagues resolved the heterogeneity without alerting the result ($n = 2338$; MD − 1.97 days; 95% CI − 2.27 to − 1.68; $I^2 = 0\%$; $P < 0.00001$) [24, 31–34, 37, 39].

Procalcitonin-guided initiation of antibiotics

Three studies examined the efficacy of PCT-guided initiation of antibiotics [13, 30, 36]. Only one study examined the efficacy of PCT-guided initiation of antibiotics. In this case, antibiotic consumption was comparable between groups with the treatment days represented 62.6% and 57.7% of ICU stays in the PCT and standard care groups, respectively ($P = 0.11$) [36]. There was no statistically significant difference between groups in the

Table 1 Characteristics of included studies

Study/year	Trial design	Population	Type of ICU	N PCT/Ctrl	PCT-guided group protocol	Control group protocol	PCT assay
Svoboda et al. [30]	SC, P, R, OL	Postoperative severe sepsis	Surgical	38/34	AI: prompted change of ABT and catheter (≥ 2 ng/ml), prompted to repeated radiographic and/or surgical evaluation (< 2 ng/ml)	Standard evaluation by consultant surgeon	PCT-Q
Schroeder et al. [31]	SC, P, R, OL	Postoperative severe sepsis	Surgical	14/13	AD: if clinic signs and symptoms improved and PCT < 1 ng/ml or 25–35% of baseline	According to clinical signs and empiric rules	LIA
Nobre et al. [32]	SC, P, R, OL	Sepsis	Mixed	39/40	AD: if baseline PCT > 1 µg/L, re-evaluation at day 5. ABT discontinuation if PCT < 0.25 µg/L or PCT dropped by > 90% from the baseline peak level. If baseline PCT < 1 µg/L, re-evaluation at day 3. ABT discontinuation if PCT < 0.1 µg/L and careful clinical evaluation	Regimens according to guidelines	Kryptor
Hochreiter et al. [33]	SC, P, R, OL	Infection	Surgical	53/57	AD: if clinic signs and symptoms improved and PCT < 1 ng/ml or 25–35% of initial value over 3 days	Standard regimen over 8 days	LIA
Stolz et al. [34]	MC, P, R, OL	Ventilator-associated pneumonia	Mixed	51/50	AD: strongly encouraged (< 0.25 µg/L), encouraged (0.25–0.5 µg/L or a decrease ≥ 80%), discouraged (0.5–1.0 µg/L or a decrease < 80%) or strongly discouraged (> 1.0 µg/L)	According to clinical signs and empiric rules	Kryptor
Bouadma et al. [35]	MC, P, R, OL	Bacterial infection or sepsis	Mixed	311/319	AI: ABT was strongly discouraged (< 0.25 µg/L), discouraged (0.25–0.49 µg/L), encouraged (0.5–0.99 µg/L) or strongly encouraged (≥ 1 µg/L). AD: strongly encouraged (< 0.25 µg/L), encouraged (0.25–0.49 µg/L), continuing of ABT was encouraged (0.25–0.5 µg/L or > 80% peak) and change of ABT (> peak concentration and > 0.5 µg/L)	Regimens according to international and local guidelines	Kryptor
Jensen et al. [13]	MC, P, R, OL	Severe sepsis/septic shock	Mixed	212/247	AI: if PCT ≥ 1 µg/L that was not decreasing by at least 10% from previous day: increasing the antimicrobial spectrum and intensifying diagnostic efforts to find uncontrolled sources of infection	According to current guidelines	Kryptor
Layios et al. [36]	SC, P, R, OL	Infection	Mixed	258/251	AI: ABT was strongly discouraged (< 0.25 µg/L), discouraged (0.25–0.5 µg/L), encouraged (0.5–1.0 µg/L) or strongly encouraged (> 1.0 µg/L)	No reports	Kryptor
Annane et al. [38]	MC, P, R, OL	Septic shock	Mixed	31/31	AI/AD: ABT was not to be started or was to be discontinuation (< 0.25 µg/L); strongly discouraged (≥ 0.25 to < 0.5 µg/L); was recommended (≥ 0.5 to < 5 µg/L) and was strongly recommended (≥ 5 µg/L). For patients enrolled ≤ 48 h after surgery, the respective PCT cut-offs were < 4 µg/L, 4–9 µg/L and ≥ 9 µg/L	ABT at the discretion of the patient's physician	Kryptor

Table 1 continued

Study/year	Trial design	Population	Type of ICU	N PCT/Ctrl	PCT-guided group protocol	Control group protocol	PCT assay
Deliberato et al. [39]	SC, P, R, OL	Sepsis	Mixed	42/39	AD: if PCT dropped > 90% from the peak level or the absolute value < 0.5 ng/ml	The possible source of infection and local susceptibility profile	Vidas
Shehabi et al. [23]	MC, P, R, SB	Bacterial infection or sepsis	Mixed	200/200	AD: cease ABT when PCT < 0.1 ng/ml or PCT was 0.1–0.25 ng/ml and infection is highly unlikely or PCT level decreased > 90% from baseline	According to the ABT guidelines	Automated immunoassay analysers
De Jong et al. [24]	MC, P, R, OL	Infection	Mixed	776/799	AD: if PCT value decreased over 80% or PCT value lower than 0.5 μg/L	Guidelines and the discretion of attending physicians	Vidas, Roche or Kryptor machine
Bloos et al. [37]	MC, P, R, OL	Severe sepsis/septic shock	Mixed	587/593	AD: stopping ABT if PCT level on day 7 or later < 1 ng/ml r or dropped > 50% from the previous value	According to the local sepsis guidelines	Kryptor

ABT antibiotics, *AD* antibiotic discontinuation, *AI* antibiotic initiation, *Ctrl* control, *ICU* intensive care unit, *LIA* immunoluminometric assay, *MC* multi-centre, *Mixed* surgical and medical intensive care unit, *OL* open label, *P* prospective, *PCT* procalcitonin, *PCT-Q* procalcitonin immunochromatographic technology, *R* RCT, *SC* single centre

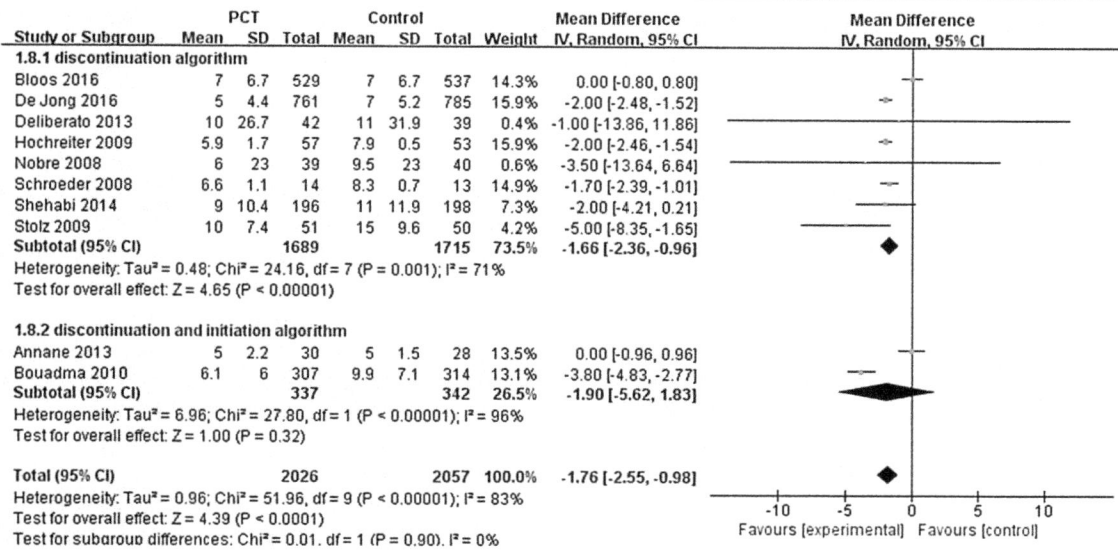

Fig. 2 Effects of PCT-guided antimicrobial strategies on total days of antibiotics

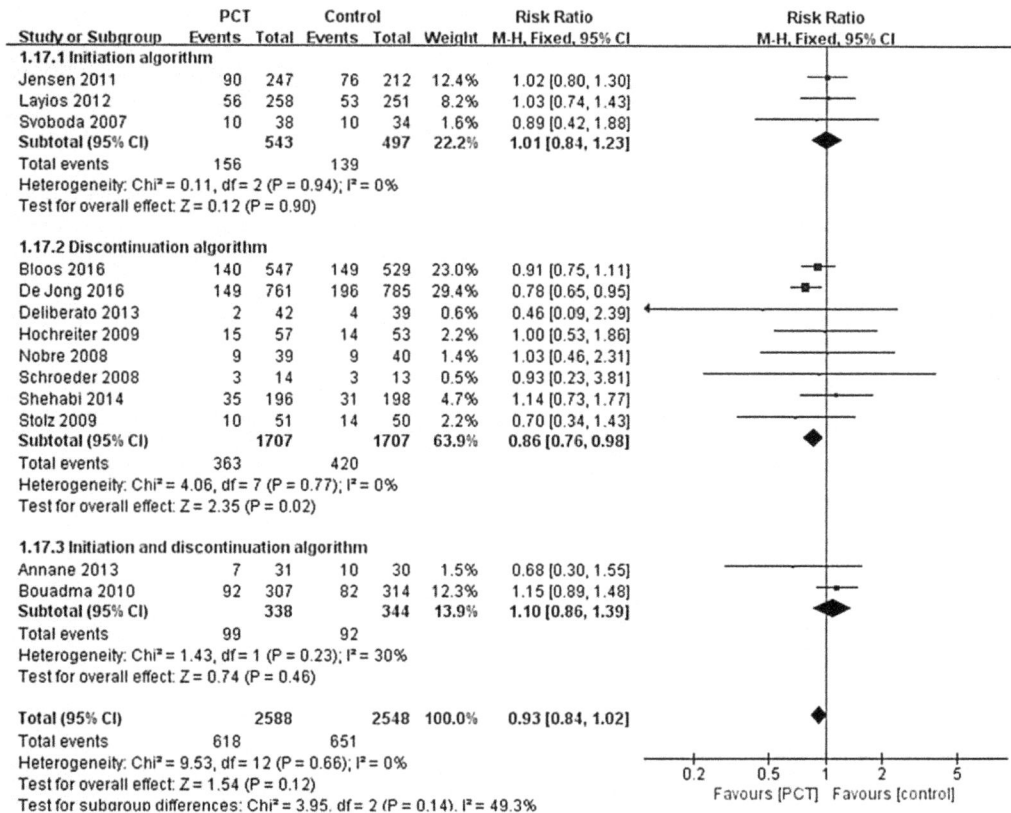

Fig. 3 Effects PCT-guided antimicrobial strategies on short-term mortality

risk of short-term mortality ($n = 1040$; RR 1.01; 95% CI 0.84–1.23; $I^2 = 0\%$; $P = 0.90$) [13, 30, 36] (Fig. 3) or ICU LOS ($n = 581$; MD − 1.22 days; 95% CI − 4.34 to 1.90; $I^2 = 60\%$; $P = 0.44$) [30, 36].

Procalcitonin-guided antibiotic initiation and discontinuation

Two studies employed a PCT-guided strategy of antibiotic initiation and discontinuation [35, 38]. No differences were observed between the PCT and standard care group in total days with antibiotics ($n = 679$; MD − 1.90 days, 95% CI − 5.62 to 1.83; $I^2 = 96\%$; $P = 0.32$) (Fig. 2), antibiotic-free days ($n = 679$; MD 1.31 days; 95% CI − 1.34 to 3.95; $I^2 = 90\%$; $P = 0.33$), short-term mortality ($n = 682$; RR 1.10; 95% CI 0.86–1.39; $I^2 = 30\%$; $P = 0.46$) (Fig. 3), the ICU LOS ($n = 682$; MD − 1.45 days; 95% CI − 0.91 to 3.80; $I^2 = 0\%$; $P = 0.23$), and hospital LOS ($n = 679$; MD − 0.43 days; 95% CI − 3.36 to 2.49; $I^2 = 0\%$; $P = 0.77$) [35, 38].

Summary of findings for the effect of PCT-guided strategy antibiotic on predefined outcomes in ICU patients is described in Table 2. We did not assess the publication bias because of the limited number of studies included in each analysis.

Discussion

PCT-guided strategies had been examined in multiple studies to optimize antibiotic treatment, with conflicting results. The current meta-analysis justified a low PCT level to discontinue antibiotic treatment, which would result in a shorter duration of antibiotic treatment of about 1.67 days, as well as lower short-term mortality compared with standard care. Due to the insufficient evidence, a baseline PCT value should not be used as a marker to guide antibiotic initiation.

Our study had several strengths. The current meta-analysis provided robust evidence to support and expand the weak suggestion in the 2016 SSC guidelines, i.e. use of low PCT level to assist the clinician in the discontinuation of empiric antibiotic [12]. In addition to those RCTs in previous meta-analyses, we had included three additional RCTs recently published, and this added to the statistical power by having 3414 cases to evaluate the primary outcome. Moreover, we had stratified enrolled RCTs according to different PCT-guided strategies, in order to eliminate the potential confounding factors caused by different strategies. Though significant heterogeneity was observed among these studies, our sensitivity analyses demonstrated that the heterogeneity was resulted from the trial by Bloss et al. [23]. This study was different from the other trials in some aspects. On the one hand, it was designed as a 2 × 2 factorial trial and the interaction between the two treatment factors was unclear; on the other hand, in the trial [23], the clinicians used a 50% decrease from previous value as a stopping rule, which was lower than that of other studies. As a result, we also demonstrated a significant improvement in short-term mortality associated with PCT-guided antibiotic discontinuation. This had added robustness to findings of reduction in antibiotics usage, since studies have demonstrated

Table 2 Summary of findings for the effect of procalcitonin-guided strategy on predefined outcomes in intensive care unit patients

PCT-guided strategy	Predefined outcome	Number of trials	N	Estimated benefit with antibiotic	I^2 (%)	P value
ABT discontinuation	Duration of antibiotic use	8	3404	− 1.66 days (− 2.36, − 0.96)	71	P < 0.0001
	Antibiotic-free days	4	2120	2.26 days (1.40, 3.12)	0	P < 0.0001
	Short-term mortality	8	3414	0.86 (0.76, 0.98)	0	0.02
	Length of stay in ICU	7	3326	− 0.00 days (− 0.58, 0.58)	0	0.99
	Length of stay in hospital	6	3290	0.43 days (− 0.83, 1.70)	30	0.50
ABT initiation	Duration of antibiotic use	–	–	–	–	–
	Antibiotic-free days	–	–	–	–	–
	Short-term mortality	3	1040	1.01 (0.84, 1.23)	0	0.90
	Length of stay in ICU	2	581	− 1.22 days (− 4.34, 1.90)	60	0.44
	Length of stay in hospital	–	–	–	–	–
ABT initiation and discontinuation	Duration of antibiotic use	2	679	− 1.90 days (− 5.62, 1.83)	96	0.32
	Antibiotic-free days	2	679	1.31 days (− 1.34, 3.95)	90	0.33
	Short-term mortality	2	682	1.10 (0.86, 1.39)	30	0.46
	Length of stay in ICU	2	682	− 1.45 days (− 0.91, 3.80)	0	0.23
	Length of stay in hospital	2	750	− 0.43 days (− 3.36, 2.49)	0	0.77

ABT antibiotics, *PCT* procalcitonin, *ICU* intensive care unit

that strategies aiming at restricting antibiotic overuse could help improve survival [40, 41]. Our findings that short-term mortality was significantly reduced in the PCT-guided discontinuation group contrasted those of previous meta-analyses. Despite the fact that no heterogeneity was detected, the beneficial effect was clearly driven by the study results of de Jong et al. [24]. However, as the authors acknowledged, this study was a non-inferiority study; therefore, the beneficial effect of mortality in PCT-guided group was unexpected, which merited cautious interpretation and further validation.

As for a PCT strategy that combined initiation and discontinuation of antibiotics, we found no beneficial effect with regard to any predefined outcomes. The reason for this failure may be that only two trials (one positive [35] and one negative [38]) investigated the combined strategies varying in objective and the methodology. On the other hand, reported non-compliance rate was high. For example, in a prospective, multicenter, open-label randomized trial (PRORATA trial) involving 630 non-surgical patients with suspected bacterial infections [35], patients in the PCT group had significantly more antibiotic-free days. However, the algorithm-guided treatment recommendation was not strictly followed in 53% of patients in the PCT group. Moreover, this trial [35] reported a higher standard deviation with regard to duration of antibiotic treatment as well as antibiotic-free days (possibly due to reported higher non-compliance rate), compared to that in the negative trial [38], which weaken its statistic weight in the meta-analysis. Interestingly, it was noteworthy that initial antibiotic prescription rate was similar in PCT and standard care groups, suggesting that the improvement in antibiotic-free days was more likely the result of antibiotic discontinuation, while it was less likely due to exclusion of potential infection.

In our study, we could not verify the efficacy of PCT-based antibiotic initiation strategy because we found only three RCT through the literature search [13, 30, 36]. Of these trials, only the trial by Layios and coworkers reported the antibiotics exposure and concluded that PCT measuring for the initiation of antibiotics failed to decrease the antibiotic consummation [36]. The reasons for this failure may be that almost half of PCT serum samples were > 1 μg/L, thus encouraging the antibiotic treatment, and the relative low proportion of patient-days with antibiotic treatment in the control group (57%). Another reason could be related to the high non-compliance rate with the PCT-guided antibiotic initiation strategy described in the study. The authors reported that nearly 64% of patients in the PCT group received antibiotics regardless of a normal PCT level (< 0.5 μg/L).

The incidence of non-compliance with the recommendations based on PCT algorithm, as reported in some, but not all RCTs, showed significant variability, ranging from 0 to 59%. In most case of non-compliance, physicians were reluctant to stop antibiotics, even with a very low PCT level (Additional file 4: Table S4), possibly due to the concerns about the accuracy of single PCT value as a biomarker of infection [42, 43]. This might lead to unnecessarily prolonged exposure of antibiotics, which supported the robustness of our findings that implementation of PCT algorithm was associated with shorter duration of antibiotic treatment and longer antibiotic-free days.

Our meta-analysis has some limitations. First, studies examining the PCT-guided strategies other than discontinuation of antibiotic treatment were scarce, with limited number of studies available as well as small number of enrolled patients. As such, data on these strategies were insufficient to draw solid conclusions. Second, the high exclusion rate of screened patients in the included studies (such as immunosuppressed patients and those requiring long-term antibiotic therapy) precluded generalization of the study results. Third, antibiotic strategy in the control group (indications to initiate and discontinue antibiotics) was not specified in most studies. Whether the variation in antibiotic strategy, if any, in the control group might have affected the results of our meta-analysis is unclear. Thus, a more uniform approach to evaluating and reporting standard care related to antibiotic use would be needed in future studies. Fourth, the uneven distribution of different underlying diseases among included studies might also exert a prognostic value. Of note, in the two recently published systematic reviews and individual patient data meta-analysis [44, 45], Schuetz et al. demonstrated with sufficient evidence that PCT-guided antibiotic treatment in patients with acute respiratory infections reduced antibiotic exposure and side effects and improved survival. Finally, different cut-off values of PCT and different PCT measurements were reported across included studies, which might also lead to bias in our results. We had originally tried to perform subgroup analyses exploring studies according to all the diversities. However, there were insufficient data.

Conclusions

In summary, based on the results of our meta-analysis, we recommend use of PCT to guide antibiotic discontinuation, which was associated with a reduction in antibiotic exposure and lower short-term mortality. Further studies are needed to define the optimal cut-off value of PCT for antibiotic discontinuation and to generalize our findings in other patient population including immunocompromised patients and those received long-term antibiotic therapy in ICU.

Abbreviations

CI: confidence interval; ICU: intensive care unit; IQR: interquartile range; LOS: length of stay; MD: mean difference; PCT: procalcitonin; RR: risk ratio; RCTs: randomized controlled trials; SD: standard deviations; VAP: ventilator-associated pneumonia.

Authors' contributions

H-BH contributed to the conception of the study, data collection, analysis, and drafting of the article. WJ and C-YW contributed to data collection and analysis. LW and J-MP contributed to design and revisions of this manuscript. BD was responsible for the integrity of the work as a whole, from inception to publication of the article. All authors read and approved the final manuscript.

Author details

[1] Medical ICU, Peking Union Medical College Hospital, Peking Union Medical College and Chinese Academy of Medical Sciences, 1 Shuai Fu Yuan, Beijing 100730, People's Republic of China. [2] Department of Critical Care Medicine, The First Affiliated Hospital of Fujian Medical University, Fuzhou, China.

Acknowledgements

We thank Jing-Chao Luo, MD, for his assistance in searching the literature.

Competing interests

The authors declare that they have no competing interests.

Funding

Cams Innovation Fund for Medical Sciences (2016-12M-1-014).

References

1. Braykov NP, Morgan DJ, Schweizer ML, et al. Assessment of empirical antibiotic therapy optimisation in six hospitals: an observational cohort study. Lancet Infect Dis. 2014;14(14):1220–7.
2. Llor C, Bjerrum L. Antimicrobial resistance: risk associated with antibiotic overuse and initiatives to reduce the problem. Ther Adv Drug Saf. 2014;5(6):229–41.
3. Dellit TH, Owens RC, McGowan JE Jr, et al. Infectious Diseases Society of America and the Society for Healthcare Epidemiology of America guidelines for developing an institutional program to enhance antimicrobial stewardship. Clin Infect Dis. 2007;44(4):263–4.
4. Dimopoulos G, Poulakou G, Pneumatikos IA, Armaganidis A, Kollef MH, Matthaiou DK. Short- vs long-duration antibiotic regimens for ventilator-associated pneumonia: a systematic review and meta-analysis. Chest. 2013;144(6):1759–67.
5. Najafi A, Khodadadian A, Sanatkar M, et al. The comparison of procalcitonin guidance administer antibiotics with empiric antibiotic therapy in critically ill patients admitted in intensive care unit. Acta Medica Iranica. 2015;53(9):562–7.
6. Evans HL, Lefrak SN, Lyman J, et al. Cost of gram-negative resistance. Crit Care Med. 2007;35(1):89–95.
7. Vincent JL, Rello J, Marshall J, et al. International study of the prevalence and outcomes of infection in intensive care units. J Am Med Assoc. 2009;302(21):2323–9.
8. Luyt CE, Combes A, Reynaud C, et al. Usefulness of procalcitonin for the diagnosis of ventilator-associated pneumonia. Intensive Care Med. 2008;34(8):1434–40.
9. Simon L, Lacroix J. Serum procalcitonin and C-reactive protein levels as markers of bacterial infection: a systematic review and meta-analysis. Clin Infect Dis. 2004;39:206–17.
10. Wacker C, Prkno A, Brunkhorst FM, Schlattmann P. Procalcitonin as a diagnostic marker for sepsis: a systematic review and meta-analysis. Lancet Infect Dis. 2013;13(5):426–35.
11. Schuetz P, Muller B, Christ-Crain M, et al. Procalcitonin to initiate or discontinue antibiotics in acute respiratory tract infections. Evid Based Child Health. 2013;8:1297–371.
12. Rhodes A, Evans LE, Alhazzani W, et al. Surviving sepsis campaign: international guidelines for management of sepsis and septic shock. Crit Care Med. 2017;45(3):486–552.
13. Jensen JU, Hein L, Lundgren B, et al. Procalcitonin-guided interventions against infections to increase early appropriate antibiotics and improve survival in the intensive care unit: a randomized trial. Crit Care Med. 2011;39(9):2048–58.
14. Kopterides P, Siempos II, Tsangaris I, Tsantes A, Armaganidis A. Procalcitonin-guided algorithms of antibiotic therapy in the intensive care unit: a systematic review and meta-analysis of randomized controlled trials. Crit Care Med. 2010;38(11):2229–41.
15. Heyland DK, Johnson AP, Reynolds SC, Muscedere J. Procalcitonin for reduced antibiotic exposure in the critical care setting: a systematic review and an economic evaluation. Crit Care Med. 2011;39(7):1792–9.
16. Agarwal R, Schwartz DN. Procalcitonin to guide duration of antimicrobial therapy in intensive care units: a systematic review. Clin Infect Dis. 2011;53(4):379–87.
17. Schuetz P, Chiappa V, Briel M, Greenwald JL. Procalcitonin algorithms for antibiotic therapy decisions: a systematic review of randomized controlled trials and recommendations for clinical algorithms. Arch Intern Med. 2011;171(15):1322–31.
18. Soni NJ, Pitrak DL, Aronson N, Samson DJ, Galaydick JL, Vats V. Procalcitonin-guided antibiotic therapy. Agency for Healthcare Research and Quality. 2012.
19. Matthaiou DK, Ntani G, Kontogiorgi M, Poulakou G, Armaganidis A, Dimopoulos G. An ESICM systematic review and meta-analysis of procalcitonin-guided antibiotic therapy algorithms in adult critically ill patients. Intensive Care Med. 2012;38(6):940–9.
20. Tang H, Huang T, Jing J, Shen H, Cui W. Effect of procalcitonin-guided treatment in patients with infections: a systematic review and meta-analysis. Infection. 2009;37(6):497–507.
21. Prkno A, Wacker C, Brunkhorst FM, Schlattmann P. Procalcitonin-guided therapy in intensive care unit patients with severe sepsis and septic shock—a systematic review and meta-analysis. Crit Care. 2013;17(6):R291.
22. Westwood M, Ramaekers B, Whiting P, et al. Procalcitonin testing to guide antibiotic therapy for the treatment of sepsis in intensive care settings and for suspected bacterial infection in emergency department settings a systematic review and cost-effectiveness analysis. Health Technol Assess. 2015;19(96):1–236.
23. Bloos F, Trips E, Nierhaus A, et al. Effect of sodium selenite administration and procalcitonin-guided therapy on mortality in patients with severe sepsis or septic shock: a randomized clinical trial. JAMA Intern Med. 2016;176(9):1266–76.
24. de Jong E, van Oers JA, Beishuizen A, et al. Efficacy and safety of procalcitonin guidance in reducing the duration of antibiotic treatment in critically ill patients: a randomised, controlled, open-label trial. Lancet Infect Dis. 2016;16(7):819–27.
25. Moher D, Liberati A, Tetzlaff J, Altman DG, Group TP. Preferred reporting items for systematic reviews and meta-analyses: the PRISMA statement. J Chin Integr Med. 2010;8(5):336–41.
26. Huang H, Li Y, Ariani F, Chen X, Lin J. Timing of tracheostomy in critically ill patients: a meta-analysis. PLoS ONE. 2014;9(3):e92981.
27. Wang F, Wu Y, Bo L, et al. The timing of tracheotomy in critically ill patients undergoing mechanical ventilation: a systematic review and meta-analysis of randomized controlled trials. Chest. 2011;140(140):1456–65.
28. Higgins JP, Altman DG, Gotzsche PC, et al. The Cochrane Collaboration's tool for assessing risk of bias in randomised trials. BMJ. 2011;343(oct18 2):d5928.
29. Wan X, Wang W, Liu J, Tong T. Estimating the sample mean and standard deviation from the sample size, median, range and/or interquartile range. BMC Med Res Methodol. 2014;14(8):735–46.
30. Svoboda P, Kantorová I, Scheer P, Radvanova J, Radvan M. Can procalcitonin help us in timing of re-intervention in septic patients after multiple trauma or major surgery? Hepatogastroenterology. 2007;54(74):359–63.

31. Schroeder S, Hochreiter M, Koehler T, et al. Procalcitonin (PCT)-guided algorithm reduces length of antibiotic treatment in surgical intensive care patients with severe sepsis: results of a prospective randomized study. Langenbecks Arch Surg. 2009;394(2):221–6.

32. Nobre V, Harbarth S, Graf JD, Rohner P, Pugin J. Use of procalcitonin to shorten antibiotic treatment duration in septic patients: a randomized trial. Am J Respir Crit Care Med. 2008;177(5):498–505.

33. Hochreiter M, Kohler T, Schweiger AM, et al. Procalcitonin to guide duration of antibiotic therapy in intensive care patients: a randomized prospective controlled trial. Crit Care. 2009;13(3):R83.

34. Stolz D, Smyrnios N, Eggimann P, et al. Procalcitonin for reduced antibiotic exposure in ventilator-associated pneumonia: a randomised study. Eur Respir J. 2009;34(6):1364–75.

35. Bouadma L, Luyt CE, et al. Use of procalcitonin to reduce patients' exposure to antibiotics in intensive care units (PRORATA trial): a multicentre randomised controlled trial. Lancet. 2010;375(9713):463–74.

36. Layios N, Lambermont B, Canivet JL, et al. Procalcitonin usefulness for the initiation of antibiotic treatment in intensive care unit patients. Crit Care Med. 2012;40(8):2304–9.

37. Shehabi Y, Sterba M, Garrett PM, et al. Procalcitonin algorithm in critically ill adults with undifferentiated infection or suspected sepsis. A randomized controlled trial. Am J Respir Crit Care Med. 2014;190(10):1102–10.

38. Annane D, Maxime V, Faller JP, et al. Procalcitonin levels to guide antibi-otic therapy in adults with non-microbiologically proven apparent severe sepsis: a randomised controlled trial. BMJ Open. 2013;3(2):e002186.

39. Deliberato RO, Marra AR, Sanches PR, et al. Clinical and economic impact of procalcitonin to shorten antimicrobial therapy in septic patients with proven bacterial infection in an intensive care setting. Diagn Microbiol Infect Dis. 2013;76(3):266–71.

40. Levy SB, Marshall B. Antibacterial resistance worldwide: causes, challenges and responses. Nat Med. 2004;10(12 suppl):S122–9.

41. Cohen ML. Epidemiology of drug resistance: implications for a post-antimicrobial era. Science. 1992;257(257):1050–5.

42. Schuetz P, Affolter B, Hunziker S, et al. Serum procalcitonin, C-reactive protein and white blood cell levels following hypothermia after cardiac arrest: a retrospective cohort study. Eur J Clin Invest. 2010;40(4):376–81.

43. Jung B, Molinari N, Nasri M, et al. Procalcitonin biomarker kinetics fails to predict treatment response in perioperative abdominal infection with septic shock. Crit Care. 2013;17(5):R25.

44. Schuetz P, Wirz Y, Sager R, et al. Procalcitonin to initiate or discontinue antibiotics in acute respiratory tract infections. Cochrane Database Syst Rev. 2017;10:CD007498.

45. Schuetz P, Wirz Y, Sager R et al. Effect of procalcitonin-guided antibiotic treatment on mortality in acute respiratory infections: a patient level meta-analysis. Lancet Infect Dis. 2017. https://doi.org/10.1016/S1473-3099(17)30592-3.

The host response in critically ill sepsis patients on statin therapy: a prospective observational study

Maryse A. Wiewel[1,2]*[iD], Brendon P. Scicluna[1,2,3], Lonneke A. van Vught[1,2], Arie J. Hoogendijk[1,2], Aeilko H. Zwinderman[3], René Lutter[4], Janneke Horn[5], Olaf L. Cremer[6], Marc J. Bonten[7,8], Marcus J. Schultz[5] and Tom van der Poll[1,2,9]

Abstract

Background: Statins can exert pleiotropic anti-inflammatory, vascular protective and anticoagulant effects, which in theory could improve the dysregulated host response during sepsis. We aimed to determine the association between prior statin use and host response characteristics in critically ill patients with sepsis.

Methods: We performed a prospective observational study in 1060 patients admitted with sepsis to the mixed intensive care units (ICUs) of two hospitals in the Netherlands between January 2011 and July 2013. Of these, 351 patients (33%) were on statin therapy before admission. The host response was evaluated by measuring 23 biomarkers providing insight into key pathways implicated in sepsis pathogenesis and by analyzing whole-blood leukocyte transcriptomes in samples obtained within 24 h after ICU admission. To account for indication bias, a propensity score-matched cohort was created ($N = 194$ in both groups for protein biomarkers and $N = 95$ in both groups for gene expression analysis).

Results: Prior statin use was not associated with an altered mortality up to 90 days after admission (38.0 vs. 39.7% in the non-statin users in the propensity-matched analysis). Statin use did not modify systemic inflammatory responses, activation of the vascular endothelium or the coagulation system. The blood leukocyte genomic response, characterized by over-expression of genes involved in inflammatory and innate immune signaling pathways as well as under-expression of genes associated to T cell function, was not different between patients with and without prior statin use.

Conclusions: Statin therapy is not associated with a modified host response in sepsis patients on admission to the ICU.

Keywords: Statins, Sepsis, Host response, Biomarkers, Mortality

Background

Sepsis is the consequence of a deregulated host response to infection, featured by disproportionate pro- and anti-inflammatory mechanisms and disturbed vascular responses, including increased leukocyte adhesion, vasodilation, and loss of endothelial barrier function [1, 2]. In addition, obstruction of microvessel lumens by microthrombi and plugs of white and red blood cells, fibrin deposition and impaired anticoagulant mechanisms are other important elements of sepsis-induced organ dysfunction.

Statins, or HMG-CoA reductase inhibitors, are widely used to lower blood cholesterol levels. Besides decreasing cholesterol concentrations, statins have multiple additional effects that might influence the host response during sepsis, including inhibition of proinflammatory

*Correspondence: m.a.wiewel@amc.uva.nl
[1] Center for Experimental and Molecular Medicine, Academic Medical Center, University of Amsterdam, Meibergdreef 9, Room G2-130, 1105 AZ Amsterdam, The Netherlands

cytokine release and endothelial cell activation, reduction of endothelial dysfunction and attenuation of coagulation activation [3–6]. Several, but not all, observational studies have shown a survival benefit for patients with sepsis on statin therapy, with recent meta-analyses reporting an overall lower risk of sepsis and infection-associated death in chronic statin users [7, 8]. Considering the abundant literature on pleiotropic non-lipid lowering properties of statins, we investigated the association between prior statin use and potential host response alterations in this population of critically ill patients with sepsis. For this, we measured 23 biomarkers indicative of systemic inflammation, and activation of the vascular endothelium and the coagulation system, and in an unbiased approach analyzed whole-blood leukocyte transcriptomes in sepsis patients stratified according to prior statin use.

Methods

Study design, patients and definitions

This study was conducted as part of the "Molecular Diagnosis and Risk Stratification of Sepsis" (MARS) project, a prospective observational study in the mixed ICUs of two tertiary teaching hospitals (Academic Medical Center in Amsterdam and University Medical Center Utrecht) in the Netherlands [9–11]. Trained physicians prospectively collected the following data: demographics, comorbidities, chronic medication use, ICU admission characteristics, daily physiological measurements, severity scores, antibiotic use, and culture results. The plausibility of infection was post hoc scored based on all available evidence and classified on a 4-point scale (none, possible, probable or definite) according to Center for Disease Control and Prevention [15] and International Sepsis Forum consensus definitions [16], as described in detail previously [9]. For the current analysis, we selected all patients included in the MARS-study between January 2011 and July 2013 with sepsis, diagnosed within 24 h after admission, defined by the presence of a definite or probable infection [9] combined with at least one of general, inflammatory, hemodynamic, organ dysfunction or tissue perfusion parameters derived from the 2001 International Sepsis Definitions Conference [17]. Readmissions and patients transferred from another ICU were excluded, except for patients referred to one of the study centers on the day of admission. Organ failure was defined as a score of 3 or greater on the SOFA score, except for cardiovascular failure for which a score of 1 or more was used [12]. Shock was defined as use of vasopressors (noradrenaline) for hypotension in a dose of 0.1 mcg/kg/min during at least 50% of the ICU day. Patients were assessed daily for the presence of acute kidney injury and acute lung injury using strict preset criteria [13, 14]. Left-over plasma (obtained from blood drawn for patient care) was obtained within 24 h of admission to the ICU and stored within 4 h at − 80 °C. The Medical Ethical Committees of both study centers gave approval for an opt-out consent method (IRB no. 10-056C) [9, 10]. The Municipal Personal Records Database was queried to determine survival up to 1 year after ICU admission.

Biomarker assays

All measurements were performed in EDTA anticoagulated plasma obtained on admission. Tumor necrosis factor alpha (TNF-α), interleukin-1beta (IL-1β), IL-6, IL-8, IL-10, IL-13, interferon-γ, granulocyte-macrophage colony-stimulating factor (GM-CSF), soluble intercellular adhesion molecule-1 (ICAM-1), soluble E-selectin and fractalkine were measured using FlexSet cytometric bead arrays (BD Bioscience, San Jose, CA) using a FACS Calibur (Becton Dickenson, Franklin Lakes, NJ, USA). Angiopoietin-1, angiopoietin-2, protein C, antithrombin, matrix metalloproteinase (MMP)-8, tissue inhibitor of metalloproteinase (TIMP)-1 (R&D systems, Abingdon, UK), and D-dimer (Procartaplex, eBioscience, San Diego, CA) were measured by Luminex multiplex assay using a BioPlex 200 (BioRad, Hercules, CA). C-reactive protein (CRP) was determined by an immunoturbidimetric assay (Roche diagnostics). Platelet counts were determined by hemocytometry, prothrombin time (PT) and activated partial thromboplastin time (aPTT) by using a photometric method with Dade Innovin Reagent or by Dade Actin FS Activated PTT Reagent, respectively (both Siemens Healthcare Diagnostics). Normal biomarker values were acquired from 27 age- and gender-matched healthy volunteers, from whom written informed consent was obtained, except for CRP, platelet counts, PT and aPTT (routine laboratory reference values).

Blood gene expression microarrays

Whole blood was collected in PAXgene™ tubes (Becton–Dickinson, Breda, the Netherlands) within 24 h after ICU admission. PAXgene blood samples were also obtained from 42 healthy controls [median age 35 (interquartile range 30–63) years; 57% male] after providing written informed consent. Total RNA was isolated using the PAXgene blood mRNA kit (Qiagen, Venlo, the Netherlands) in combination with QIAcube automated system (Qiagen, Venlo, the Netherlands), according to the manufacturer's instructions. RNA (RNA integrity number > 6.0) was processed and hybridized to the Affymetrix Human Genome U219 96-array and scanned by using the GeneTitan instrument at the Cologne Center for Genomics (CCG), Cologne, Germany, as described by the manufacturer (Affymetrix).

Raw data scans (.CEL files) were read into the R language and environment for statistical computing (version

2.15.1; R Foundation for Statistical Computing, Vienna, Austria; http://www.R-project.org/). Pre-processing and quality control was performed by using the Affy package version 1.36.1. Array data were background corrected by robust multi-array average, quantiles-normalized and summarized by median polish using the expresso function (Affy package). The resultant 49,386 log-transformed probe intensities were filtered by means of a 0.5 variance cutoff using the genefilter method [18] to recover 24,646 expressed probes in at least one sample. The occurrence of non-experimental chip effects was evaluated by means of the Surrogate Variable Analysis (R package version 3.4.0) and corrected by the empirical Bayes method ComBat [19, 20]. The non-normalized and normalized MARS gene expression data sets are available at the Gene Expression Omnibus public repository of NCBI under accession number GSE65682. The 24,646 probes were assessed for differential abundance across healthy subject and patient samples by means of the limma method (version 3.14.4) [21]. Supervised analysis (comparison between pre-defined groups) was performed by moderated t statistics. Throughout Benjamini–Hochberg (BH) multiple comparison adjusted probabilities, correcting for the 24,646 probes (false discovery rate < 5%), defined significance. Ingenuity Pathway Analysis (Ingenuity Systems IPA, http://www.ingenuity.com) was used to identify the associating canonical signaling pathways stratifying genes by over- and under-expressed patterns. The ingenuity gene knowledgebase was selected as reference and human species specified. All other parameters were default. Multiple comparison adjusted Fisher test probabilities < 0.05 defined significance.

Statistical analysis

Data analyses were performed in R (v3.1.1) [22]. Baseline characteristics of study groups were compared with Chi-square test for categorical variables and t-test for continuous variables. Non-normally distributed continuous variables, including biomarker levels, were analyzed with Wilcoxon rank sum test. To account for differential likelihood of receiving statins, we constructed a propensity score [23], using logistic regression, including variables associated with use of statins and variables that we considered of relevance to our outcome. This score included age, gender, weight, race (white), cerebrovascular disease, chronic cardiovascular insufficiency, chronic renal insufficiency, congestive heart failure, chronic obstructive pulmonary disease (COPD), diabetes mellitus, hematologic malignancy, hypertension, metastatic malignancy, history of myocardial infarction, ACE-inhibitors/ARBs, antiplatelet drugs, beta-blockers, oral antidiabetic drugs, and site of infection (pulmonary, abdominal, urinary). Subjects were 1:1 matched by the estimated propensity

score using nearest neighbor matching with a caliper of 0.2SD of the logit of the propensity score, using R package "MatchIt". Patients whose plasma samples were not collected for biomarker analyses within 24 h of ICU admission and were excluded from the matching procedure. In addition, matching for analyses of gene expression profiles was done using only patients from whom gene expression data were available. Standardized differences were calculated to determine balance between the propensity-matched groups [24]. In order to retain enough power to detect differences in biomarker levels, we accepted standardized differences between propensity-matched groups for comorbidities and chronic medication up to 20%. To investigate the independent association between statin use and 30-day mortality in our propensity-matched plasma biomarker cohort, we performed logistic regression including statin use, variables associated with mortality and comorbidities not optimally matched between users and non-users. P values below 0.05 were considered statistically significant. In host response biomarker comparisons, a Bonferroni-corrected P value of 0.002 was taken as cutoff to define statistical significance.

Results

Study population

From January 2011 until July 2013, 6994 admissions were included in the MARS-study, of which 1483 involved an admission diagnosis of sepsis (Additional file 1: Figure 1). Transfers from other ICUs and readmissions were excluded (129 and 250, respectively). Prior use of medication could not be traced in 44 cases. As a result, 1060 patients were included for analysis, of whom 351 (33.1%) used statins (Table 1). Simvastatin was the most common statin prescribed (53.8%), followed by atorvastatin (21.4%), pravastatin (14%) and rosuvastatin (8%). Patients who used statins were older, more frequently men, and had higher body mass indexes. As expected, statin users were more often suffering from diabetes, hypertension, cerebrovascular disease, chronic renal insufficiency, congestive heart failure, COPD and peripheral vascular disease; statin users had a lower prevalence of malignancy. In accordance with these differences in comorbid conditions, statin users more often used a variety of other types of chronic medication, including ACE inhibitors, ARBs, antiplatelet drugs, beta-blockers, insulin, and oral antidiabetic drugs. Statin use was associated with a lower prevalence of alcohol or drug abuse. Considering the large differences in demographics and comorbidities between users and non-users of statins at baseline, we constructed propensity score-matched cohorts to correct for these pre-admission dissimilarities [23]. Nine patients (1%) could not be assigned a propensity score due to

Table 1 Baseline characteristics of sepsis patients admitted to the ICU stratified according to prior use of statins

Characteristics	Unmatched cohort			Propensity-matched cohort		
	Statins N = 351	No statins N = 709	p	Statins N = 194	No statins N = 194	p
Demographics						
Age, years, mean [SD]	67.0 [9.9]	58.7 [15.6]	< .0001	66.7 [10.5]	65.8 [13.2]	.43
Gender, male (%)	238 (67.8)	402 (56.7)	.002	123 (63.4)	121 (62.4)	.93
Race, white (%)	315 (89.7)	619 (87.3)	.19	175 (90.2)	175 (90.2)	1
BMI, kg/m^2, mean [SD]	26.8 [6.2]	25.6 [6.1]	.002	26.6 [6.09]	27.0 [6.95]	.49
Comorbidities						
Cerebrovascular disease (%)	58 (16.5)	43 (6.1)	< .001	32 (16.5)	24 (12.4)	.31
Chronic cardiovascular insufficiency (%)	22 (6.3)	17 (2.4)	.002	11 (5.7)	10 (5.2)	1
Chronic renal insufficiency (%)	88 (25.1)	67 (9.4)	< .001	46 (23.7)	38 (19.6)	.38
Congestive heart failure (%)	29 (8.3)	23 (3.2)	.002	10 (5.2)	10 (5.2)	1
COPD (%)	70 (19.9)	89 (12.6)	.005	32 (16.5)	36 (18.6)	.70
Diabetes mellitus (%)	133 (37.9)	89 (12.6)	< .001	60 (30.9)	48 (24.7)	.19
Hematologic malignancy (%)	9 (2.6)	70 (9.9)	.001	7 (3.6)	6 (3.1)	1
Hypertension (%)	174 (49.6)	159 (22.4)	< .001	81 (41.8)	76 (39.2)	.68
Immune deficiency (%)	72 (20.5)	158 (22.3)	.52	38 (19.6)	43 (22.2)	.63
Metastatic malignancy (%)	6 (1.7)	39 (5.5)	.004	3 (1.5)	1 (0.5)	.62
Myocardial infarction (history of) (%)	70 (19.9)	30 (4.2)	< .001	29 (14.9)	22 (11.3)	.38
Non-metastatic malignancy (%)	62 (17.7)	89 (12.6)	.03	43 (22.2)	33 (17)	.24
Peripheral vascular disease (%)	82 (23.4)	50 (7.1)	< .001	46 (23.7)	26 (13.4)	.01
Alcohol or drug abuse (%)	17 (4.8)	60 (8.5)	.04	11 (5.7)	17 (8.8)	.33
Chronic medication						
ACE inhibitors and ARBs (%)	192 (54.7)	134 (18.9)	< .001	90 (46.4)	76 (39.2)	.19
Anticoagulants (%)	72 (20.5)	97 (13.7)	.009	45 (23.2)	44 (22.7)	1
Antiplatelet drugs (%)	203 (57.8)	91 (12.8)	< .001	91 (46.9)	69 (35.6)	.03
Beta-blockers (%)	215 (61.3)	135 (19)	< .001	100 (51.5)	86 (44.3)	.18
Calcium channel blockers (%)	108 (30.8)	79 (11.1)	< .001	54 (27.8)	46 (23.7)	.42
Corticosteroids (%)	54 (15.4)	109 (15.4)	1	28 (14.4)	37 (19.1)	.27
Insulin (%)	77 (21.9)	51 (7.2)	< .001	43 (22.2)	28 (14.4)	.05
Oral antidiabetic drugs (%)	91 (25.9)	47 (6.6)	< .001	38 (19.6)	27 (13.9)	.18
Other antiarrhythmic drugs (%)	27 (7.7)	28 (3.9)	.008	17 (8.8)	17 (8.8)	1
Statins						
Simvastatin (%)	189 (53.8)	–		109 (56.2)	–	
Atorvastatin (%)	75 (21.4)	–		37 (19.1)	–	
Pravastatin (%)	49 (14)	–		27 (13.9)	–	
Rosuvastatin (%)	28 (8)	–		15 (7.7)	–	
Fluvastatin (%)	8 (2.3)	–		4 (2.1)	–	
Unknown statin (%)	2 (0.6)	–		2 (1)	–	
Site of infection						
Pulmonary (%)	137 (39)	326 (46)	.04	75 (38.7)	79 (40.7)	.77
Abdominal (%)	63 (17.9)	140 (19.7)	.50	39 (20.1)	31 (16)	.37
Urinary tract (%)	45 (12.8)	64 (9)	.07	25 (12.9)	24 (12.4)	1
Other (%)[a]	64 (18.2)	101 (14.2)	.11	33 (17)	38 (19.6)	.60
Co-infection (%)	42 (12)	78 (11)	.69	22 (11.3)	22 (11.3)	1
Admission type, medical (%)	253 (72.1)	531 (74.9)	.34	135 (69.6)	155 (79.9)	.02
Causative pathogens[b]						
Gram-positive (%)	184 (52.4)	327 (46)	.34	88 (45.4)	85 (43.8)	.79
Gram-negative (%)	220 (62.7)	395 (55.7)	.31	119 (61.3)	111 (57.2)	.49

Table 1 continued

Characteristics	Unmatched cohort			Propensity-matched cohort		
	Statins N = 351	No statins N = 709	p	Statins N = 194	No statins N = 194	p
Yeast/fungi (%)	38 (10.8)	79 (11.1)	.68	20 (10.3)	25 (12.9)	.54
Other (%)	39 (11.1)	94 (13.3)	.21	25 (12.9)	24 (12.4)	.89
Unknown (%)	51 (14.5)	124 (17.5)	.14	26 (13.4)	34 (17.5)	.35
Severity of disease in first 24 h						
APACHE IV Score, median [IQR]	83 [67–103]	78 [61–101]	.04	85 [66–103]	83 [66–106]	.95
Acute physiology score, median [IQR]	68 [51–86]	65 [51–85]	.45	71 [52–87]	67 [53–92]	,91
SOFA score, median [IQR][c]	8 [6–10]	7 [5–9]	.007	8 [6–10]	7 [5–9.75]	.38
Organ failure (%)	295 (84)	600 (84.6)	.09	169 (87.1)	174 (89.7)	.79
Shock (%)	119 (33.9)	240 (33.9)	1	73 (37.6)	77 (39.7)	.75
Acute lung injury (%)	89 (25.4)	202 (28.5)	.30	53 (27.3)	50 (25.8)	.82
Acute kidney injury (%)	157 (44.7)	271 (38.2)	.04	81 (41.8)	90 (46.4)	.41
Mechanical ventilation (%)	272 (77.5)	549 (77.4)	1	153 (78.9)	155 (79.9)	.90
Renal replacement therapy (%)	48 (13.7)	61 (8.6)	.02	32 (16.5)	19 (9.8)	.05
Lactate max. (mmol/l), median [IQR][d]	2.6 [1.7–4.9]	2.6 [1.6–4.77]	.57	2.5 [1.6–4.6]	2.9 [1.8–4.6]	.41

ACE angiotensin-converting-enzyme, *APACHE* acute physiology and chronic health evaluation, *ARBs* angiotensin receptor blockers, *BMI* body mass index, *COPD* chronic obstructive pulmonary disease, *IQR* interquartile range, *NSAIDs* non-steroidal anti-inflammatory drugs, *SD* standard deviation, *SOFA* sequential organ failure assessment

[a] Site of infection: "other" includes cardiovascular infection, mediastinitis and skin infection

[b] Percentages represent the proportion of cases caused by the particular pathogen. In some cases multiple causative pathogens were isolated

[c] Central nervous system not included in score, due to large number of sedated patients

[d] Lactate levels were absent in 220 patients

missing data. In total, 194 of 351 statin users could be matched to non-users (Table 1 and Additional file 1: Figure 2). Yet, a higher prevalence peripheral vascular disease and use of antiplatelet drugs remained in the statin group after propensity score matching.

Statin use and sepsis presentation and outcome

In the unmatched comparison, statins users presented with higher median APACHE IV (median 83 vs. 78, $P = 0.04$) and SOFA scores (median 8 vs. 7, $P = 0.007$). Acute kidney injury was more frequently observed in statin users (44.7%) compared to non-users (38.2%, $P = 0.04$) and renal replacement therapy more often required (13.7 vs. 8.6%, $P = 0.02$). Sites of infection were largely similar between groups, besides a pulmonary source of infection, which was less frequently recorded in the statin group (39.0 vs. 46.0%, $P = 0.04$). Following propensity score matching on pre-admission variables, none of these differences in sepsis presentation and severity were present anymore.

Statin users were similar to non-users with regard to ICU or hospital length of stay, development of ICU-acquired complications or mortality up to up to 90 days after ICU admission, in either the unmatched or the matched cohort (Table 2). The association of statin use with 30-day mortality was further studied

using logistic regression in the propensity-matched cohort, which revealed a survival benefit for prior statin users (odds ratio 0.58, 95% confidence intervals 0.36–0.93; Table 3).

Statin use and systemic host response biomarkers

We measured 23 biomarkers indicative of host response pathways implicated in sepsis pathogenesis in plasma or blood obtained < 24 h after ICU admission (Additional file 1: Table 1 for unmatched cohort; Figures 1–3 for matched cohort). Relative to healthy controls, patients with sepsis displayed signs of systemic inflammation, as reflected by a profound activation of the cytokine network (elevated plasma levels of IL-6, IL-8 and IL-10), elevated levels of MMP-8 and TIMP-1 and an increased acute phase protein response (elevated plasma CRP concentrations) (Fig. 1). In addition, sepsis was associated with activation of the vascular endothelium (elevated plasma concentrations of soluble E-selectin, soluble ICAM-1, fractalkine and angiopoietin-2, and reduced levels of angiopoietin-1) (Fig. 2) and the coagulation system (elevated D-dimer levels, prolonged PT and aPTT, and reduced levels of the anticoagulant proteins protein C and antithrombin) (Fig. 3). Platelet counts were not significantly altered in patients with sepsis relative to healthy controls.

Table 2 Outcomes of sepsis patients admitted to the ICU stratified according to prior use of statins

Outcomes	Unmatched cohort			Propensity-matched cohort		
	Statins N = 351	No statins N = 709	p	Statins N = 194	No statins N = 194	p
Length of stay ICU, median, days [IQR]	4 [2–9]	5 [2–10]	.28	4 [2–11]	5 [2–11]	.58
Organ failure during admission (%)	307 (87.5)	634 (89.4)	.32	175 (90.2)	180 (92.8)	1
Shock during admission (%)	150 (42.7)	296 (41.7)	.80	93 (47.9)	97 (50)	.76
Acute lung injury during admission (%)	107 (30.5)	232 (32.7)	.49	66 (34)	55 (28.4)	.29
Acute kidney injury during admission (%)	183 (52.1)	327 (46.1)	.07	99 (51)	106 (54.6)	.53
Mortality						
ICU mortality (%)	65 (18.5)	149 (21)	.36	35 (18)	48 (24.7)	.13
Hospital mortality (%)	106 (30.2)	226 (31.9)	.58	62 (32)	73 (37.6)	.31
30-day mortality (%)	92 (26.2)	198 (27.9)	.60	48 (24.7)	67 (34.5)	.051
60-day mortality (%)	112 (31.9)	235 (33.1)	.71	61 (31.4)	74 (38.1)	.24
90-day mortality (%)	129 (36.8)	255 (36)	.84	74 (38.1)	77 (39.7)	.83

ICU intensive care unit, *IQR* interquartile range

Table 3 Association of statin use with 30-day mortality using logistic regression in propensity-matched cohort

	Odds ratio	95% confidence interval	p
Statins	0.58	0.36–0.93	.02
APACHE IV score	1.02	1.01–1.03	< .0001
Age	1.04	1.01–1.06	.002
Hematologic malignancy	1.61	0.46–5.64	.45
Non-metastatic malignancy	0.93	0.52–1.66	.79
Peripheral vascular disease	1.93	1.09–3.44	.02
Diabetes mellitus	0.89	0.53–1.51	.68

None of these responses differed between statin users and statin non-users, in either the unmatched cohort (Additional file 1: Table 1) or the matched cohort (Figs. 1, 2, 3). The plasma concentrations of TNF-α, interferon-γ, IL-1β, IL-13 and GM-CSF were undetectable or very low in the vast majority of patients and not different between groups (data not shown).

Statin use and the blood leukocyte genomic response

Using an unbiased approach we compared the blood leukocyte transcriptome of sepsis patients who were on statin therapy ($N = 157$) versus those who were not ($N = 337$). With this method, we studied gene expression genome-wide (i.e., contrasting with a biased approach in which a particular signaling pathway is studied). This analysis comprised the subgroup of patients enrolled during the first 1.5 years of this study. At first, genome-wide blood gene expression profiles of statin users and statin non-users were compared to 42 healthy controls. Pronounced alterations in gene expression were

detected in both patient groups, which were strongly correlated (Additional file 1: Figure 3). Elevated expression of genes involved in typical pro-, anti-inflammatory, innate immune and metabolic pathways concomitant with decreased expression of predominantly T cell signaling pathways characterized this previously reported common host response [11]. Comparing the leukocyte transcriptomes of patients with statin therapy to those patients who did not revealed no statistically significant differences. We subsequently compared leukocyte transcriptomes of patients in the matched cohort [statin therapy ($N = 95$) and no statin therapy ($N = 95$)] (Fig. 4). Clinical characteristics of matched patients are shown in Additional file 1: Tables 2 and 3. Again, similar alterations in leukocyte transcriptomes of both patient groups were uncovered relative to health, with strongly correlated gene expression changes. No differences in leukocyte transcriptomes were uncovered when comparing patients with statin therapy to those patients who did not receive statin therapy in this matched cohort.

Discussion

In a number of randomized trials in infectious/inflammatory conditions such as ventilator-associated pneumonia and acute respiratory distress syndrome, conducted over the past years, statins failed to improve outcome [25–27]. The majority of earlier observational studies, however, reported improved outcome of statin users with sepsis [7, 8]. In accordance, by using logistic regression analysis in the propensity-matched cohort, we found a survival benefit for prior statin users. The primary objective of this study was to compare the host response between prior users and non-users of statins in sepsis patients upon admission to the ICU. We measured 23 biomarkers,

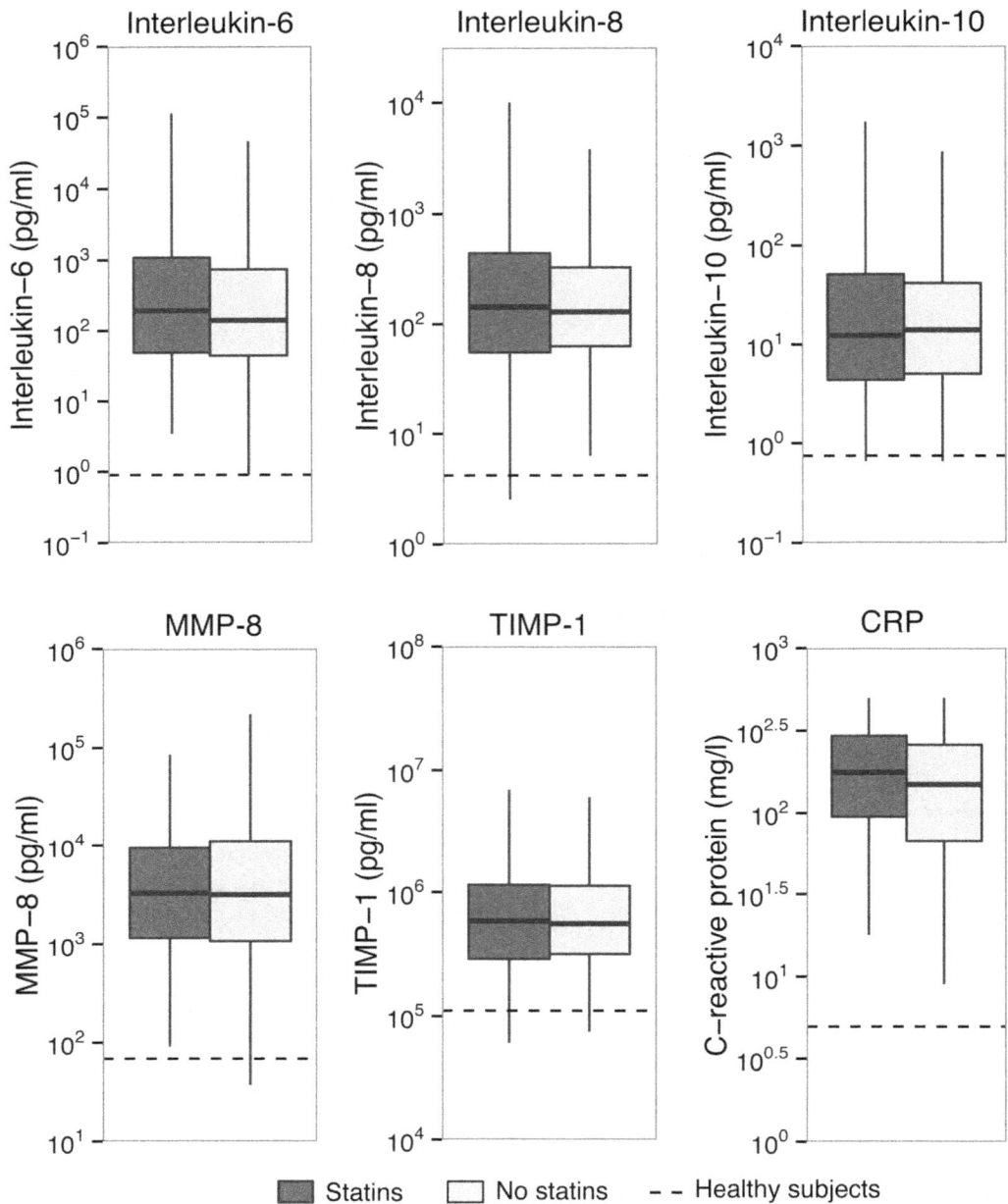

Fig. 1 Inflammatory responses in sepsis patients on ICU admission stratified according to statin use in the propensity-matched cohort. Data are expressed as box-and-whisker diagrams depicting the median and lower quartile, upper quartile and their respective 1.5IQR as whiskers (as specified by Tukey). CRP levels were missing in 104 cases. Differences between groups were not significant. Dashed lines represent median levels in 27 healthy volunteers

providing insight into systemic inflammatory reactions, activation of the endothelium and the coagulation system, and studied whole genome expression profiles in blood leukocytes, and compared these between sepsis patients who were on statin therapy prior to admission and those who were not, in both an unmatched and a propensity score-matched cohort. We defined sepsis

using the 2001 consensus definition [17]; the vast majority of MARS patients included in this analysis had a SOFA score ≥ 2 at ICU admission, which approximates the most recent consensus definitions for sepsis [28]. Our results strongly suggest that prior statin therapy does not influence the host response to sepsis in patients requiring intensive care.

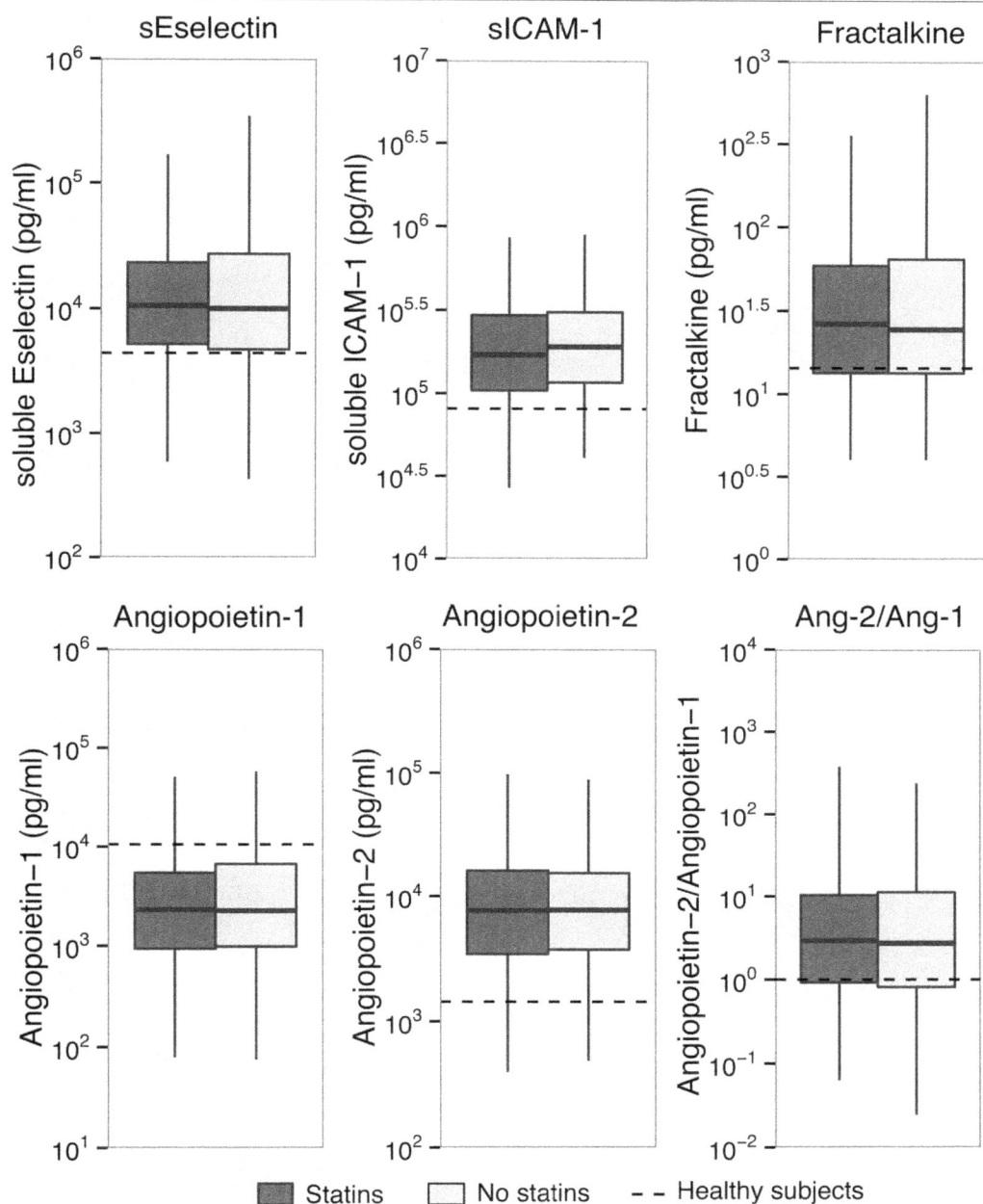

Fig. 2 Endothelial cell activation in sepsis patients on ICU admission stratified according to statin use in the propensity-matched cohort. Data are expressed as box-and-whisker diagrams depicting the median and lower quartile, upper quartile and their respective 1.5IQR as whiskers (as specified by Tukey). Dashed lines represent median levels in 27 healthy volunteers. Differences between groups were not significant. ICAM-1 = intercellular adhesion molecule-1

Previous studies in patients with infection and/or sepsis reporting on an association between statin use and host response biomarkers were small or limited to a few biomarkers. To our knowledge, only one earlier study focused on sepsis patients admitted to the ICU: in a randomized trial of 250 critically ill patients with severe sepsis, prior statin users had lower baseline levels of IL-6 compared to statin-naïve patients; treatment with atorvastatin during admission did not alter IL-6 levels compared to placebo in either prior statin users or statin-naïve patients [29]. In a targeted approach, we measured a series of biomarkers that were selected because

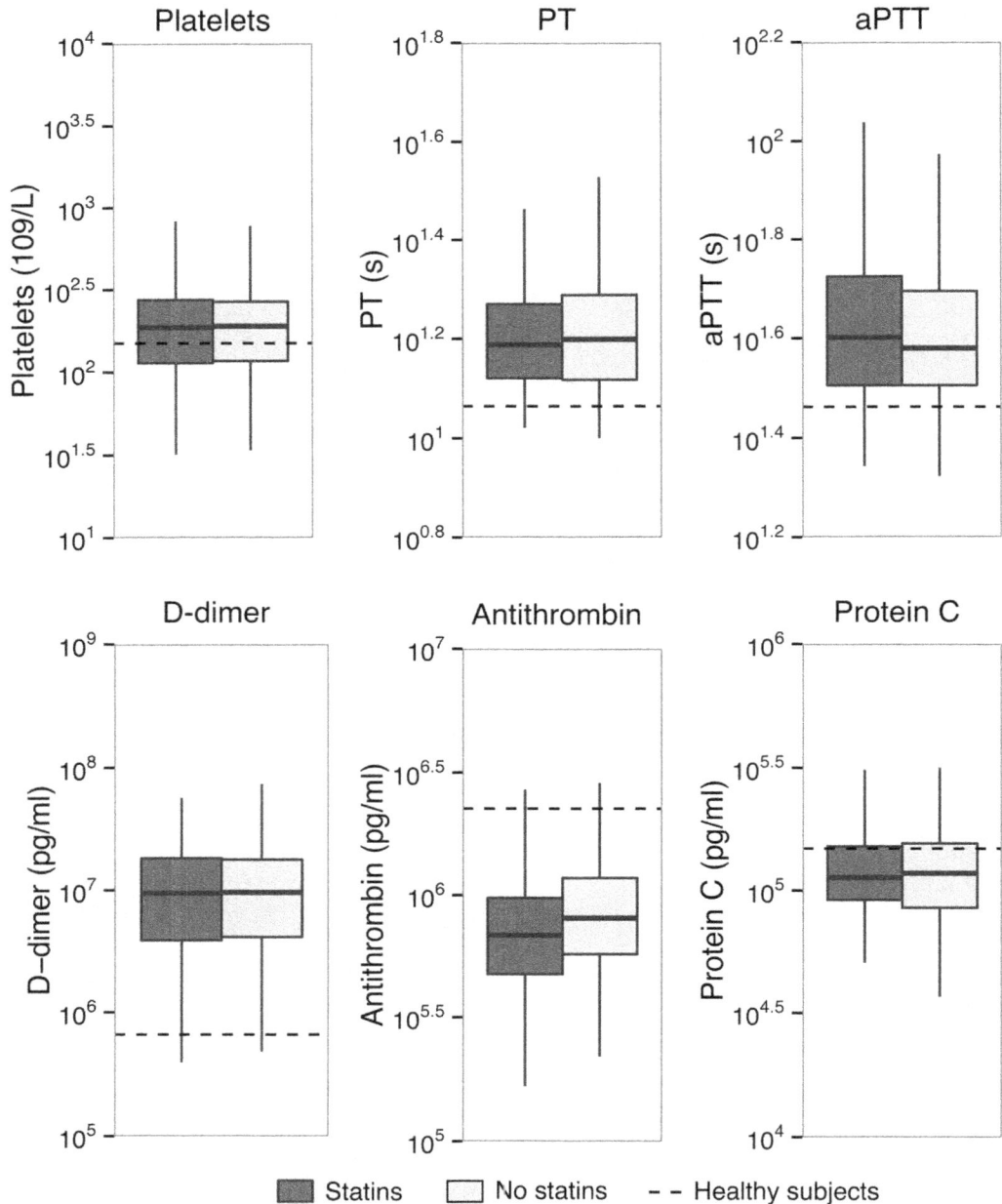

Fig. 3 Coagulation activation in sepsis patients on ICU admission stratified according to statin use in the propensity-matched cohort. Data are expressed as box-and-whisker diagrams depicting the median and lower quartile, upper quartile and their respective 1.5IQR as whiskers (as specified by Tukey). Dashed lines represent median levels in 27 healthy volunteers, except for platelets, prothrombin time and activated partial thromboplastin time, which represents the clinical laboratory lower and upper reference values, respectively. APTT was missing in 127 cases, PT in 10 and platelet count in 1 patient. Differences between groups were not significant

they provide insight into host response pathways implicated in the pathogenesis of sepsis [1, 2] and because statins have been shown to exert inhibitory effects on these mechanisms [3–6]. None of the biomarkers determined were different between prior statin users and non-users. Our results are in accordance with a study in 1895 patients with community-acquired pneumonia, in whom prior statin use did not influence cytokine release or coagulation activation, except for a modest increase in antithrombin levels [30]. This latter study is different from our cohort, as it was conducted in emergency departments with less than 20% of patients requiring

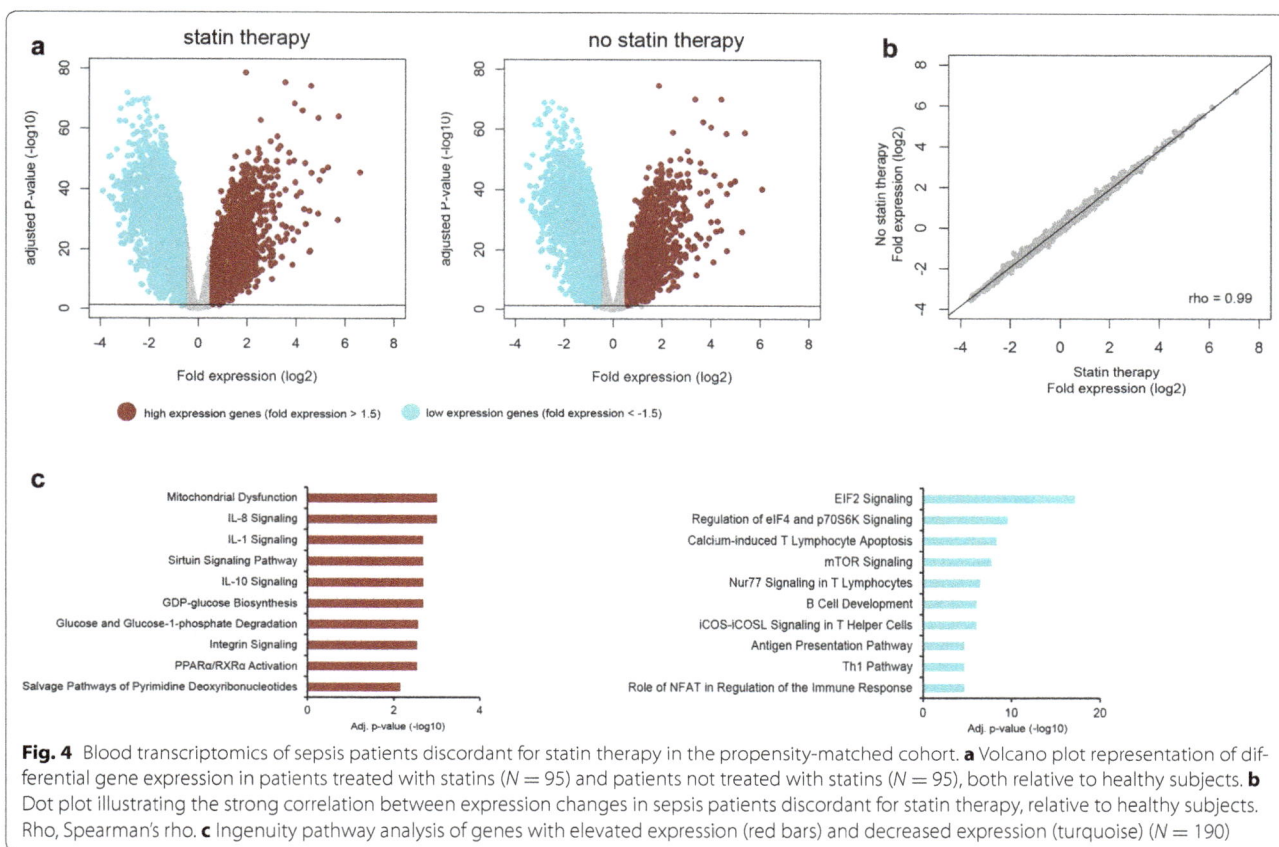

Fig. 4 Blood transcriptomics of sepsis patients discordant for statin therapy in the propensity-matched cohort. **a** Volcano plot representation of differential gene expression in patients treated with statins (N = 95) and patients not treated with statins (N = 95), both relative to healthy subjects. **b** Dot plot illustrating the strong correlation between expression changes in sepsis patients discordant for statin therapy, relative to healthy subjects. Rho, Spearman's rho. **c** Ingenuity pathway analysis of genes with elevated expression (red bars) and decreased expression (turquoise) (N = 190)

intensive care and only encompassed patients with community-acquired pneumonia. Two smaller investigations in non-ICU patients reported on the association between statin use and the host response during suspected or documented infection: in a randomized trial involving 84 hospitalized patients who were not using statins prior to admission TNF-α and IL-6 levels were significantly reduced in patients after treatment with simvastatin [31]; in an observational study in 209 hospitalized patients prior statin use was not associated with altered C-reactive protein levels upon admission [32]. Taken together, these and our study suggest that statin use prior to admission has little if any impact on the host response to infection in patients admitted to either a general hospital ward or the ICU.

Statins have been reported to modulate the host response in controlled models of human inflammation induced by intravenous or intrabronchial administration of lipopolysaccharide (LPS). Simvastatin attenuated pro-inflammatory cytokine release, procoagulant responses and vascular hyporeactivity induced by intravenous LPS injection into healthy humans [33, 34], and reduced neutrophil influx and the release of myeloperoxidase, TNF-α and metalloproteinases (including MMP-9) in

bronchoalveolar lavage fluid after an intrabronchial challenge with LPS [35]. While these data are in accordance with the immune modulatory properties of statins in various experimental settings [3–6], our results indicate that the potential anti-inflammatory and anticoagulant effects of statins do not influence the rigorous and unbalanced host response in a heterogeneous population of critically ill patients with sepsis.

This study has limitations. First, our study was observational; the findings cannot prove cause and effect. Second, this study was underpowered to detect small differences; nevertheless, the clinical relevance of such minor differences would be unclear. Third, although propensity score matching is an elegant way to adjust for multiple baseline differences between the investigational groups, bias can occur as a result of unmeasured confounders. Furthermore, unbalanced clinical baseline conditions remained in our propensity-matched cohort; however, in separate analyses diabetes, oral antidiabetic or antiplatelet drugs did not influence sepsis outcome or host response [36, 37]. Samples from healthy volunteers were taken as controls for biomarker analysis; hence, the change in biomarker levels cannot be specifically attributed to sepsis but may, in part, be related to an inflammatory response to acute severe disease. Although we have determined a variety of systemic host response protein biomarkers, aiming to characterize relevant pathways in sepsis pathogenesis, some biomarkers of interest were not measured, including those providing insight in the function of the glycocalyx. An additional limitation is the lack of information about the duration and adherence to statins. Strengths of our study are its prospective nature, in which consecutively admitted patients were included and disease presentation, course and outcome were meticulously documented.

In conclusion, prior statin therapy was not associated with an altered host response in patients with sepsis upon admission to the ICU.

Abbreviations
APACHE: acute physiology and chronic health evaluation; aPTT: activated partial thromboplastin time; COPD: chronic obstructive pulmonary disease; CRP: C-reactive protein; ICAM: intercellular adhesion molecule; ICU: intensive care unit; IL: interleukin; GM-CSF: granulocyte-macrophage colony-stimulating factor; MMP: matrix metalloproteinase; PT: prothrombin time; SOFA: sequential organ failure assessment; TIMP: tissue inhibitor of metalloproteinase; TNF: tumor necrosis factor.

Authors' contributions
MAW designed the study, acquired patient data, performed laboratory experiments, analyzed data and drafted the manuscript; TvdP designed the study and drafted the manuscript; BPS performed laboratory experiments, analyzed data and drafted the manuscript; AJH and RL performed laboratory experiments; LAvV, JH, OLC, MJS, MJB were involved in acquisition of patient data and substantially contributed to the design of the study; AHZ assisted with statistical analyses; all authors reviewed and revised the manuscript critically for important intellectual content. All authors read and approved the final manuscript.

Author details
[1] Center for Experimental and Molecular Medicine, Academic Medical Center, University of Amsterdam, Meibergdreef 9, Room G2-130, 1105 AZ Amsterdam, The Netherlands. [2] The Center for Infection and Immunity Amsterdam, Academic Medical Center, University of Amsterdam, Meibergdreef 9, 1105 AZ Amsterdam, The Netherlands. [3] Department of Clinical Epidemiology, Bioinformatics, and Biostatistics, Academic Medical Center, University of Amsterdam, Meibergdreef 9, 1105 AZ Amsterdam, The Netherlands. [4] Department of Respiratory Medicine and Experimental Immunology, Academic Medical Center, University of Amsterdam, Meibergdreef 9, 1105 AZ Amsterdam, The Netherlands. [5] Department of Intensive Care, Academic Medical Center, University of Amsterdam, Meibergdreef 9, 1105 AZ Amsterdam, The Netherlands. [6] Department of Intensive Care Medicine, University Medical Center Utrecht, Heidelberglaan 100, 3584 CX Utrecht, The Netherlands. [7] Julius Center for Health Sciences and Primary Care, University Medical Center Utrecht, Heidelberglaan 100, 3584 CX Utrecht, The Netherlands. [8] Department of Medical Microbiology, University Medical Center Utrecht, Heidelberglaan 100, 3584 CX Utrecht, The Netherlands. [9] Division of Infectious Diseases, Academic Medical Center, University of Amsterdam, Meibergdreef 9, 1105 AZ Amsterdam, The Netherlands.

Acknowledgements
The authors acknowledge all members of the MARS consortium for the participation in data collection and especially acknowledge: Friso M. de Beer, MD, Lieuwe D. J. Bos, PhD, Gerie J. Glas, MD, Roosmarijn T. M. van Hooijdonk, MD, PhD (Department of Intensive Care, Academic Medical Center, University of Amsterdam), Mischa A. Huson, MD, PhD (Center for Experimental and Molecular Medicine, Academic Medical Center, University of Amsterdam), Peter M.C. Klein Klouwenberg, MD, PharmD, PhD, David S. Y. Ong, MD, PharmD, PhD (Department of Intensive Care Medicine, Julius Center for Health Sciences and Primary Care and Department of Medical Microbiology, University Medical Center Utrecht, Utrecht, the Netherlands), Laura R. A. Schouten, MD (Department of Intensive Care, Academic Medical Center, University of Amsterdam), Marleen Straat, MD, PhD Esther Witteveen, MD, and Luuk Wieske, MD, PhD (Department of Intensive Care, Academic Medical Center, University of Amsterdam).

Competing interests
The authors declare that they have no competing interests.

Funding
This work was supported by the framework of CTMM, the Center for Translational Molecular Medicine (http://www.ctmm.nl), project MARS (grant 04I-201). The sponsor CTMM was not involved in the design and conduction of the study; nor was the sponsor involved in collection, management, analysis, and interpretation of the data or preparation, review or approval of the manuscript. Decision to submit the manuscript was not dependent on the sponsor.

References
1. Gotts JE, Matthay MA. Sepsis: pathophysiology and clinical management. BMJ. 2016;353:i1585.
2. Angus DC, van der Poll T. Severe sepsis and septic shock. N Engl J Med. 2013;369:840–51.
3. Zhou Q, Liao JK. Pleiotropic effects of statins. Basic research and clinical perspectives. Circ J. 2010;74:818–26.
4. Bedi O, Dhawan V, Sharma PL, Kumar P. Pleiotropic effects of statins: new therapeutic targets in drug design. Naunyn-Schmiedeberg's Arch Pharmacol. 2016;389:695–712.
5. Undas A, Brummel-Ziedins KE, Mann KG. Anticoagulant effects of statins and their clinical implications. Thromb Haemost. 2014;111:392–400.
6. Terblanche M, Almog Y, Rosenson RS, Smith TS, Hackam DG. Statins and sepsis: multiple modifications at multiple levels. Lancet Infect Dis. 2007;7:358–68.
7. Ma Y, Wen X, Peng J, Lu Y, Guo Z, Lu J. Systematic review and meta-analysis on the association between outpatient statins use and infectious disease-related mortality. PLoS ONE. 2012;7:e51548.
8. Wan YD, Sun TW, Kan QC, Guan FX, Zhang SG. Effect of statin therapy on mortality from infection and sepsis: a meta-analysis of randomized and observational studies. Crit Care. 2014;18:R71.
9. Klein Klouwenberg PM, Ong DS, Bos LD, de Beer FM, van Hooijdonk RT, Huson MA, et al. Interobserver agreement of Centers for Disease Control and Prevention criteria for classifying infections in critically ill patients. Crit Care Med. 2013;41:2373–8.
10. Scicluna BP, Klein Klouwenberg PM, van Vught LA, Wiewel MA, Ong DS, Zwinderman AH, et al. A molecular biomarker to diagnose community-acquired pneumonia on intensive care unit admission. Am J Respir Crit Care Med. 2015;192:826–35.
11. van Vught LA, Klein Klouwenberg PM, Spitoni C, Scicluna BP, Wiewel MA, Horn J, et al. Incidence, risk factors, and attributable mortality of secondary infections in the intensive care unit after admission for sepsis. JAMA. 2016;315:1469–79.
12. Kaukonen KM, Bailey M, Suzuki S, Pilcher D, Bellomo R. Mortality related to severe sepsis and septic shock among critically ill patients in Australia and New Zealand, 2000–2012. JAMA. 2014;311:1308–16.
13. Bellomo R, Ronco C, Kellum JA, Mehta RL, Palevsky P. Acute renal failure—definition, outcome measures, animal models, fluid therapy and information technology needs: the Second International Consensus Conference of the Acute Dialysis Quality Initiative (ADQI) Group. Crit Care. 2004;8:R204–12.
14. Force ADT, Ranieri VM, Rubenfeld GD, Thompson BT, Ferguson ND, Caldwell E, et al. Acute respiratory distress syndrome: the Berlin definition. JAMA. 2012;307:2526–33.

15. Garner JS, Jarvis WR, Emori TG, Horan TC, Hughes JM. CDC definitions for nosocomial infections, 1988. Am J Infect Control. 1988;16:128–40.

16. Calandra T, Cohen J. The international sepsis forum consensus conference on definitions of infection in the intensive care unit. Crit Care Med. 2005;33:1538–48.

17. Levy MM, Fink MP, Marshall JC, Abraham E, Angus D, Cook D, et al. 2001 SCCM/ESICM/ACCP/ATS/SIS international sepsis definitions conference. Intensive Care Med. 2003;29:530–8.

18. Bourgon R, Gentleman R, Huber W. Independent filtering increases detection power for high-throughput experiments. Proc Natl Acad Sci U S A. 2010;107:9546–51.

19. Leek JT, Storey JD. Capturing heterogeneity in gene expression studies by "surrogate variable analysis". PLoS Genet. 2005;preprint:e161.

20. Johnson WE, Li C, Rabinovic A. Adjusting batch effects in microarray expression data using empirical Bayes methods. Biostatistics. 2007;8:118–27.

21. van Lieshout MH, Scicluna BP, Florquin S, van der Poll T. NLRP3 and ASC differentially affect the lung transcriptome during pneumococcal pneumonia. Am J Respir Cell Mol Biol. 2014;50:699–712.

22. R Core Team. R: a language and environment for statistical computing. Vienna: R Foundation for Statistical Computing; 2015. http://www.R-project.org.

23. Rubin DB. Estimating causal effects from large data sets using propensity scores. Ann Intern Med. 1997;127:757–63.

24. Austin PC. Balance diagnostics for comparing the distribution of baseline covariates between treatment groups in propensity-score matched samples. Stat Med. 2009;28:3083–107.

25. National Heart L, Blood Institute ACTN, Truwit JD, Bernard GR, Steingrub J, Matthay MA, et al. Rosuvastatin for sepsis-associated acute respiratory distress syndrome. N Engl J Med. 2014;370:2191–200.

26. Papazian L, Roch A, Charles P-E, Penot-Ragon C, Perrin G, Roulier P, et al. Effect of statin therapy on mortality in patients with ventilator-associated pneumonia: a randomized clinical trial. JAMA J Am Med Assoc. 2013;310:1692–700.

27. Craig TR, Duffy MJ, Shyamsundar M, McDowell C, O'Kane CM, Elborn JS, et al. A randomized clinical trial of hydroxymethylglutaryl- coenzyme a reductase inhibition for acute lung injury (the HARP study).

28. Singer M, Deutschman CS, Seymour CW, Shankar-Hari M, Annane D, Bauer M, et al. The third international consensus definitions for sepsis and septic shock (sepsis-3). JAMA. 2016;315:801–10.

29. Kruger PS, Harward ML, Jones MA, Joyce CJ, Kostner KM, Roberts MS, et al. Continuation of statin therapy in patients with presumed infection: a randomized controlled trial. Am J Respir Crit Care Med. 2011;183:774–81.

30. Yende S, Milbrandt EB, Kellum JA, Kong L, Delude RL, Weissfeld LA, et al. Understanding the potential role of statins in pneumonia and sepsis. Crit Care Med. 2011;39:1871–8.

31. Novack V, Eisinger M, Frenkel A, Terblanche M, Adhikari NK, Douvdevani A, et al. The effects of statin therapy on inflammatory cytokines in patients with bacterial infections: a randomized double-blind placebo controlled clinical trial. Intensive Care Med. 2009;35:1255–60.

32. Shankar-Hari M, Donnelly A, Pinto R, Salih Z, McKenzie C, Terblanche M, et al. The influence of statin exposure on inflammatory markers in patients with early bacterial infection: pilot prospective cohort study. BMC Anesthesiol. 2014;14:106.

33. Pleiner J, Schaller G, Mittermayer F, Zorn S, Marsik C, Polterauer S, et al. Simvastatin prevents vascular hyporeactivity during inflammation. Circulation. 2004;110:3349–54.

34. Steiner S, Speidl WS, Pleiner J, Seidinger D, Zorn G, Kaun C, et al. Simvastatin blunts endotoxin-induced tissue factor in vivo. Circulation. 2005;111:1841–6.

35. Shyamsundar M, McKeown ST, O'Kane CM, Craig TR, Brown V, Thickett DR, et al. Simvastatin decreases lipopolysaccharide-induced pulmonary inflammation in healthy volunteers. Am J Respir Crit Care Med. 2009;179:1107–14.

36. Wiewel MA, de Stoppelaar SF, van Vught LA, Frencken JF, Hoogendijk AJ, Klein Klouwenberg PM, et al. Chronic antiplatelet therapy is not associated with alterations in the presentation, outcome, or host response biomarkers during sepsis: a propensity-matched analysis. Intensive Care Med. 2016;42:352–60.

37. van Vught LA, Scicluna BP, Hoogendijk AJ, Wiewel MA, Klein Klouwenberg PM, Cremer OL, et al. Association of diabetes and diabetes treatment with the host response in critically ill sepsis patients. Crit Care. 2016;20:252.

5

Sodium lactate improves renal microvascular thrombosis compared to sodium bicarbonate and 0.9% NaCl in a porcine model of endotoxic shock: an experimental randomized open label controlled study

Thibault Duburcq[1]*[iD], Arthur Durand[1,6], Antoine Tournoys[4], Viviane Gnemmi[4], Valery Gmyr[2,3], François Pattou[2,3], Mercedes Jourdain[1,2,3], Fabienne Tamion[5], Emmanuel Besnier[5], Sebastien Préau[1], Erika Parmentier-Decrucq[1], Daniel Mathieu[1], Julien Poissy[1] and Raphaël Favory[1,6]

Abstract

Background: Sodium lactate seemed to improve fluid balance and avoid fluid overload. The objective of this study was to determine if these beneficial effects can be at least partly explained by an improvement in disseminated intravascular coagulation (DIC)-associated renal microvascular thrombosis.

Methods: Ancillary work of an interventional randomized open label controlled experimental study. Fifteen female "Large White" pigs (2 months old) were challenged with intravenous infusion of *E. coli* endotoxin. Three groups of five animals were randomly assigned to receive different fluids: a treatment group received sodium lactate 11.2% (SL group); an isotonic control group received 0.9% NaCl (NC group); a hypertonic control group, with the same amount of osmoles and sodium than SL group, received sodium bicarbonate 8.4% (SB group). Glomerular filtration rate (GFR) markers, coagulation and inflammation parameters were measured over a 5-h period. Immediately after euthanasia, kidneys were withdrawn for histological study. Statistical analysis was performed with nonparametric tests and the Dunn correction for multiple comparisons. A $p < 0.05$ was considered significant.

Results: The direct immunofluorescence study revealed that the percentage of capillary sections thrombosed in glomerulus were significantly lesser in SL group [5 (0–28) %] compared to NC [64 (43–79) %, $p = 0.01$] and SB [64 (43–79), $p = 0.03$] groups. Alterations in platelet count and fibrinogen level occurred earlier and were significantly more pronounced in both control groups compared to SL group ($p < 0.05$ at 210 and 300 min). The increase in thrombin–antithrombin complexes was significantly higher in NC [754 (367–945) µg/mL; $p = 0.03$] and SB [463 (249–592) µg/mL; $p = 0.03$] groups than in SL group [176 (37–265) µg/mL]. At the end of the experiment, creatinine clearance was significantly higher in SL group [55.46 (30.07–67.85) mL/min] compared to NC group [1.52 (0.17–27.67) mL/min, $p = 0.03$].

Conclusions: In this study, we report that sodium lactate improves DIC-associated renal microvascular thrombosis and preserves GFR. These findings could at least partly explain the better fluid balance observed with sodium lactate infusion.

*Correspondence: thibault.duburcq@chru-lille.fr
[1] Centre de Réanimation - Rue Emile Laine, CHU de Lille – Hôpital R Salengro, 59037 Lille Cedex, France
Full list of author information is available at the end of the article

Keywords: Septic shock, Fluid resuscitation, Lactate infusion, Glomerular filtration rate, Disseminated intravascular coagulation, Renal histology

Background

Sepsis, considered today as a syndrome of physiologic, pathologic and biochemical abnormalities induced by infection [1], is a major public health concern responsible for considerable morbidity and mortality [2]. Sepsis is frequently complicated by acute kidney injury, which is associated with higher risk of in-hospital mortality [3, 4], and by disseminated intravascular coagulation (DIC) due to a massive activation of the coagulation system [5, 6]. Many studies imply that DIC is an important mediator in both microvascular thrombosis, multiple organ failure syndrome development [7] and mortality in patients with serious infections [8].

Sepsis is also associated with deficit in effective blood volume. Large amounts of intravenous fluids are commonly used to increase cardiac output and improve peripheral blood flow [9]. First, mounting evidence suggests that resuscitation fluids contribute, in varying degrees, to clinically relevant renal [10, 11] and haemostatic disturbances, particularly if artificial colloids such as hydroxyethyl starch (HES) and gelatine or saline preparations are used. The undesirable consequences of using HES resulted in a strong recommendation [9] against the use of HES in resuscitation of patients with sepsis [12, 13]. Moreover, saline with the presence of supraphysiological concentrations of chloride may increase the incidence of acute kidney injury and the use of renal replacement therapy [14–16]. Secondly, aggressive use of large-volume intravenous fluids induces fluid overload which is associated with renal failure [17, 18] and leads to hemodilution, which in turn may exacerbate coagulopathy [19]. In order to reduce the volume of intravenous solutions, the concept of small volume resuscitation with hypertonic saline and/or hypertonic saline–HES or dextran has been widely studied during trauma resuscitation [20, 21]. The potential of these hypertonic fluids to modulate the coagulation cascade is less well known, as data are limited and contradictory [22]. Anyway, hypertonic solutions containing HES and/or saline could increase acute kidney injury in sepsis as far as isotonic fluids. Hence, in an attempt to avoid the detrimental effects of chloride anion and/or HES, the use of metabolized anions such as lactate could be more suitable. The use of lactate, as a resuscitation fluid-based energetic substrate, is an interesting alternative because this anion is well metabolized [23] even in poor hemodynamic conditions [24].

We previously observed that sodium lactate infusion enhanced fluid balance in pig endotoxic shock [25, 26]. This beneficial effect of sodium lactate could not be totally explained neither by its hyperosmolar or alkalizing effects [25] nor by its energy load or its effect on the chloride balance [26]. Finally, two additional mechanisms have been hypothesized: first, lactate infusion is better metabolized in poor hemodynamic conditions than glucose, and second, lactate could decrease proinflammatory response and/or improve endothelial barrier function. Interestingly, it is well known that proinflammatory response and endothelial dysfunction exacerbate the endotoxin-induced DIC [27, 28]. So, in order to better understand the beneficial effect of sodium lactate on fluid balance, we conducted an ancillary work focused on DIC and renal histology.

The main objective of the present study was to determine if sodium lactate improve DIC-associated renal microvascular thrombosis. The secondary objective was to explore the glomerular filtration rate (GFR).

Methods

This is an ancillary work of a recent experimental study on the beneficial hemodynamic and metabolic effects of sodium lactate infusion in endotoxic shock [26]. The experimental protocol (CEEA No. 132012) received the approval of the Nord-Pas-de-Calais Animal Ethics Committee (Comité d'Ethique en Expérimentation Animale Nord-Pas-de-Calais; C2EA-75) and the French Ministry of Education and Research. Care and handling of the animals were in accordance with the experimental animal use guidelines of the French Ministry of Agriculture and Food.

Animal preparation

For the experiment, animals were premedicated with intramuscular injection of ketamine (Kétalar®, Virbac, France, 2.5 mg/kg of body weight) and xylazine (Sédaxylan®, CEVA Santé Animale, France, 2.5 mg/kg of body weight). Then, we used isoflurane (AErrane®, Baxter, France) for the intubation process, and maintenance of anaesthesia was performed with a continuous infusion of midazolam (Hypnovel®, Roche, France, 1 mg/kg body weight/h) for the whole experiment. All animals were mechanically ventilated (Osiris 2®, Taema, France) with a tidal volume of 8 mL/kg, a positive end-expiratory pressure set at 4 cm H_2O to limit cardiovascular effects,

FiO_2 0.6 to prevent fatal hypoxaemia during the study, and respiratory rate 20–24 breaths/min only adjusted to maintain normocapnia (40–45 mmHg) at baseline. We chose to maintain ventilation similar in all animals during the experiment. No recruitment manoeuvres were done. Muscle relaxation was obtained by a continuous intravenous infusion of cisatracurium besylate (Nimbex®, Hospira, France, 2 mg/kg body weight/h). Analgesia was achieved by a subcutaneous injection of buprenorphine (Vetergesic®, Sogeval, France, 0.1 mg/kg body weight). After dissection of neck vessels, catheters were inserted in the right carotid artery for continuous blood pressure monitoring and blood sampling. To monitor urine output, a suprapubic urinary catheter was inserted.

Study design

Fifteen female "Large White" pigs (2 months old) were used in this study. The study was carried out as depicted in Fig. 1. During preparation period, animals received 25 mL/kg 0.9% NaCl to prevent hypovolemia. Measurements were taken over a 5-h period: at baseline after the stabilization period (T0) and at 60 (T60), 120 (T120), 210 (T210) and 300 (T300) minutes. All animals were administered 5 µg/kg/min Escherichia coli lipopolysaccharide (LPS) (serotype 055:B5; Sigma Chemical Co., St. Louis, MO, USA). The endotoxin was diluted in 50 ml of 0.9% NaCl and infused over a 30-min period intravenously. We studied three groups receiving 450 mL (from T30 to T300) of different fluids as follows: a treatment group ($n = 5$) receiving 11.2% hypertonic sodium lactate AP-HP® (AGEPS, Paris, France) (**SL group**) containing 90 g (1000 mmol) of lactate and 23 g (1000 mmol) of sodium per litre and two control groups; one isotonic control group ($n = 5$) receiving 0.9% NaCl (**NC group**), and one hypertonic control group ($n = 5$) receiving 8.4% hypertonic sodium bicarbonate (**SB group**) containing 61 g (1000 mmol) of bicarbonate and 23 g (1000 mmol) of sodium per litre. Sodium bicarbonate provided the same amount of sodium (450 mmol) and osmoles (900 mosm), and the same alkalizing effect than sodium lactate [25]. The SL group received 40.5 g lactate (3.61 kcal/g). NC and SB groups received an equivalent energy supply: 39 g glucose (3.75 kcal/g) as 780 mL 5% glucose solution (Baxter SAS, Guyancourt, France) from T30 to T300. Finally, the SL group received 780 mL sterile water for injection (Baxter SAS, Guyancourt, France) in place of the 5% glucose solution to ensure the same fluid intake in the three groups. The only resuscitation endpoint was mean arterial pressure (MAP). If MAP felt below 65 mmHg, 2.5 mL/kg infusion of NaCl 0.9% was given as rescue therapy every 15 min. Bolus infusions were performed to maintain MAP above 65 mmHg as recommended by Sepsis Surviving Campaign [9]. At the end of the study period, all animals were sacrificed with T61 administration (T61, 0.3 mL/kg of body weight, Intervet International GmbH, Köln, Germany).

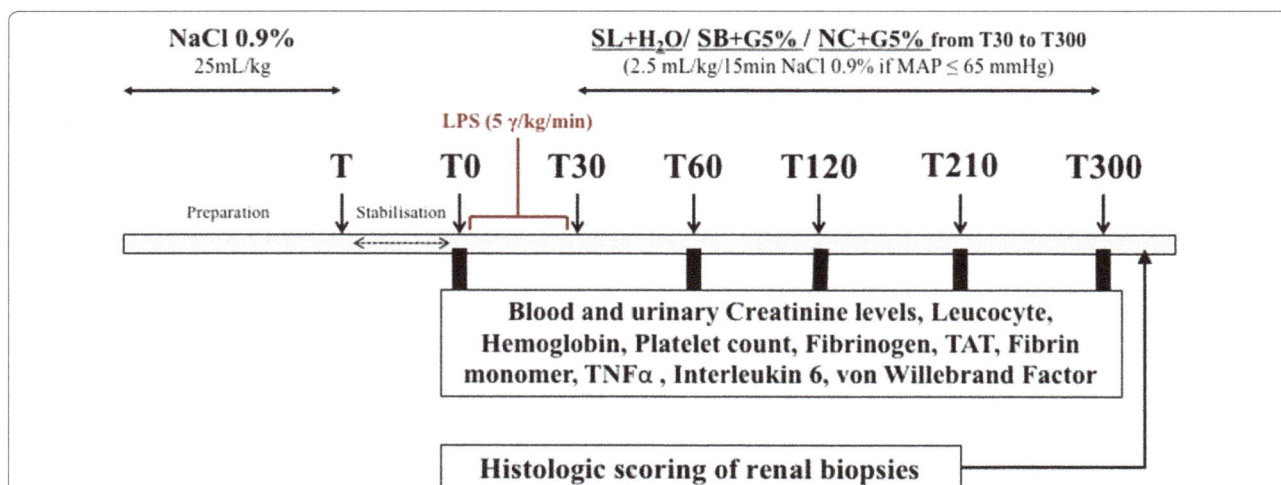

Fig. 1 Study design. During preparation period, all animals received 25 mL/kg 0.9% NaCl to prevent hypovolemia. Measurements were taken over a 5-h period: at baseline (T0) and at 60 (T60), 120 (T120), 210 (T210) and 300 (T300) minutes. All animals were administered 5 µg/kg/min Escherichia coli lipopolysaccharide (LPS). The endotoxin was infused over a 30-min period intravenously. The SL group received 40.5 g lactate (3.61 kcal/g). NC and SB groups received an equivalent energy supply: 39 g glucose (3.75 kcal/g) as 780 mL 5% glucose solution from T30 to T300. To ensure the same fluid intake, the SL group received 780 mL sterile water for injection. If mean arterial pressure (MAP) felt below 65 mmHg, 2.5 mL/kg infusion of NaCl 0.9% was given as rescue therapy every 15 min. At the end of the study period, all animals were sacrificed with T61 administration. Immediately after euthanasia, renal biopsies were performed

Histological analysis

At the end of the experiment and immediately after euthanasia, kidneys were withdrawn for histological study. After macroscopic examination, a part of the samples from each kidney were fixed with acidified formal alcohol (AFA) and another part of the sample was frozen by liquid nitrogen and stored at − 80 °C. The samples fixed in AFA were embedded in paraffin and sectioned (3–4 μm width). After deparaffinization and rehydration, sections were stained with Masson's trichrome, Periodic acid–Schiff (PAS) and hematoxylin eosin safran (HES) and evaluated in light microscopy. On frozen tissue, cryosections of 5 μm were cut on a cryostat and incubated 30 min with an antifibrinogen antibody directly conjugated with fluorescein for a direct immunofluorescence. The antibody was a polyclonal rabbit antibody, which recognized fibrinogen (ref. F0111, Dako SA, Trappes, France). We established two semiquantitative scores for histological abnormalities defined as: score (%) = (number of glomeruli damaged)/(number of glomeruli examined) and (number of capillary sections thrombosed)/(number of capillary sections examined) per damaged glomeruli. At least 50 glomeruli were observed in each sample. The pathologist was blinded to the groups examined.

Biological methods

Leucocyte, haemoglobin and platelet counts were obtained on EDTA anticoagulated blood. For coagulation assays, blood (four parts) was collected in tubes containing 3.8% sodium citrate (one part). Fibrinogen levels were rapidly measured by standard procedures. Immunoassay methods were used to determine quantitative thrombin–antithrombin complexes (TAT) (Enzygnost® TAT micro, Siemens, Munich, Germany). Fibrin monomer (Liatest FM® Stago, Asnières, France) was performed by immunoturbidimetric assay. The quantitative determination of vWF antigen (Ag) was measured by turbidimetric assay (vWF Ag® Reagent, Siemens, Nederland) ($n = 70$–100%).

TNFα and interleukin-6 (Il-6) were measured in serum. Plasma levels were detected by ELISA method with porcine anti-TNFα antibodies (Quantikine® Porcine TNFα, R&D Systems, USA) and anti-Il-6 antibodies (Quantikine® Porcine Il-6, R&D Systems, USA).

Blood and urinary creatinine levels (Cobas® 8000 modular analyser, Roche Diagnostics, Switzerland) were measured at each time except T30. We computed creatinine clearance, a surrogate marker of GFR, with standard formula [creatinine clearance (CrCl) = (creatinine urinary concentration × rate of urine formation)/Creatinine plasma concentration]. Diuresis, a marker of both GFR and tubular function, was measured at each time except T30.

Data analysis

We considered that the sample size of five animals per group would be sufficient to show a statistical difference if any based on a previous work on the same model [27]. Statistical analysis was performed with GraphPad Prism 6 software (San Diego, California). As the distribution was not normal (Shapiro–Wilk test), quantitative data were expressed using median and interquartile range. Considering the differences between groups for some parameters at baseline, values are expressed as a percentage of the first value. For multiple intergroup testing, we used Kruskal–Wallis test with Dunn's multiple comparisons test and Mann–Whitney U test. Intragroup comparisons were realized by Friedman test with Dunn's multiple comparisons test and Wilcoxon matched-pairs signed rank test. The two-tailed significance level was set at $p < 0.05$.

Results

Median weight was similar in the three groups of animals: 22.5 (18.25–23.75) kg in NC group, 23 (21.75–23.5) kg in SB group and 23 (20.5–24) kg in SL group.

The endotoxin challenge resulted in hypodynamic shock with a decreased of cardiac index in all animals. As already described, the infusion of sodium lactate infusion enhanced hemodynamics with a limitation of fluid overload [26].

Histological results

Kidneys appeared macroscopically enlarged and swollen in the three groups. Glomeruli showed signs of oedema uniformly, and fibrin thrombi were mainly observed in glomerular capillaries (Fig. 2). Percentage of thrombosed glomeruli and percentage of thrombosed capillary in glomerulus were significantly higher in control groups compared to SL group (Table 1) and consistent with an increased amount of microthrombosis.

Percentage of thrombosed glomeruli (%) = (number of glomeruli damaged)/(number of glomeruli examined) and percentage of capillary sections thrombosed (%) = (number of capillary sections thrombosed)/(number of capillary sections examined) per damaged glomeruli. Results are expressed as median with interquartile ranges. Kruskal–Wallis test with Dunn's multiple comparisons test and Mann–Whitney U test were used for intergroup comparisons.

Coagulation and endothelial parameters

Changes in leucocyte, platelet count, fibrinogen, haemoglobin, TAT and vWF in the three groups are illustrated in Fig. 3. As expected, we observed a dramatic procoagulant response. Alterations in platelet count and fibrinogen level occurred earlier and were significantly

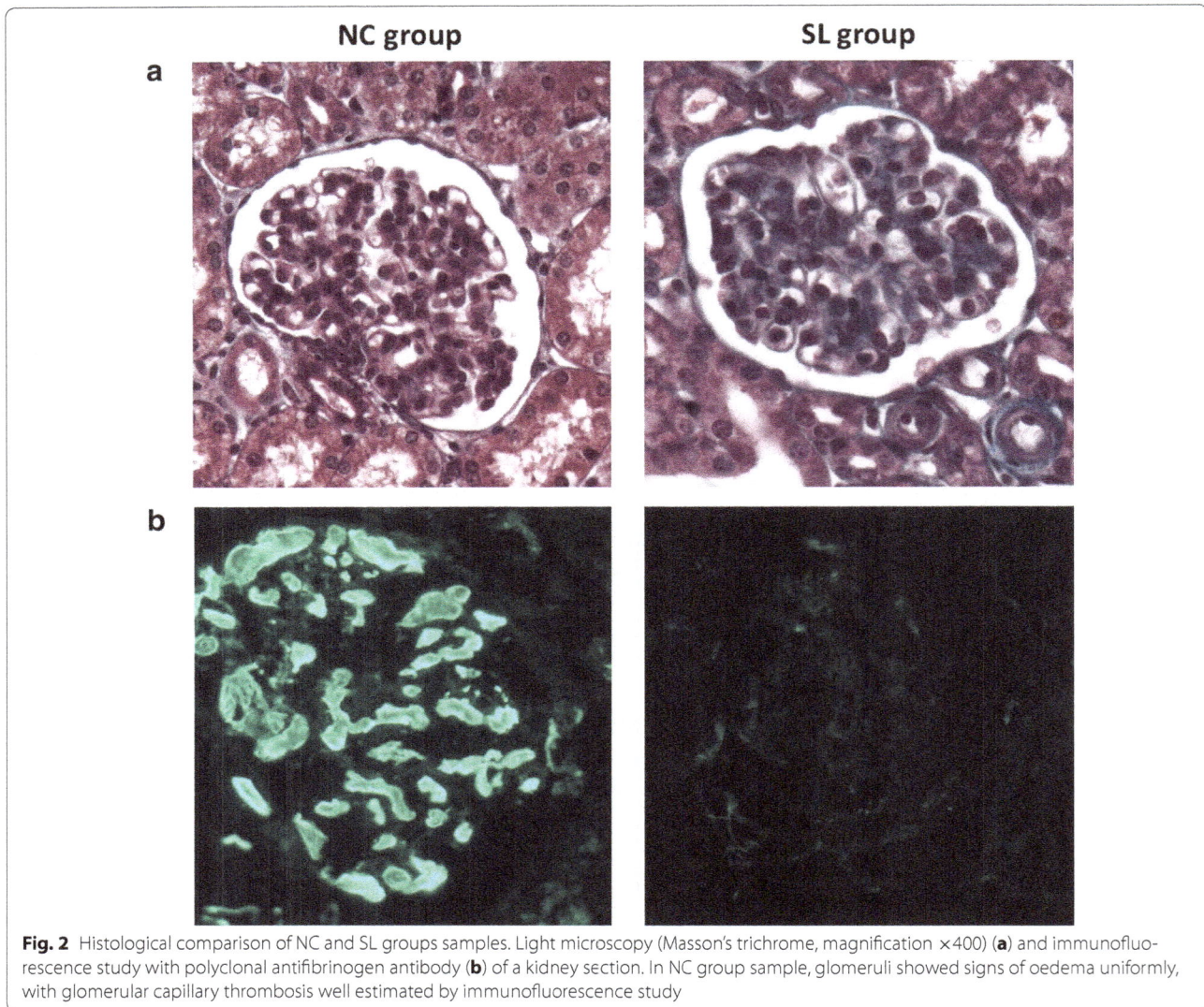

Fig. 2 Histological comparison of NC and SL groups samples. Light microscopy (Masson's trichrome, magnification ×400) (**a**) and immunofluorescence study with polyclonal antifibrinogen antibody (**b**) of a kidney section. In NC group sample, glomeruli showed signs of oedema uniformly, with glomerular capillary thrombosis well estimated by immunofluorescence study

Table 1 Semiquantitative histological scores

Groups	Percentage of thrombosed glomeruli		Percentage of capillary sections thrombosed	
	Light microscopy	Immunofluorescence	Light microscopy	Immunofluorescence
NC	95 (42–100)	96 (54–100)	58 (31–69)	64 (43–79)
SB	96 (41–100)	94 (46–100)	57 (39–75)	68 (31–77)
SL	14 (0–43)	10 (0–49.20)	5 (0–32)	5 (0–28)
p				
NC versus SB	Ns	Ns	Ns	Ns
SL versus NC	$p = 0.03$	$p = 0.03$	$p = 0.04$	$p = 0.01$
SL versus SB	$p = 0.03$	$p = 0.03$	$p = 0.02$	$p = 0.03$

more pronounced in both control groups compared to SL group. Circulating platelets significantly declined at T300 in NC [28 (24–45) %; $p = 0.03$ compared to baseline] and SB [38 (24–50) %; $p = 0.03$ compared to baseline] groups, while in SL group, the decrease in the platelet count was less important [67 (48–74) %; $p = 0.06$ compared to

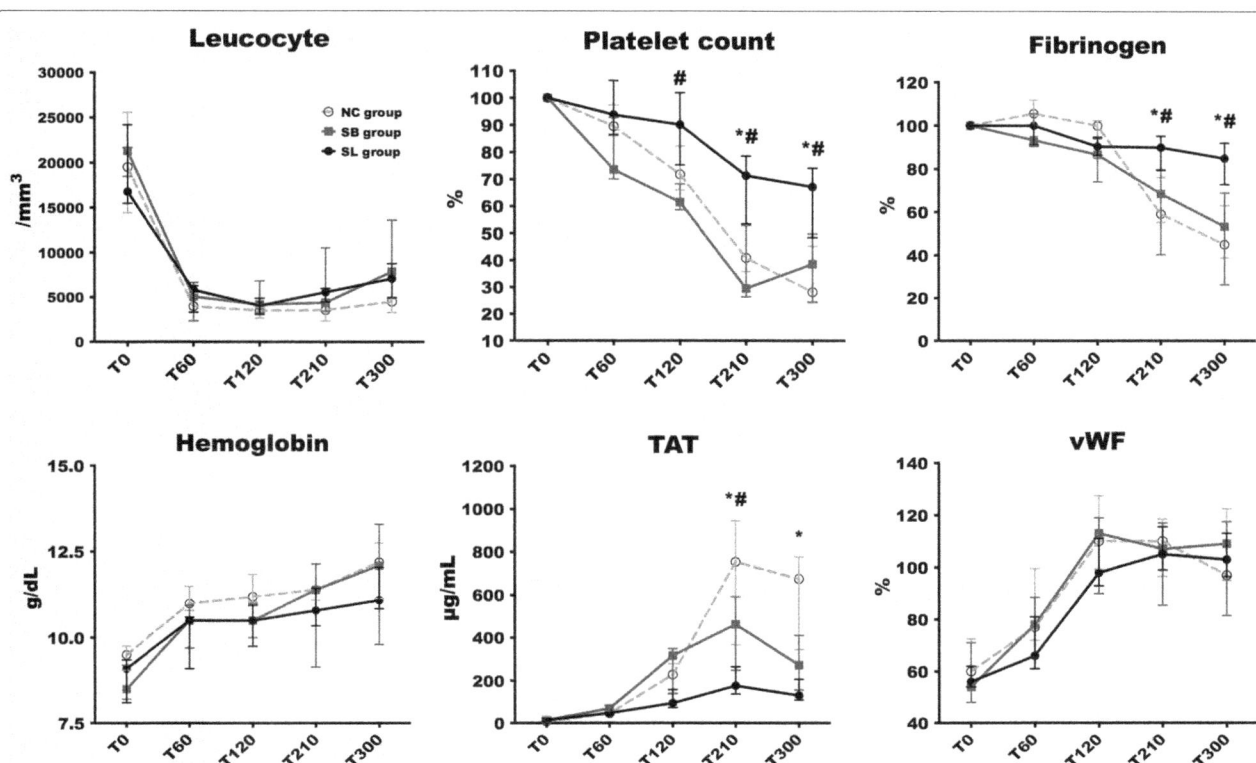

Fig. 3 Changes in leucocyte, platelet count, fibrinogen, haemoglobin, TAT and vWF in the three groups. Considering the differences between groups for platelet count and fibrinogen at baseline, values are expressed as a percentage of the first value. Open circles and dotted line: NC group ($n = 5$); squares and grey line: SB group ($n = 5$); closed circles and black line: SL group ($n = 5$). Results are expressed as median with interquartile ranges. *$p < 0.05$, NC versus SL. #$p < 0.05$, SB versus SL. &$p < 0.05$, NC versus SB

baseline]. In the same way, the activation of the coagulation cascade was illustrated by a decrease in circulating fibrinogen. Fibrinogen level significantly declined at T300 in NC [45 (39–63) %; $p = 0.03$ compared to baseline] and SB [53 (26–69) %; $p = 0.03$ compared to baseline] groups, while it remained stable in SL group [85 (73–92) %; $p = 0.06$ compared to baseline]. The increase in fibrin monomer started earlier and was significantly higher at T120 in NC [104 (82–175) µg/mL; $p = 0.01$] and SB groups [161 (69–200) µg/mL; $p = 0.03$] compared to SL group [28 (19–74) µg/mL]. Unfortunately, we could not interpret the results at 210 and 300 min in the three groups because some values were over 200 µg/mL, the upper limit of measurement, despite dilutions (data not shown). Thrombin–antithrombin complex (TAT) concentrations started to increase at T60 to achieve a maximum level at T210. The increase in TAT complexes was earlier and significantly higher in NC [754 (367–945) µg/mL; $p = 0.03$] and SB [463 (249–592) µg/mL; $p = 0.03$] groups than in SL group [176 (37–265) µg/mL]. Von Willebrand factor (vWF) increased in all animals without any significant difference between groups.

Inflammation parameters

Changes in interleukin-6 and TNFα in the three groups are illustrated in Fig. 4. We observed a same evolution of TNFα levels in the three groups without any significant differences. TNFα increased rapidly, peaked at T120 in both hypertonic groups and at T210 in NC group, and subsequently decreased until the end of the experiment without returning to baseline levels. Il-6 was significantly higher in NC group [22,938 (16,619–29,613) pg/mL at T210 and 25,687 (18,617–42,792) pg/mL at T300] compared to SL group [7904 (4838–9310) pg/mL at T210, $p = 0.02$ and 6148 (4216–13,445) at T300, $p = 0.03$] and SB group [9234 (8108–10,869) pg/mL at T210, $p = 0.02$ and 8433 (5174–11,961) at T300, $p = 0.02$]. No significant differences were seen on Il-6 evolution between SB and SL groups at any time.

Glomerular filtration rate (GFR) markers

Creatinine clearance (CrCl) and diuresis in the three groups are illustrated in Fig. 5. At the end of the experiment (between T210 and T300), diuresis was significantly higher in SL group [150 (125–245) mL] compared to NC

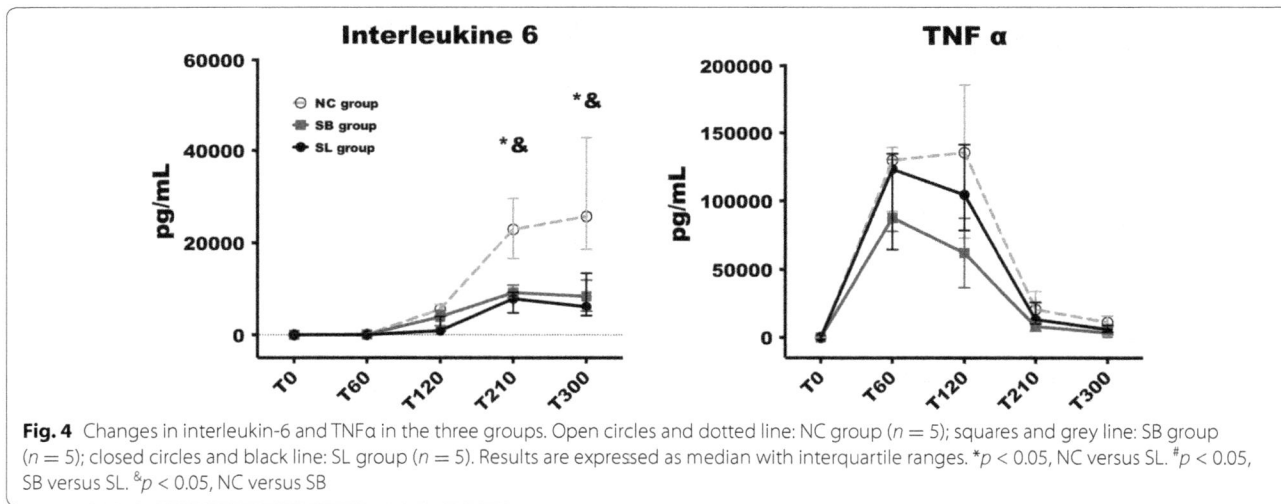

Fig. 4 Changes in interleukin-6 and TNFα in the three groups. Open circles and dotted line: NC group (*n* = 5); squares and grey line: SB group (*n* = 5); closed circles and black line: SL group (*n* = 5). Results are expressed as median with interquartile ranges. *$p < 0.05$, NC versus SL. #$p < 0.05$, SB versus SL. &$p < 0.05$, NC versus SB

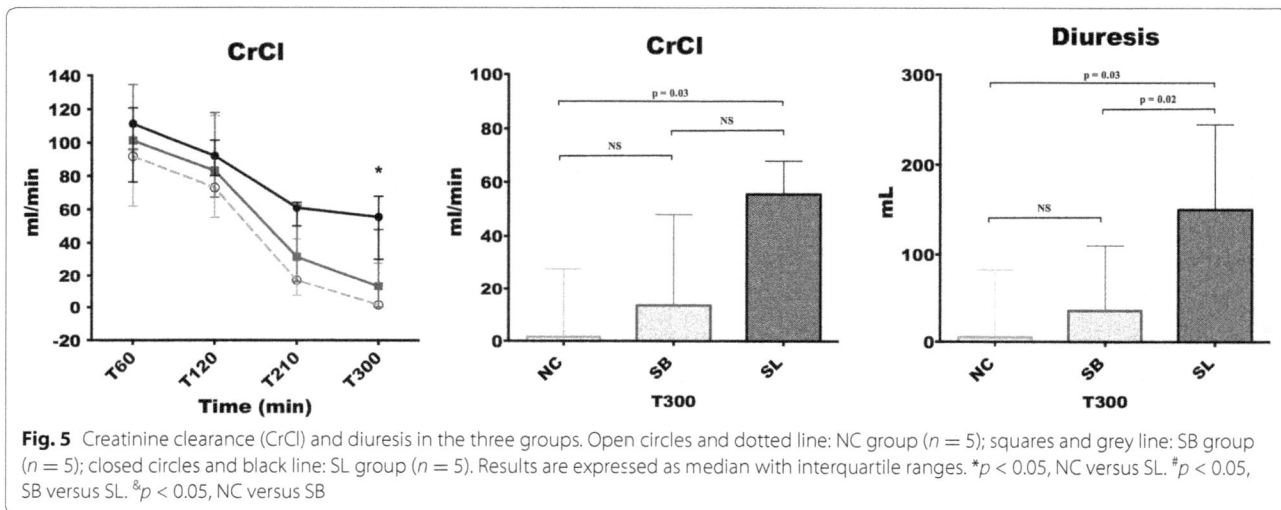

Fig. 5 Creatinine clearance (CrCl) and diuresis in the three groups. Open circles and dotted line: NC group (*n* = 5); squares and grey line: SB group (*n* = 5); closed circles and black line: SL group (*n* = 5). Results are expressed as median with interquartile ranges. *$p < 0.05$, NC versus SL. #$p < 0.05$, SB versus SL. &$p < 0.05$, NC versus SB

[5 (2.5–82.5) mL, $p = 0.03$] and SB groups [35 (1–110), $p = 0.02$]. Creatinine clearance was higher in SL group [55.46 (30.07–67.85) mL/min] compared to NC [1.52 (0.17–27.67) mL/min, $p = 0.03$] and SB groups [13.46 (0.31–47.99) mL/min, $p = 0.09$].

Discussion

In the present study, we compare hypertonic sodium lactate with two different therapeutic regimens; (1) a standard fluid therapy with isotonic crystalloids (0.9% NaCl, the most commonly used crystalloid). Although comparing hypertonic with isotonic formulations could appear misleading, it seemed necessary to have a control group corresponding to the usual clinical practice. (2) a non-conventional hypertonic fluid therapy. Due to

an acidifying effect on pH and an elevated chloride concentration, hypertonic saline was not close enough to hypertonic sodium lactate. Conversely, sodium bicarbonate provided the same alkalizing effect and the same amount of sodium and osmoles than sodium lactate. Thereby, this comparison allows extracting clear conclusions and physiological assumptions. We report here that sodium lactate infusion improves DIC-associated renal microvascular thrombosis. The decrease in renal microvascular thrombosis in SL group could be at least partly explained by the delayed and attenuated procoagulant response (sodium lactate infusion resulted in a significant smaller decrease in platelets and fibrinogen concentrations and a significant smaller increase in plasma levels of TAT). It is known that glomerular thrombosis and vascular thrombosis due to the activation of inflammation and coagulation pathway contribute to the occurrence of acute renal failure in sepsis [5, 29]. Indeed, glomerular thrombosis and microvascular fibrin thrombosis compromise glomerular capillary flow, leading to focal ischaemia and necrosis, which is considered to be the main pathogenesis of LPS-induced acute renal failure [29, 30].

We first hypothesized that sodium lactate infusion may reduce the endothelial dysfunction and therefore restrict the coagulation cascade. In fact, it is known that endothelial dysfunction precedes derangement of platelet function or coagulation parameters and drives a pre-DIC-associated microvascular thrombosis in endotoxemia [28]. In paediatric severe Dengue infection, hypertonic sodium lactate induced a partial recovery from endothelial dysfunction, as indicated by a significant decrease in sVCAM-1 [31]. Moreover, lactate as a metabolizable anion may lead to chloride egress from endothelial cells, causing reduction in swelling and improvement in barrier function [32]. In our model, we already observed that sodium lactate infusion seemed to reduce capillary leakage [26]. In the same way, we observed a non-significant lesser haemoconcentration with lactate infusion in the present study. However, the evolution of von Willebrand factor, a marker of endothelial dysfunction, was not different between groups. Finally, further investigations focused on endothelial function are warranted to explore the sodium lactate impact on capillary leak.

An other explanation of the beneficial effect of sodium lactate on DIC could be an anti-inflammatory effect. It is known that excessive inflammatory mediators play a central role in the development of endotoxin-induced DIC. TNFα plays an important part in the early activation of the haemostatic mechanism and in the pathogenesis of DIC [33]. Indeed, a TNFα inhibitor can act as a protective drug in lipopolysaccharide-induced DIC in a dose-dependent manner [34]. Then, it is known that plasma IL-6 is higher in patients with DIC than in those without DIC. Some data suggest that increases in IL-6 might give rise to hypercoagulable and hypofibrinolytic states. IL-6 could be a cause of DIC and be related to prognosis and organ failure [35]. At last, immunoglobulin, in LPS-induced DIC model, could significantly decreased plasma levels of TNFα and IL-6 and improved haemostatic abnormality [36]. Experimental studies of sepsis showed beneficial effects of hyperosmolar solutions modulating inflammatory response, as for instance the expression and release of cytokines TNFα and IL-6 [37–39]. The use of hypertonic saline solution has also demonstrated potential anti-inflammatory effects related to neutrophil activation [40]. Hypertonic solution acts on polymorphonuclear A2 adenosine receptors and causes

a feedback mechanism that stimulates cAMP and PKA release, thus blocking neutrophil activation [41, 42]. Nevertheless, the therapeutic window for a beneficial effect of fluid resuscitation with hypertonic fluid seemed to be very narrow [43] and may be related to leukocyte activation at the time of fluid use [44]. Our study confirms the beneficial impact of hypertonic solutions on the IL-6 release but not on TNFα. These results could explain part of the beneficial impact of sodium lactate infusion compared to saline. However, it does not elucidate the difference on coagulation status between SL and SB groups. In this way, another explanation could be that lactate by itself has important other anti-inflammatory properties. Binding of lactate on a specific membrane receptor (the plasma membrane GPR81) recruits the intracellular adaptor molecule ARRB2 to the receptor with subsequent inhibition of the NLRP3 inflammasome leading to a reduction in the Il-1β-mediated proinflammatory response [45]. Systemic LPS administration induced high levels of proinflammatory cytokines Il-1β, which contribute to the increased leukocyte–endothelium interaction and promote coagulation cascade [46].

Pigs were chosen as a clinically relevant species, resembling to humans in coagulation reactions [47]. Nevertheless, our model presents some limits. The length of evaluation is short, only 5 h. Bolus injection of endotoxin induces initial characteristics of human sepsis such as activation of innate immune system and rises in TNFα. Its short-term effects on the inflammatory cascade and the lack of an active nidus do not allow to study the compensatory anti-inflammatory phase often leading to immunosuppression. Nevertheless, endotoxin challenge is still a way to explore the very beginning of sepsis and the better resuscitation fluid strategy in this initial phase. Endotoxic model is not a model of hyperdynamic septic shock. Our model was a hypodynamic shock with a pronounced pulmonary vascular response. However, it reproduces some main alterations of inflammatory states, e.g. macrocirculatory and microcirculatory dysfunctions, coagulopathy, organs failure. We used the intravenous route for sepsis induction while patients are often infected by *natural route*. The temporal evolution of the aggression was imposed when the pathological process of patients following an individual natural progression. The endotoxin challenge is responsible for a more explosive proinflammatory response than in a septic shock. These limits, without questioning the validity of our pathophysiological model, could impair the comparability with DIC observed in human septic shock.

In this study, we also reported that sodium lactate preserves GFR. This finding could be at least partly explained by the slightest renal microvascular thrombosis but also by the hemodynamics and microcirculation improvements previously described [25, 26]. Two limits must be reported; (1) GFR do not accurately assess kidney function. Moreover, there is a dependence between diuresis and CrCl calculation which might have participated to the improvement in CrCl. (2) The mean arterial target threshold of 65 mmHg was not reached for two animals in isotonic saline group and one animal in sodium bicarbonate group. This may have impacted negatively the renal perfusion pressure during the resuscitation phase independently from the type of fluid resuscitation. Nevertheless, low blood pressure (< 65 mmHg) occurred only at the end of the experiment, and we already found severe oligo-anuria in these animals before mean arterial pressure falls below 65 mmHg.

Conclusions

In conclusion, sodium lactate improves DIC-associated renal microvascular thrombosis and preserves GFR in our model of endotoxic shock. In the same way as hemodynamics improvement previously observed, these findings could at least partly explain the preservation of fluid balance with sodium lactate.

In our model, the beneficial effect of sodium lactate on DIC-associated renal microvascular thrombosis could be related to an anti-inflammatory effect (e.g. blockage of the NLRP3 inflammasome). Further investigations are warranted to explain the underlying mechanisms and to assess the potential clinical benefits of sodium lactate resuscitation in human sepsis.

Abbreviations

SL: Sodium lactate; SB: Sodium bicarbonate; NC: NaCl 0.9%; MAP: Mean arterial pressure; TAT: Thrombin–antithrombin complex; vWF: von Willebrand factor; TNFα: Tumour necrosis factor α; Il-6: Interleukin 6; Il-1β: Interleukin 1β; *E. coli*: *Escherichia coli*; LPS: Lipopolysaccharide; AKI: Acute kidney injury; CrCl: Creatinin clearance; GFR: Glomerular filtration rate.

Authors' contributions

TD involved in conception and design, logistics, data acquisition and analysis, drafting of manuscript, manuscript writing and final approval of the manuscript. AD contributed to data acquisition, logistics and final approval of the manuscript, and AT contributed to data acquisition and final approval of the manuscript. VG involved in histology analysis and final approval of the manuscript and also in logistics and data analysis. FP, FT, SP, EB and EP-D involved in conception and design and final approval of the manuscript. MJ contributed to logistics and final approval of the manuscript. DM involved in conception and design, data analysis and final approval of the manuscript. JP contributed to conception and design, data analysis and final approval of the manuscript. RF involved in conception and design, data acquisition and analysis, drafting of manuscript, manuscript writing and final approval of the manuscript. All authors read and approved the final manuscript.

Author details

[1] Centre de Réanimation - Rue Emile Laine, CHU de Lille – Hôpital R Salengro, 59037 Lille Cedex, France. [2] INSERM U1190 Translational Research for Diabetes, Univ Lille, 59000 Lille, France. [3] European Genomic Institute for Diabetes, 59000 Lille, France. [4] Centre de Biologie Pathologie, CHU Lille, 59000 Lille, France. [5] Medical Intensive Care Unit, Rouen University Hospital, Rouen, France. [6] LIRIC Inserm U995 Glycation: From Inflammation to Aging, 59000 Lille, France.

Acknowledgements

We thank M.H. Gevaert and R.M. Siminski (Laboratory of Histology, UNIVERSITE de LILLE, F-59000 Lille, France) for the technical support.

Competing interests

The authors declare that they have no competing interests.

Funding

All authors report no funding for support of this work.

References

1. Singer M, Deutschman CS, Seymour CW, Shankar-Hari M, Annane D, Bauer M, et al. The third international consensus definitions for sepsis and septic shock (sepsis-3). JAMA. 2016;315:801–10.
2. Fleischmann C, Scherag A, Adhikari NKJ, Hartog CS, Tsaganos T, Schlattmann P, et al. Assessment of global incidence and mortality of hospital-treated sepsis. Current estimates and limitations. Am J Respir Crit Care Med. 2016;193:259–72.
3. Bellomo R, Kellum JA, Ronco C, Wald R, Martensson J, Maiden M, et al. Acute kidney injury in sepsis. Intensive Care Med. 2017;43:816–28.
4. Bagshaw SM, Uchino S, Bellomo R, Morimatsu H, Morgera S, Schetz M, et al. Septic acute kidney injury in critically ill patients: clinical characteristics and outcomes. Clin J Am Soc Nephrol. 2007;2:431–9.
5. Levi M, Ten Cate H. Disseminated intravascular coagulation. N Engl J Med. 1999;341:586–92.
6. Bakhtiari K, Meijers JCM, de Jonge E, Levi M. Prospective validation of the International Society of Thrombosis and Haemostasis scoring system for disseminated intravascular coagulation. Crit Care Med. 2004;32:2416–21.
7. Gando S. Microvascular thrombosis and multiple organ dysfunction syndrome. Crit Care Med. 2010;38:S35–42.
8. Angstwurm MWA, Dempfle C-E, Spannagl M. New disseminated intravascular coagulation score: a useful tool to predict mortality in comparison with Acute Physiology and Chronic Health Evaluation II and Logistic Organ Dysfunction scores. Crit Care Med. 2006;34:314–20.
9. Rhodes A, Evans LE, Alhazzani W, Levy MM, Antonelli M, Ferrer R, et al. Surviving sepsis campaign: international guidelines for management of sepsis and septic shock: 2016. Intensive Care Med. 2017;43:304–77.
10. Mårtensson J, Bellomo R. Does fluid management affect the occurrence of acute kidney injury? Curr Opin Anaesthesiol. 2017;30:84–91.
11. Severs D, Hoorn EJ, Rookmaaker MB. A critical appraisal of intravenous fluids: from the physiological basis to clinical evidence. Nephrol Dial Transplant Off Publ Eur Dial Transpl Assoc Eur Ren Assoc. 2015;30:178–87.
12. Rochwerg B, Alhazzani W, Sindi A, Heels-Ansdell D, Thabane L, Fox-Robichaud A, et al. Fluid resuscitation in sepsis: a systematic review and network meta-analysis. Ann Intern Med. 2014;161:347–55.
13. Haase N, Perner A, Hennings LI, Siegemund M, Lauridsen B, Wetterslev M, et al. Hydroxyethyl starch 130/0.38–0.45 versus crystalloid or albumin in patients with sepsis: systematic review with meta-analysis and trial sequential analysis. BMJ. 2013;346:f839.
14. Yunos NM, Bellomo R, Hegarty C, Story D, Ho L, Bailey M. Association between a chloride-liberal vs chloride-restrictive intravenous fluid administration strategy and kidney injury in critically ill adults. JAMA. 2012;308:1566–72.
15.. Semler MW, Wanderer JP, Ehrenfeld JM, Stollings JL, Self WH, Siew ED, et al. Balanced crystalloids versus saline in the intensive care unit: the SALT randomized trial. Am J Respir Crit Care Med. 2017;195:1362–72.
16. Krajewski ML, Raghunathan K, Paluszkiewicz SM, Schermer CR, Shaw AD. Meta-analysis of high- versus low-chloride content in perioperative and critical care fluid resuscitation. Br J Surg. 2015;102:24–36.
17. Prowle JR, Kirwan CJ, Bellomo R. Fluid management for the prevention and attenuation of acute kidney injury. Nat Rev Nephrol. 2014;10:37–47.
18. Ostermann M, Straaten HMO, Forni LG. Fluid overload and acute kidney injury: cause or consequence? Crit Care. 2015;27(19):443.
19. Paydar S, Bazrafkan H, Golestani N, Roozbeh J, Akrami A, Moradi AM. Effects of intravenous fluid therapy on clinical and biochemical parameters of trauma patients. Emerg Tehran Iran. 2014;2:90–5.
20. Feinman M, Cotton BA, Haut ER. Optimal fluid resuscitation in trauma: type, timing, and total. Curr Opin Crit Care. 2014;20:366–72.

21. Gantner D, Moore EM, Cooper DJ. Intravenous fluids in traumatic brain injury: what's the solution? Curr Opin Crit Care. 2014;20:385–9.

22. Kaczynski J, Wilczynska M, Hilton J, Fligelstone L. Impact of crystalloids and colloids on coagulation cascade during trauma resuscitation-a literature review. Emerg Med Health Care. 2013;1:1–6.

23. Chioléro R, Schneiter P, Cayeux C, Temler E, Jéquier E, Schindler C, et al. Metabolic and respiratory effects of sodium lactate during short iv nutrition in critically ill patients. JPEN J Parenter Enteral Nutr. 1996;20:257–63.

24. Chioléro RL, Revelly JP, Leverve X, Gersbach P, Cayeux MC, Berger MM, et al. Effects of cardiogenic shock on lactate and glucose metabolism after heart surgery. Crit Care Med. 2000;28:3784–91.

25. Duburcq T, Favory R, Mathieu D, Hubert T, Mangalaboyi J, Gmyr V, et al. Hypertonic sodium lactate improves fluid balance and hemodynamics in porcine endotoxic shock. Crit Care. 2014;18:467.

26. Duburcq T, Durand A, Dessein A-F, Vamecq J, Vienne J-C, Dobbelaere D, et al. Comparison of fluid balance and hemodynamic and metabolic effects of sodium lactate versus sodium bicarbonate versus 0.9% NaCl in porcine endotoxic shock: a randomized, open-label, controlled study. Crit Care. 2017;21:113.

27. Duburcq T, Tournoys A, Gnemmi V, Hubert T, Gmyr V, Pattou F, et al. Impact of obesity on endotoxin-induced disseminated intravascular coagulation. Shock. 2015;44:341–7.

28. De Ceunynck KEP, Higgins SJ, Chaudhry SA, Parikh S, Flaumenhaft RC. Dysfunctional endothelium drives a Pre-DIC state in endotoxemia. Blood. 2016;128:3725.

29. Schrier RW, Wang W. Acute renal failure and sepsis. N Engl J Med. 2004;351:159–69.

30. Hertig A, Rondeau E. Role of the coagulation/fibrinolysis system in fibrin-associated glomerular injury. J Am Soc Nephrol JASN. 2004;15:844–53.

31. Somasetia DH, Setiati TE, Sjahrodji AM, Idjradinata PS, Setiabudi D, Roth H, et al. Early resuscitation of Dengue Shock Syndrome in children with hyperosmolar sodium-lactate: a randomized single blind clinical trial of efficacy and safety. Crit Care. 2014;18:466.

32. Hoffmann EK, Lambert IH, Pedersen SF. Physiology of cell volume regulation in vertebrates. Physiol Rev. 2009;89:193–277.

33. van der Poll T, Büller HR, ten Cate H, Wortel CH, Bauer KA, van Deventer SJ, et al. Activation of coagulation after administration of tumor necrosis factor to normal subjects. N Engl J Med. 1990;322:1622–7.

34. Yamamoto N, Sakai F, Yamazaki H, Nakahara K, Okuhara M. Effect of FR167653, a cytokine suppressive agent, on endotoxin-induced disseminated intravascular coagulation. Eur J Pharmacol. 1996;314(1–2):137–42.

35. Hoppensteadt D, Tsuruta K, Hirman J, Kaul I, Osawa Y, Fareed J. Dysregulation of inflammatory and hemostatic markers in sepsis and suspected disseminated intravascular coagulation. Clin Appl Thromb Off J Int Acad Clin Appl Thromb. 2015;21:120–7.

36. Asakura H, Takahashi Y, Kubo A, Ontachi Y, Hayashi T, Omote M, et al. Immunoglobulin preparations attenuate organ dysfunction and hemostatic abnormality by suppressing the production of cytokines in lipopolysaccharide-induced disseminated intravascular coagulation in rats. Crit Care Med. 2006;34:2421–5.

37. Theobaldo MC, Llimona F, Petroni RC, Rios ECS, Velasco IT, Soriano FG. Hypertonic saline solution drives neutrophil from bystander organ to infectious site in polymicrobial sepsis: a cecal ligation and puncture model. PLoS ONE. 2013;8:e74369.

38. Theobaldo MC, Barbeiro HV, Barbeiro DF, Petroni R, Soriano FG. Hypertonic saline solution reduces the inflammatory response in endotoxemic rats. Clin Sao Paulo Braz. 2012;67:1463–8.

39. Coelho AMM, Jukemura J, Sampietre SN, Martins JO, Molan NAT, Patzina RA, et al. Mechanisms of the beneficial effect of hypertonic saline solution in acute pancreatitis. Shock. 2010;34:502–7.

40. Angle N, Hoyt DB, Cabello-Passini R, Herdon-Remelius C, Loomis W, Junger WG. Hypertonic saline resuscitation reduces neutrophil margination by suppressing neutrophil L selectin expression. J Trauma. 1998;45:7–13.

41. Pascual JL, Khwaja KA, Ferri LE, Giannias B, Evans DC, Razek T, et al. Hypertonic saline resuscitation attenuates neutrophil lung sequestration and transmigration by diminishing leukocyte-endothelial interactions in a two-hit model of hemorrhagic shock and infection. J Trauma. 2003;54:121–32.

42. Inoue Y, Tanaka H, Sumi Y, Woehrle T, Chen Y, Hirsh MI, et al. A3 adenosine receptor inhibition improves the efficacy of hypertonic saline resuscitation. Shock. 2011;35:178–83.

43. Petroni RC, Biselli PJC, de Lima TM, Velasco IT, Soriano FG. Impact of time on fluid resuscitation with hypertonic saline (NaCl 7.5%) in rats with LPS-induced acute lung injury. Shock. 2015;44:609–15.

44. Ciesla DJ, Moore EE, Zallen G, Biffl WL, Silliman CC. Hypertonic saline attenuation of polymorphonuclear neutrophil cytotoxicity: timing is everything. J Trauma. 2000;48:388–95.

45. Hoque R, Farooq A, Ghani A, Gorelick F, Mehal WZ. Lactate reduces liver and pancreatic injury in Toll-like receptor- and inflammasome-mediated inflammation via GPR81-mediated suppression of innate immunity. Gastroenterology. 2014;146:1763–74.

46. Zhou J, Schmidt M, Johnston B, Wilfart F, Whynot S, Hung O, et al. Experimental endotoxemia induces leukocyte adherence and plasma extravasation within the rat pial microcirculation. Physiol Res. 2011;60:853–9.

47. Hildebrand F, Andruszkow H, Huber-Lang M, Pape H-C, van Griensven M. Combined hemorrhage/trauma models in pigs-current state and future perspectives. Shock. 2013;40:247–73.

6

Risk stratification using SpO_2/FiO_2 and PEEP at initial ARDS diagnosis and after 24 h in patients with moderate or severe ARDS

Luigi Pisani[1,8*†] ⓘ, Jan-Paul Roozeman[1†], Fabienne D. Simonis[1,2†], Antonio Giangregorio[1], Sophia M. van der Hoeven[1,2], Laura R. Schouten[1,4], Janneke Horn[1], Ary Serpa Neto[1,6], Emir Festic[7], Arjen M. Dondorp[1,8], Salvatore Grasso[3], Lieuwe D. Bos[1,2,5], Marcus J. Schultz[1,2,8] and for the MARS consortium

Abstract

Background: We assessed the potential of risk stratificat on of ARDS patients using SpO_2/FiO_2 and positive end-expiratory pressure (PEEP) at ARDS onset and after 24 h.

Methods: We used data from a prospective observational study in patients admitted to a mixed medical–surgical intensive care unit of a university hospital in the Netherlands. Risk stratification was by cutoffs for SpO_2/FiO_2 and PEEP. The primary outcome was in-hospital mortality. Patients with moderate or severe ARDS with a length of stay of > 24 h were included in this study. Patients were assigned to four predefined risk groups: group I ($SpO_2/FiO_2 \geq 190$ and PEEP < 10 cm H_2O), group II ($SpO_2/FiO_2 \geq 190$ and PEEP $\geq$ 10 cm), group III ($SpO_2/FiO_2 < 190$ and PEEP < 10 cm H_2O) and group IV ($SpO_2/FiO_2 < 190$ and PEEP $\geq$ 10 cm H_2O).

Results: The analysis included 456 patients. SpO_2/FiO_2 and PaO_2/FiO_2 had a strong relationship ($P < 0.001$, $R_2 = 0.676$) that could be described in a linear regression equation ($SpO_2/FiO_2 = 42.6 + 1.0 * PaO_2/FiO_2$). Risk stratification at initial ARDS diagnosis resulted in groups that had no differences in in-hospital mortality. Risk stratification at 24 h resulted in groups with increasing mortality rates. The association between group assignment at 24 h and outcome was confounded by several factors, including APACHE IV scores, arterial pH and plasma lactate levels, and vasopressor therapy.

Conclusions: In this cohort of patients with moderate or severe ARDS, SpO_2/FiO_2 and PaO_2/FiO_2 have a strong linear relationship. In contrast to risk stratification at initial ARDS diagnosis, risk stratification using SpO_2/FiO_2 and PEEP after 24 h resulted in groups with worsening outcomes. Risk stratification using SpO_2/FiO_2 and PEEP could be practical, especially in resource-limited settings.

Keywords: Acute respiratory distress syndrome (ARDS), Pulse oximetry, Blood gas analysis, Positive end-expiratory pressure (PEEP), Classification, Risk stratification, Outcome, Mortality

Introduction

In the Berlin definition for acute respiratory distress syndrome (ARDS), risk stratification was suggested by categorizing patients as having 'mild,' 'moderate' or 'severe' ARDS based on the ratio of the arterial oxygen tension (PaO_2) to the fraction of inspired oxygen (FiO_2) at initial diagnosis [1]. This approach knows several challenges. First, it requires invasive and expensive arterial blood sampling and analysis that is frequently not available, in particular in resource-limited settings. Second, the robustness of this way of classifying patients was not confirmed by external validation [2]. Most important, though, is that the level of positive end-expiratory pressure (PEEP) may affect the PaO_2/FiO_2 [3] and that PaO_2/FiO_2 and PEEP collected at later time points, for instance 24 h after the initial ARDS diagnosis, largely improve risk stratification [4, 5].

*Correspondence: luigipisani@gmail.com
†Luigi Pisani, Jan-Paul Roozeman, and Fabienne D. Simonis contributed equally to this work
[1] Department of Intensive Care, Academic Medical Center, Meibergdreef 9, 1105 AZ Amsterdam, The Netherlands

Due to the sigmoidal nature of the oxyhemoglobin dissociation curve, the pulse oximetry saturation (SpO_2) may serve as a reliable alternative for the PaO_2 in patients with SpO_2 levels lower than 97% [6]. Indeed, patients with ARDS diagnosed by means of the SpO_2/FiO_2 have similar characteristics and outcomes as patients in whom ARDS is diagnosed using the PaO_2/FiO_2 [7], and persistence of a high oxygen saturation index at 24 h has been found to be associated with worse outcomes in cases of pediatric ARDS [8]. As pulse oximetry is noninvasive, inexpensive and widely available, SpO_2/FiO_2 could serve as an attractive alternative for PaO_2/FiO_2 in risk stratification of ARDS patients.

The overarching aim of the present investigation was to determine whether classification of patients using SpO_2/FiO_2 and PEEP at initial ARDS diagnosis and after 24 h could be used to stratify for risk of mortality. Specifically, we hypothesized that the SpO_2/FiO_2 could serve as an alternative for the PaO_2/FiO_2 in risk classification and that re-classification using SpO_2/FiO_2 and PEEP after 24 h improves risk stratification in a cohort of consecutive adult patients with moderate or severe ARDS in an intensive care unit (ICU) in the Netherlands.

Methods
Study design
We used data from a prospective observational conveniently sized cohort of well-defined critically ill patients admitted to the mixed surgical–medical intensive care unit of one university hospital in the Netherlands [9]. These data were matched with nurse-validated oxygenation data at baseline and after 24 h that was retrospectively collected from the patient data management system (Metavision®, iMDSoft, Tel Aviv, Israel). The Institutional Review Board of the Academic Medical Center approved the parent study protocol and use of an 'opt-out' consent method (IRB no. 10-056C).

Inclusion and exclusion criteria
A team of trained ICU researchers scored patients for the absence or presence of ARDS according to the criteria stated by the American–European Consensus Conference on ARDS [10]. Although this study started in 2011 (i.e., before publication of the Berlin definition for ARDS [1]), all patients diagnosed with ARDS fulfilled the criteria of the latest definition for ARDS. Patients with mild ARDS were excluded as were patients discharged or transferred to another ICU before 24 h after the initial ARDS diagnosis.

Outcomes
The primary outcome was all-cause in-hospital mortality. Secondary outcomes included ICU mortality,

30- and 90-day, and 1-year mortality, and the number of ventilator-free days and alive at day 28 (VFD-28), defined as the number of days from days 1 to 28 that the patient is alive and breathing without invasive assistance of the mechanical ventilator for at least 24 consecutive hours.

Data collection
At initial ARDS diagnosis and after 24 h, pulse oximetry results were retrospectively collected, and the corresponding SpO_2/FiO_2 was calculated. For this, we first collected ten successive nurse-validated SpO_2 and FiO_2 values over 10 min directly preceding, and at the time, an arterial blood sample was drawn for blood gas analysis. The median of these ten SpO_2 and FiO_2 values was used to calculate the SpO_2/FiO_2 to alleviate potential artifactual SpO_2 values. In all patients, pulse oximetry was measured by conventional two-wavelength finger pulse oximeters. The local protocol dictated a change in finger position every 3–4 h to avoid decubitus lesions and to use alternative probes, such as nose and forehead probes, only in patients in whom no adequate signal could be obtained with a conventional pulse oximeter on a finger. In addition to this, PaO_2 and $PaCO_2$ levels, pH levels and body temperature were collected, and it was determined whether or not patients received treatment with vasopressors at both time points.

Baseline data collected from the original database included demographic and ventilator data, comorbidities, admission type, patient category and cause of ARDS. The Acute Physiology and Chronic Health Evaluation (APACHE) IV score [11], the Lung Injury Prediction Score [12] and Charlson comorbidity score [13] were calculated.

Analysis plan
The correlation between SpO_2/FiO_2 and PaO_2/FiO_2 was studied only using SpO_2/FiO_2 and PaO_2/FiO_2 at initial ARDS diagnosis. SpO_2 values of > 97% were excluded from the correlation analysis as the oxyhemoglobin dissociation curve flattens above this level and large changes in the PaO_2 may result in little or no change in the SpO_2, in line with previous investigations that analyzed this relationship [6, 14, 15]. A nonlinear equation (the 'Ellis formula') was also used to estimate PaO_2/FiO_2 from SpO_2 and FiO_2 values [16, 17].

Next, we classified all patients at initial ARDS diagnosis and re-classified patients after 24 h, into four risk groups based on predefined SpO_2/FiO_2 and PEEP cutoffs. As two recent studies of risk stratification of ARDS patients used a cutoff for the PaO_2/FiO_2 of 150 mmHg [4, 5], which corresponds to a SpO_2/FiO_2 of 190 [6], we used this value as a cutoff for SpO_2/FiO_2 in the present analysis. We used the same cutoff for PEEP as in two previous studies [4, 5]. Accordingly, we created four groups: $SpO_2/FiO_2 \geq 190$ and PEEP < 10 cm H_2O (group I); $SpO_2/FiO_2 \geq 190$ and PEEP $\geq$ 10 cm (group II); SpO_2/FiO_2 < 190 and PEEP < 10 cm H_2O (group III); and SpO_2/FiO_2 < 190 and PEEP $\geq$ 10 cm H_2O (group IV). The comparison among groups included all pairwise comparisons across the four risk groups.

Statistical analysis

Data were expressed as mean $\pm$ standard deviation (SD), median with interquartile range (IQR) or number with percentage, where appropriate.

A two-way scatterplot and Pearson correlation analysis were used to characterize the relationship between SpO_2/FiO_2 (linear and nonlinear estimations) and PaO_2/FiO_2. Linear regression allowed quantification of the best regression line and derive a predictive equation for the relationship. Hence, based on the derived regression equation, we obtained the SpO_2/FiO_2 values that correspond to PaO_2/FiO_2 ratio values of 100, 150 and 200 mmHg. $PaCO_2$, arterial pH, body temperature, PEEP and use of vasopressors were tested as interaction terms in the model to evaluate moderation of the association between SpO_2/FiO_2 and PaO_2/FiO_2. The area under the receiver operating characteristic (ROC) curve evaluated the applicability of SpO_2/FiO_2 in discriminating moderate from severe ARDS.

Differences between risk groups were tested with the Pearson Chi-square or Fisher exact test for categorical variables and with one-way ANOVA or Kruskal–Wallis test for continuous variables. In-hospital mortality and other mortality endpoints were calculated for each of the four groups, and a P value for trend was calculated from a chi-squared test for trend in proportions (i.e., the Cochrane–Armitage test), testing the null hypothesis that the proportions in several groups are the same. A pairwise comparison at ARDS diagnosis and after 24 h was performed using a contrast matrix predictor approach in which odd ratios (ORs) and 95% confidence intervals are generated for each mutual comparison between groups.

Post hoc analyses

Several post hoc analyses were performed. First, we evaluated whether transforming the data to fractions ($1/PaO_2/FiO_2$ and $1/SpO_2/FiO_2$) improved the fit between SpO_2/FiO_2 and PaO_2/FiO_2, as previously reported [18].

Second, risk classification using the Berlin definition threshold for severe ARDS (i.e., 100 mm Hg) [6] was performed.

Third, in the last post hoc analysis we analyzed whether the association between risk stratification and in-hospital mortality was confounded by factors such as disease severity, and other readily available parameters in the database,

such as arterial pH and plasma lactate levels, blood pressure levels and vasopressor therapy. For this analysis, a multivariable logistic regression model was built to assess the confounding effect of these variables on the association between risk groups and the primary outcome.

All analyses were performed in R via the R-studio interface (R version 3.0, www.r-project.org). A P value below 0.05 was considered significant.

Results

Patients

Of 554 patients with ARDS, 456 were classified as having moderate or severe ARDS according to the Berlin definition and had complete datasets. Of them, 382 could be used for the correlation analyses, and all patients for the classification and re-classification analyses (Fig. 1). Pneumonia, sepsis, major surgery and trauma were the most common causes of ARDS (Table 1). At baseline, there were no differences between survivors and non-survivors with regard to oxygenation parameters, tidal volume size, the Lung Injury Prediction Score and the etiology of ARDS. Also, there were no differences with regard to the comorbidity score. Overall all-cause in-hospital mortality rate was 39.7%. Non-survivors were older, had a lower arterial pH levels at ARDS diagnosis, were ventilated at higher respiratory rates and had higher disease severity scores. Berlin definition class distribution was not different between survivors and non-survivors.

Relationship between SpO_2/FiO_2 and PaO_2/FiO_2

The correlation between SpO_2/FiO_2 and PaO_2/FiO_2 was strong (P < 0.001, $R^2 = 0.676$; Fig. 2) and could be described in a linear regression equation:

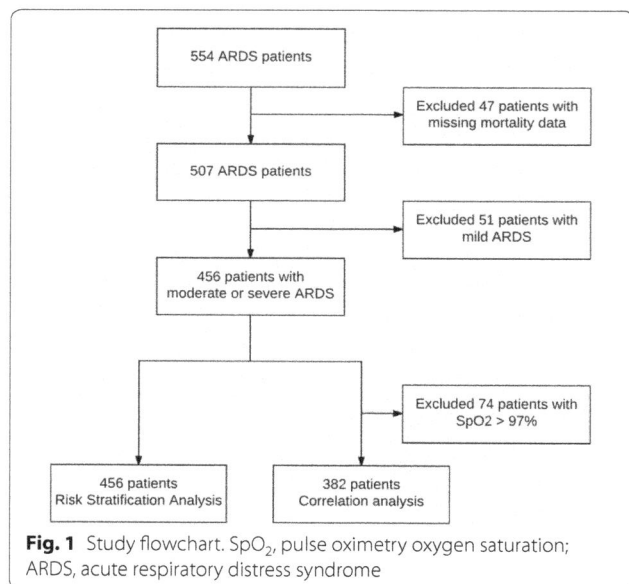

Fig. 1 Study flowchart. SpO_2, pulse oximetry oxygen saturation; ARDS, acute respiratory distress syndrome

Table 1 Baseline characteristics of 456 survivors and non-survivors with moderate and severe ARDS

Variables	All patients	Survivors $N = 275$	Non-survivors $N = 181$	P value
Age, years	62 (51–72)	60 (48–70)	63 (55–72)	0.008
Female		113 (41.1)	59 (32.6)	0.075
Weight, kg	80 (70–90)	80 (70–90)	80 (68–87)	0.347
APACHE IV	68 (51–89)	72 (58–95)	90 (74–113)	< 0.001
Charlson comorbidity index 2	1 (0–3)	1 (0–2)	1 (0–3)	0.103
Lung Injury Prediction Score	8.5 (7–10)	8 (6.5–10)	9 (7–10)	0.074
Tidal volume, ml/kg	6.3 (5.3–7.6)	6.3 (5.3–7.8)	6.3 (5.4–7.3)	0.412
Respiratory rate	23 (17–29)	20 (16–27)	25 (19–30)	0.001
PEEP, cmH$_2$O	10 (8–12)	10 (8–12)	10 (8–13)	0.436
FiO$_2$, %	60 (50–75)	60 (50–70)	60 (50–80)	0.462
Arterial pH	7.34 (7.26–7.41)	7.35 (7.28–7.41)	7.31 (7.22–7.39)	0.001
PaCO2, kPa	5.8 (5.1–6.9)	5.7 (5–6.9)	6 (5.2–7.3)	0.072
PaO$_2$/FiO$_2$	120 (89–149)	123 (91–149)	115 (89–149)	0.353
SpO$_2$/FiO$_2$	160 (126–190)	163 (127–191)	157 (124–190)	0.344
Vasopressor use in first 24 h	293 (64.3)	164 (59.6)	129 (71.3)	0.015
ARDS class				
Moderate ARDS	300 (65.8)	181 (65.8)	119 (65.7)	1
Severe ARDS	156 (34.2)	94 (34.2)	62 (34.3)	1
Cause of ARDS				
Pulmonary origin	325 (71.3)	200 (72.7)	125 (69.1)	0.732
Non-pulmonary origin	185 (40.6)	104 (37.8)	81 (44.8)	0.382

Categorical variables: number (percentage); continuous variables: median (25–75 percentile)

PEEP positive end-expiratory pressure, *FiO2* fraction of inspired oxygen, *PaCO$_2$* arterial carbon dioxide tension, *PaO$_2$* arterial oxygen tension, *SpO$_2$* pulse oximetry saturation, *ARDS* acute respiratory distress syndrome, *APACHE IV* acute physiology and chronic evaluation IV

$$\mathrm{SpO_2/FiO_2} = 42.6 + 1.00 * \mathrm{PaO_2/FiO_2}$$

This relationship was neither moderated by arterial PaCO$_2$ and PEEP, nor by body temperature and vasopressor therapy. There was a moderation effect by arterial pH and FiO$_2$, as the steepness of the slope between PaO$_2$/FiO$_2$ and SpO$_2$/FiO$_2$ was inclined by arterial pH (1.4, $P < 0.001$) and declined by FiO$_2$ (-0.01, $P < 0.001$).

Based on the found equation, a PaO$_2$/FiO$_2$ of 200 mm Hg corresponded to a SpO$_2$/FiO$_2$ of 243 [95% CI 220–265], a PaO$_2$/FiO$_2$ of 150 mm Hg to a SpO$_2$/FiO$_2$ of 193 [95% CI 174–211] and a PaO$_2$/FiO$_2$ of 100 mm Hg to a SpO$_2$/FiO$_2$ of 143 [95% CI 127–158].

The SpO$_2$/FiO$_2$ had an excellent ability to discriminate moderate from severe ARDS, with a ROC area under the curve of 0.928 (Fig. 3). The nonlinear formula (Ellis formula) to estimate the PaO$_2$/FiO$_2$ from the SpO$_2$ and FiO$_2$ was not superior to the linear model when SpO$_2$ $\leq$ 97% ($N = 382$, $R^2 = 0.656$).

The use of fractions (1/SpO$_2$/FiO$_2$ and 1/PaO$_2$/FiO$_2$) did not result in a stronger linear relationship ($R^2 = 0.629$). The regression equation, though, was very similar to one previously reported in pediatric patients (1/SpO$_2$/FiO$_2$ = 0.0024 + 0.46/PaO$_2$/FiO$_2$) [18].

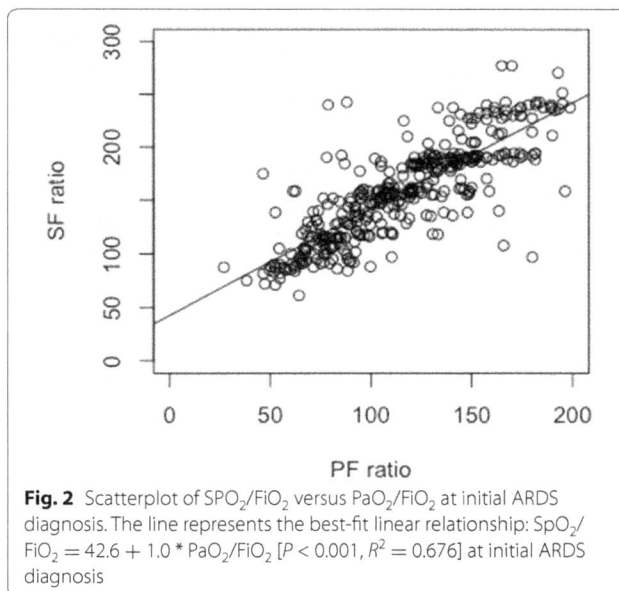

Fig. 2 Scatterplot of SPO$_2$/FiO$_2$ versus PaO$_2$/FiO$_2$ at initial ARDS diagnosis. The line represents the best-fit linear relationship: SpO$_2$/FiO$_2$ = 42.6 + 1.0 * PaO$_2$/FiO$_2$ [$P < 0.001$, $R^2 = 0.676$] at initial ARDS diagnosis

Risk stratification

The distribution and outcome data for the four risk groups are presented in Table 2. There was no trend for increasing in-hospital mortality rate among the four risk groups at baseline (P value for trend $= 0.90$). A pairwise comparison also showed no significant differences in hospital mortality between groups at ARDS diagnosis. In contrast, the same categorization after 24 h resulted in risk groups with increasing rates of in-hospital mortality (P value for trend < 0.001). A pairwise comparison showed that the differences in in-hospital mortality

between group IV and group II (OR 2.40 [1.15–4.82]; P value $= 0.012$), and between group IV and group I were significant (OR 2.47 [1.26–4.85]; P value $= 0.003$) (Table 3).

Findings were comparable for the secondary outcomes. While classification using cutoffs for SpO_2/FiO_2 and PEEP at initial ARDS diagnosis were not related to any of these outcomes, risk stratification at 24 h resulted in significant positive trends across groups, and significantly worse secondary outcomes in group IV compared to group I and to group II (Additional file 1: Table E1).

Distribution of patients in each subset noticeably changed at 24 h. Less than a quarter of patients maintained to have $SpO_2/FiO_2 < 190$; their in-hospital mortality was much higher than that of patients with a $SpO_2/FiO_2 \geq 190$ (56.1 vs. 35.2%, $P = 0.001$). Half of the patients were ventilated at PEEP < 10 cm H_2O; their in-hospital mortality was similar to that of patients who were kept at PEEP ≥ 10 cm H_2O (36.1 vs. 43.4 $P = 0.107$). When considering the characteristics of the four risk groups at 24 h, we found statistical differences in the APACHE IV score, arterial pH and FiO_2 at 24 h, maximum plasma lactate levels and vasopressor use, which could explain the significant differences in outcome (Table 3).

Post hoc analyses

The post hoc analysis with the adapted SpO_2/FiO_2 cutoff of 150, in line with the Berlin definition cutoff of PaO_2/FiO_2 of 100 mm Hg, showed similar results to the primary analysis, albeit group sizes changed. No trends in risk were observed other than for ICU mortality when

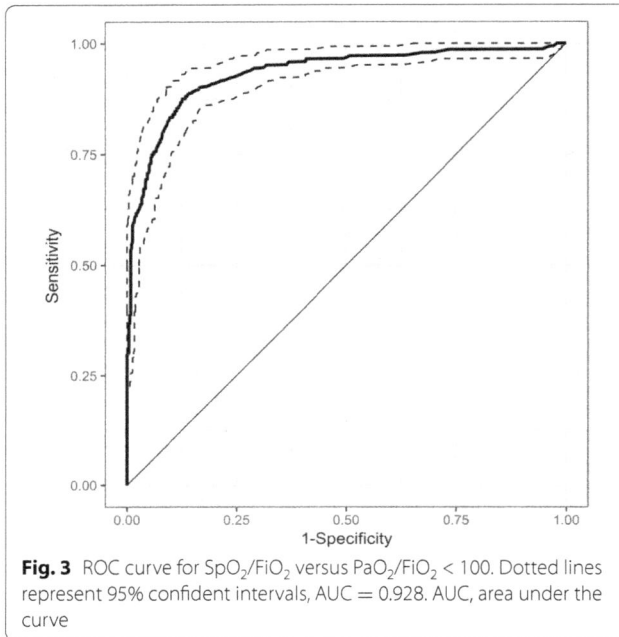

Fig. 3 ROC curve for SpO_2/FiO_2 versus $PaO_2/FiO_2 < 100$. Dotted lines represent 95% confident intervals, AUC $= 0.928$. AUC, area under the curve

Table 2 Distribution and outcomes of each subset of patients with ARDS at initial diagnosis and after 24 h

Outcome	Group I $SpO_2/FiO_2 \geq 190$ and PEEP < 10	Group II $SpO_2/FiO_2 \geq 190$ and PEEP ≥ 10	Group III $SpO_2/FiO_2 < 190$ and PEEP < 10	Group IV $SpO_2/FiO_2 < 190$ and PEEP ≥ 10	P value
At onset of ARDS (N)	87	43	100	226	
ICU mortality (%)	19.5	23.3	18.0	30.1	0.042
In-hospital mortality (%)	44.8	30.2	36.0	41.2	0.897
30-day mortality (%)	27.6	27.9	24.0	33.2	0.276
90-day mortality (%)	47.1	34.9	41.0	42.0	0.636
1-year mortality (%)	60.9	41.9	47.0	49.6	0.182
VFD (days) (IQR)	19 (7–24)	22 (6.5–25)	20.5 (6–25)	18 (0–23)	0.070
After 24 h (N)	213	145	17	81	
ICU mortality (%)	15.5	24.1	35.3	48.2	< 0.001
In-hospital mortality (%)	34.7	35.9	52.9	56.8	< 0.001
30-day mortality (%)	23.9	26.9	47.1	45.7	< 0.001
90-day mortality (%)	38.0	38.6	52.9	56.8	0.003
1-year mortality (%)	47.4	45.5	58.8	65.4	0.006
VFD 28 (days) (IQR)	23 (15–26)	18 (0–23)	6 (0–17)	0 (0–17)	< 0.001

VFD-28 ventilator-free days and alive at day 28, *IQR* interquartile range, *CI* confidence interval

Table 3 Intergroup comparisons at ARDS diagnosis and after 24 h for in-hospital mortality

Comparison	At ARDS diagnosis		After 24 h	
	OR (95% CI)	P value	OR (95% CI)	P value
Group II versus I	0.53 (0.19–1.46)	0.376	1.05 (0.59–1.86)	0.996
Group III versus I	0.69 (0.32–1.49)	0.600	2.11 (0.59–7.62)	0.433
Group IV versus I	0.86 (0.45–1.65)	0.933	2.47 (1.26–4.85)	0.003
Group III versus II	1.30 (0.48–3.53)	0.907	2.01 (0.55–7.43)	0.509
Group IV versus II	1.61 (0.65–4.03)	0.531	2.40 (1.15–4.82)	0.012
Group IV versus III	1.24 (0.66–2.34)	0.811	1.17 (0.30–4.53)	0.991

ARDS acute respiratory distress syndrome, *OR* odd ratio, *CI* confidence interval

using this cutoff at onset of ARDS, while a significant trend across the four risk groups was noted using this cutoff after 24 h (Additional file 1: Table E2). The intergroup comparisons also mirrored the primary analysis, with no significant contrasts at ARDS diagnosis, but clear contrast after 24 h (group IV vs. group I and II) (Additional file 1: Table E3).

The multivariable model showed that APACHE IV scores, plasma lactate levels and arterial pH significantly confounded the relationship between the group stratification and in-hospital mortality (Additional file 1: Table E4). The same applied when restricting this analysis to the extreme risk groups (i.e., groups I and IV), in which even vasopressor therapy was a significant confounder (Additional file 1: Table E5).

Discussion

To our best knowledge, this is the first study in which ARDS patients were classified using predefined cutoff values for SpO_2/FiO_2 and PEEP. The most relevant findings of this study are: (1) SpO_2/FiO_2 confirms to be a valid surrogate for PaO_2/FiO_2 in patients with moderate or severe ARDS; (2) re-classification after 24 h using predefined cutoffs for SpO_2/FiO_2 and PEEP improves risk stratification compared to the same cutoffs at baseline; and (3) the association between risk group and outcome, however, is confounded by disease severity, arterial pH and lactate levels, and vasopressor therapy. We believe that the approach of using SpO_2/FiO_2 and PEEP to classify patients could be useful for the implementation of an individualized approach for appropriate diagnosis and therapy in ARDS patients, in particular in settings where it is difficult, if not impossible, to perform (repeated) blood gas analyses (Table 4).

Our study has several strengths. The prospective design of the collection of data, the completeness of follow-up and the fact that the ARDS diagnosis was scored by a team of trained ICU researchers prevented against bias.

In addition, we could re-categorize patients from the criteria stated by the American–European Consensus Conference on ARDS [10] to the newer Berlin definition for ARDS [1], after we could select patients with moderate or severe ARDS. Finally, the number of participants was large, patients were homogeneous regarding their clinical characteristics as well as type of ARDS and the overall in-hospital mortality rate of our cohort was comparable to the pooled mortality for moderate and severe ARDS patients in the recently published LUNG SAFE study [19].

SpO_2/FiO_2 is an increasingly appreciated parameter in the diagnosis and management of patients with ARDS [6, 15, 17, 20, 21]. The current pediatric ARDS definition includes oximetry-based measures in preference of the PaO_2/FiO_2, captured in the oxygenation saturation index [22]. Unfortunately, mean airway pressures, necessary for calculation of the oxygenation saturation index, were not reliably captured in our cohort preventing us from comparing our results to those from previous studies in children [8, 18, 23]. We used a previously reported equation ($SpO_2/FiO_2 = 64 + (0.84 * PaO_2/FiO_2)$ [6] to convert a previously used cutoff for PaO_2/FiO_2 (i.e., 150 mm Hg) to a cutoff for SpO_2/FiO_2 of 190. Using the equation that came from our own data a very similar cutoff for SpO_2/FiO_2 would have been chosen. Due to its increased feasibility, the SpO_2/FiO_2 was actually considered for inclusion during the Berlin criteria definition process [24], but was successively excluded on the possibility that it may misclassify mild into severe ARDS patients. A cutoff for PaO_2/FiO_2 of 150 mm Hg has frequently been shown to accurately stratify for in-hospital mortality [4, 5, 25] and was also used in two of the largest, and ultimately positive, randomized controlled trials in ARDS patients [26, 27].

The present findings on the relationship between SpO_2/FiO_2 and PaO_2/FiO_2 mirror results from previous investigations in adult [6, 15] and pediatric patients [14, 18, 23, 28], albeit that a marginally different regression equation was found. One investigation did not find a strong relationship between SpO_2/FiO_2 and PaO_2/FiO_2, but in that study the data were collected from automated anesthesia information system with a very high portion of the data excluded due to high SpO_2 values [29]. Recently, the linear relation between SpO_2/FiO_2 and PaO_2/FiO_2 was re-challenged and both a fractional transformation [14] and a nonlinear imputation method [17, 30] were proposed to improve the model fit or better represent the sigmoidal shape of the oxyhemoglobin dissociation curve. Despite the clear physiological rationale, these approaches did not improve the relationship in the present dataset.

It has been described before that FiO_2 at levels > 70% alters the PaO_2/FiO_2: an increase in FiO_2 > 70% gradually

Table 4 Main characteristics of 456 patients with ARDS—classification 24 h after initial ARDS diagnosis based on SpO$_2$/ FiO$_2$ cutoff of 190 and PEEP cutoff of 10 cm H$_2$O

Variables	Group I (N = 213) SpO$_2$/FiO$_2$ ≥ 190 and PEEP < 10	Group II (N = 145) SpO$_2$/FiO$_2$ ≥ 190 and PEEP ≥ 10	Group III (N = 17) SpO$_2$/FiO$_2$ < 190 and PEEP < 10	Group IV (N = 81) SpO$_2$/FiO$_2$ < 190 and PEEP ≥ 10	P value
APACHE IV score	75 (60–93)	84 (65–108)	78 (65–112)	86 (68–110)	0.001
Age, years	63 (53–73)	60 (49–69)	57 (42–70)	59 (49–69)	0.018
Female	80 (37.6)	61 (42.1)	5 (29.4)	26 (32.1)	0.436
CCI 2	1 (0–3)	1 (0–2)	2 (0–3)	1 (0–2)	0.423
LIPS	8 (6.5–9.5)	9 (7.5–10.5)	7 (6.5–8)	9.5 (7.5–11.5)	< 0.001
Tidal volume, ml/kg	6.4 (5.3–7.7)	6.2 (5.2–7.5)	7.2 (6.5–8.2)	6.4 (5.6–7.4)	0.166
FiO$_2$, %	40 (36–40)	40 (40–50)	60 (55–60)	60 (55–65)	< 0.001
PEEP, cm H$_2$O	5 (5–8)	12 (10–13)	7 (5–8)	14 (12–15)	< 0.001
Arterial pH	7.4 (7.4–7.5)	7.4 (7.3–7.4)	7.4 (7.3–7.5)	7.3 (7.3–7.4)	< 0.001
PaCO$_2$, kPa	5.3 (4.7–6.2)	5.6 (4.9–6.2)	5.6 (5–7)	5.8 (5.1–6.6)	0.018
Plasma lactate level, mmol/l	2.4 (1.4–4.1)	3.1 (1.7–6.2)	1.6 (1.4–3.9)	5.4 (2.6–10.9)	< 0.001
Respiratory rate	22 (17–27)	24 (17.2–30)	22 (18–28)	24 (16–34)	0.183
PaO$_2$/FiO$_2$	207 (175–252)	193 (167–226)	128 (120–149)	133 (105–153)	< 0.001
SpO$_2$/FiO$_2$	243 (231–265)	232 (200–245)	165 (154–170)	158 (136–176)	< 0.001
Vasopressor use in first 24 h	100 (47.0)	102 (70.3)	6 (35.3)	67 (82.72)	< 0.001
ARDS class after 24 h					
Mild ARDS	122 (57.3)	61 (42.1)	0 0	5 (6.2)	< 0.001
Moderate ARDS	91 (42.7)	84 (57.9)	15 (88.2)	59 (72.8)	< 0.001
Severe ARDS	0 0	0 0	2 (11.8)	17 (21)	< 0.001
Cause of ARDS					
Pulmonary	156 (73.2)	99 (68.3)	12 (70.6)	58 (71.6)	0.509
Non-pulmonary	67 (31.5)	78 (53.8)	5 (29.4)	40 (49.4)	0.426

Categorical variables: number (percentage); continuous variables: median (25–75 percentile)

CCI Charlson Comorbidity Index, *LIPS* Lung Injury Prediction Score, *APACHE* acute physiology and chronic health evaluation, *PEEP* positive end-expiratory pressure, *FiO$_2$* fraction of inspired oxygen, *PaCO$_2$* arterial carbon dioxide tension, *PaO$_2$* arterial oxygen tension, *SpO$_2$* pulse oximetry oxygen saturation, *ARDS* acute respiratory distress syndrome

increases the PaO$_2$/FiO$_2$ [31], particularly at low levels of shunt fraction [32]. The effect of FiO$_2$ on SpO$_2$/ FiO$_2$, however, could be opposite as pulse oximetry has an intrinsic upper limit much tighter than PaO$_2$. An increase in FiO$_2$ will gradually decrease the SpO$_2$/FiO$_2$. This intrinsic mathematical limitation of the SpO$_2$/FiO$_2$ can possibly lead to misclassification of individual ARDS cases. Of note, FiO$_2$ > 70% was used in 25% of patients at ARDS diagnosis, and only in 3% after 24 h.

The level of PEEP is known to be particularly relevant as the evolution and prognosis of ARDS are related to changes in PaO$_2$/FiO$_2$ in response to changes in PEEP greater than or equal to 10 cm H$_2$O [3, 33, 34]. While PEEP does not affect the oxyhemoglobin curve and may not significantly alter the relationship between SpO$_2$ and PaO$_2$ [15], it may impact the SpO$_2$/FiO$_2$ ratio by improving ventilation–perfusion matching and thus was considered in our analysis. Of note, the approach of using PaO$_2$/ FiO$_2$, or SpO$_2$/FiO$_2$, and PEEP is not new. Indeed, risk

classification in the Berlin definition uses PaO$_2$/FiO$_2$ and PEEP levels [1], though only at onset of ARDS and not after 24 h of standard care. The empathic aim of the present investigation was to see whether two easy to collect and almost always-available ventilator parameters, even in resource-limited settings, i.e., SpO$_2$/FiO$_2$ and PEEP, would alter risk groups.

Despite several classification and prediction systems for ARDS patients [1, 3, 25, 33, 35–37], we still lack a proper classification system for clinical management and research purposes that can serve as a practical model for setting individual therapeutic targets. Several investigations have shown that the PaO$_2$/FiO$_2$ measured at onset of ARDS cannot be used for risk stratification in patients with moderate or severe ARDS [35, 38–41]. Recently, it was shown that standardization of ventilator settings at the moment of collecting PaO$_2$/FiO$_2$ data [33] as well as re-categorization based on both PaO$_2$/FiO$_2$ and PEEP level cutoffs, measured 24 h after the initial ARDS diagnosis, largely improves risk stratification for hospital mortality [4, 5]. The findings of the present study are in agreement with and extend these findings showing for the first time that pulse oximetry after 24 h perform better than at the initial ARDS diagnosis in short- and long-term outcome stratification in adult patients with moderate or severe ARDS. Similar findings derive from the pediatric population, where oximetry derived indexes after 24 h reliably stratified outcome while initial values were not helpful in prognostication [8].

In the studied cohort of patients with moderate or severe ARDS, improvement or worsening of the SpO_2/FiO_2 in the first 24 h was strongly associated with outcome. Group I represents the less complicated patients with ARDS and a great portion of our patients fit in this group after 24 h (46.7 vs. 19.1% at baseline), underlining the ample clinical change that characterizes the initial hours of care. Few patients (17, 3.7%) were classified after 24 h as having a $SpO_2/FiO_2 < 190$ and PEEP < 10 cm H_2O (group III), in accordance with previous observations in which only few patients with a worsening oxygenation are managed with low levels of PEEP [4]. The use of a different SpO_2/FiO_2 cutoff (150, corresponding with 100 mm Hg as used in the Berlin definition for ARDS to classify severe ARDS) did not essentially change the results. This underlines the rationale of the 24 h re-classification.

The comparisons between risk groups emphasize the improvement in risk stratification after 24 h but also suggest that the proposed classification by SpO_2/FiO_2 and PEEP in four risk groups is dependent on other factors. The fact that differences between group III and the other groups did not reach significance could be explained in part by the small number of patients in this group after 24 h. Also interestingly, differences in outcomes between groups separated by PEEP were not significant (group I vs. II and group III vs. IV). This does not weaken the improvement in risk stratification after 24 h, but probably suggests that our findings are driven more by SpO_2/FiO_2 than by PEEP. Hence, although PEEP is an attractive stratification tool due to its ubiquity, alternative variables might result in a better classification when combined to the SpO_2/FiO_2 ratio.

The high mortality rates, especially in the lower risk groups, are high, but confirm those from previous investigations [4, 5]. Re-classification after 24 h lead to lower mortality rates in the lowest risk group, but still the proportion of patients that died was high. This too is in line with findings from the earlier studies [4, 5]. Noticeable differences were seen in APACHE IV, arterial pH, plasma lactate levels in the first 24 h, and vasopressor use between the risk groups, and all could, at least in part be associated with the significant differences in mortality rates. In fact, the post hoc multivariate analysis showed that stratification based on SpO_2/FiO_2 and PEEP looses it predictive capability when controlled for APACHE IV scores, plasma lactate levels, arterial pH, blood pressure levels and vasopressor therapy. This at least suggests that persistence of hypoxemia after 24 h could be a surrogate, e.g., overall disease severity but also underlines the weakness of a simplified classification system. Nevertheless, we think that the proposed risk stratification may still be useful in settings where only pulse oximetry is available for monitoring and where laboratory examinations to compute disease severity scores are lacking.

The results of this study suggest that the SpO_2/FiO_2 can accurately surrogate the PaO_2/FiO_2 in stratifying for mortality of adult patients with established ARDS in resource-rich settings. This simple approach may in particular be useful in settings where repeated blood gas analyses are difficult to obtain or unavailable, such as in pediatric patients [23] and resource-limited settings [42]. However, it must be acknowledged that oximetry may never fully replace arterial blood gas analyses completely. Indeed, acid–base status and $PaCO_2$ levels are clinically important. However, we stress that pulse oximetry is consistently present in low-resource settings while blood gas analyzers are scarce, if not completely absent. Moreover, several point-of-care devices allow to measure capillary or venous acid–base, potentially alleviating the need for an arterial blood sample and expensive blood gas analysis devices.

The SpO_2/FiO_2 may also turn useful in identifying patients at risk for ARDS. It has already been shown to be a useful independent indicator of ARDS in the Kigali criteria for ARDS, in which SpO_2/FiO_2 and lung ultrasound were used instead of PaO_2/FiO_2 and chest radiography [42]. Further studies in resource-rich and resource-poor settings are still needed to assess the utility of these adapted criteria in patients at risk for ARDS.

Limitations of our analysis include its single-center design and the lack of standardization of the SpO_2 measurements, due to their retrospective collection. Indeed, standardization of ventilatory settings at baseline and after 24 h, and thus calculation of the PaO_2/FiO_2, may be crucial for appropriate stratification and patient selection bias minimization [43], and the same may apply for SpO_2-based markers. While we tried to minimize potential errors by increasing the number of SpO_2 values collected, we are aware that potential artifactual SpO_2 values or ones resulting from acute events unrelated to the disease process may have been included (such as patient–ventilator asynchrony, obstruction of endotracheal tubes, suctioning and hemodynamic instability). We also did not collect information on skin pigmentation, motion artifacts, skin perfusion, ambient light, methemoglobinemia and carboxyhemoglobinemia levels—factors that all may be associated with the accuracy of SpO_2 measurements. Its retrospective design allowed us neither to determine the type of pulse oximeter used nor to capture the positions of the probes used in individual patients. The minor but not quantifiable amount of measurements from a different probe or location other than the conventional finger oximeter represents a methodological weakness, but we do not believe affects the outcome or correlation analysis in an important way. We focused on only two time points, i.e., the time of initial ARDS diagnosis and after 24 h. It may be possible that SpO_2/FiO_2 and PEEP at other time points add to risk stratification. Finally, re-classification after 24 h means that patients who died in the first 24 h are missed. The same happens with the small proportion of patients who are extubated or transferred before 24 h. We also excluded patients with a $PaO_2/FiO_2 > 200$ mm Hg; however, we do not believe this weakens our results. We did this for the two following reasons. Patients classified as having mild ARDS [1] are very 'heterogeneous' with respect to outcomes. Moreover, the milder degree of oxygenation impairments in these patients increases the number of patients with SpO_2 values > 97%, above which the relationship between PaO_2 and SpO_2 becomes weak.

Conclusions

SpO_2/FiO_2 and PaO_2/FiO_2 have a strong linear relationship. In contrast to risk stratification at initial ARDS diagnosis, risk stratification using SpO_2/FiO_2 and PEEP at 24 h leads to risk groups with worsening outcomes. Despite the fact that the association between risk group assignment and outcome is confounded by several factors, risk stratification using SpO_2/FiO_2 and PEEP could be useful and practical, especially in settings where repeated blood analyses are difficult or impossible.

Abbreviations
SpO_2: peripheral capillary oxygen saturation; FiO_2: fraction of inspired oxygen; PaO_2: arterial oxygen partial pressure; PEEP: positive end-expiratory pressure; ARDS: acute respiratory distress syndrome; ICU: intensive care unit; VFD: ventilator-free days; APACHE: acute physiology and chronic health evaluation; LIPS: Lung Injury Prediction Score; ROC: receiver operating characteristic; AUC: area under the curve; AECC: American–European Consensus Conference on ARDS.

Authors' contributions
LP, FDS and MJS designed the study. LP, JPR, FDS, LRS and LDB performed the analyses. JPR and AG and members of the MARS consortium collected the data. LP, JPR, FDS, LDB, ASN and MJS drafted the manuscript. SMvdH, JH, ASN, EF, AMD, SG, MJS critically reviewed the manuscript. All authors read and approved the final version of this manuscript. LP, JPR, FDS and MJS had full access to all the data in the study and take responsibility for the integrity of the data and the accuracy of the data analysis.

Author details
[1] Department of Intensive Care, Academic Medical Center, Meibergdreef 9, 1105 AZ Amsterdam, The Netherlands. [2] Laboratory of Experimental Intensive Care and Anesthesiology (LEICA), Academic Medical Center, Amsterdam, The Netherlands. [3] Anesthesia and Intensive Care Unit, Department of Emergency and Organ Transplantation, University of Bari Aldo Moro, Bari, Italy. [4] Department of Pediatrics, Academic Medical Center, Amsterdam, The Netherlands. [5] Department of Pulmonology, Academic Medical Center, Amsterdam, The Netherlands. [6] Department of Critical Care Medicine, Hospital Israelita Albert Einstein, São Paulo, Brazil. [7] Pulmonary and Critical Care Medicine, Mayo Clinic, Jacksonville, FL, USA. [8] Mahidol–Oxford Research Unit (MORU), Faculty of Tropical Medicine, Mahidol University, Bangkok, Thailand.

Competing interests
On behalf of all authors, the corresponding author states that there is no conflict of interest.

Funding
No funding received.

MARS consortium members
Roosmarijn T. M. van Hooijdonk, Mischa A. Huson, Laura R. A. Schouten, Marleen Straat, Fabienne D. Simonis, Lieuwe D. Bos, Lonneke A. van Vught, Maryse A. Wiewel, Esther Witteveen, Gerie J. Glas, Luuk Wieske, Jos F. Frencken, Marc Bonten, Peter M. C. Klein Klouwenberg, David Ong, Brendon P Scicluna, Arjan J Hoogendijk, H Belkasim-Bohoudi, Tom van der Poll.

References
1. The ARDS Definition Task Force*, Ranieri VM, Rubenfeld GD, et al. Acute respiratory distress syndrome: the Berlin Definition. JAMA. 2012;307:1. doi:10.1001/jama.2012.5669.
2. Hernu R, Wallet F, Thiollière F, et al. An attempt to validate the modification of the American-European consensus definition of acute lung injury/acute respiratory distress syndrome by the Berlin definition in a university hospital. Intensive Care Med. 2013;39:2161–70. doi:10.1007/s00134-013-3122-6.
3. Villar J, Pérez-Méndez L, López J, et al. An early PEEP/FIO trial identifies different degrees of lung injury in patients with acute respiratory distress syndrome. Am J Respir Crit Care Med. 2007;176:795–804. doi:10.1164/rccm.200610-1534OC.
4. Villar J, Fernandez RL, Ambros A, et al. A clinical classification of the acute respiratory distress syndrome for predicting outcome and guiding medical therapy*. Crit Care Med. 2015;43:346–53. doi:10.1097/CCM.0000000000000703.
5. Bos LD, Cremer OL, Ong DSY, et al. External validation confirms the legitimacy of a new clinical classification of ARDS for predicting outcome. Intensive Care Med. 2015;41:2004–5. doi:10.1007/s00134-015-3992-x.
6. Rice TW, Wheeler AP, Bernard GR, et al. Comparison of the SpO/FIO ratio and the PaO/FIO ratio in patients with acute lung injury or ARDS. Chest. 2007;132:410–7. doi:10.1378/chest.07-0617.
7. Chen W, Janz DR, Shaver CM, et al. Clinical characteristics and outcomes are similar in ARDS diagnosed by oxygen saturation/FiO$_2$ ratio compared with PaO$_2$/FiO$_2$ ratio. Chest J. 2015;148:1477. doi:10.1378/chest.15-0169.
8. Parvathaneni K, Belani S, Leung D, et al. Evaluating the performance of the pediatric acute lung injury consensus conference definition of acute respiratory distress syndrome. Pediatr Crit Care Med. 2017;18:17–25. doi:10.1097/PCC.0000000000000945.
9. Klouwenberg PMCK, Ong DSY, Bos LDJ, et al. Interobserver agreement of centers for disease control and prevention criteria for classifying infections in critically ill patients*. Crit Care Med. 2013;41:2373–8. doi:10.1097/CCM.0b013e3182923712.
10. Bernard GR, Artigas A, Brigham KL, et al. Report of the American-European consensus conference on ARDS: definitions, mechanisms,

relevant outcomes and clinical trial coordination. Intensive Care Med. 1994;20:225–32. doi:10.1007/BF01704707.

11. Zimmerman JE, Kramer AA, McNair DS, Malila FM. Acute Physiology and Chronic Health Evaluation (APACHE) IV: hospital mortality assessment for today's critically ill patients. Crit Care Med. 2006;34:1297–310. doi:10.1097/01.CCM.0000215112.84523.F0.

12. Gajic O, Dabbagh O, Park PK, et al. Early identification of patients at risk of acute lung injury: evaluation of lung injury prediction score in a multicenter cohort study. Am J Respir Crit Care Med. 2010. doi:10.1164/rccm.201004-0549OC.

13. Quan H, Li B, Couris CM, et al. Updating and validating the Charlson comorbidity index and score for risk adjustment in hospital discharge abstracts using data from 6 countries. Am J Epidemiol. 2011;173:676–82. doi:10.1093/aje/kwq433.

14. Khemani RG, Patel NR, Bart RD, Newth CJL. Comparison of the pulse oximetric saturation/fraction of inspired oxygen ratio and the PaO_2/fraction of inspired oxygen ratio in children. Chest. 2009;135:662–8. doi:10.1378/chest.08-2239.

15. Pandharipande PP, Shintani AK, Hagerman HE, et al. Derivation and validation of SpO_2/FiO_2 ratio to impute for PaO_2/FiO_2 ratio in the respiratory component of the Sequential Organ Failure Assessment score. Crit Care Med. 2009;37:1317–21. doi:10.1097/CCM.0b013e31819cefa9.

16. Ellis RK. Determination of PO from saturation. J Appl Physiol. 1989;67:902.

17. Brown SM, Grissom CK, Moss M, et al. Non-linear imputation of PaO_2/FiO_2 from SpO_2/FiO_2 among patients with acute respiratory distress syndrome. Chest. 2016. doi:10.1016/j.chest.2016.01.003.

18. Khemani RG, Thomas NJ, Venkatachalam V, et al. Comparison of SpO_2 to PaO_2 based markers of lung disease severity for children with acute lung injury. Crit Care Med. 2012;40:1309–16. doi:10.1097/CCM.0b013e31823bc61b.

19. Bellani G, Gattinoni L, Van Haren F, et al. Epidemiology, patterns of care, and mortality for patients with acute respiratory distress syndrome in intensive care units in 50 countries. JAMA. 2016;315:2526–33.

20. Serpa Neto A, Schultz MJ, Festic E. Ventilatory support of patients with sepsis or septic shock in resource-limited settings. Intensive Care Med. 2016;42:100–3. doi:10.1007/s00134-015-4070-0.

21. Festic E, Bansal V, Kor DJ, Gajic O. SpO_2/FiO_2 ratio on hospital admission is an indicator of early acute respiratory distress syndrome development among patients at risk. J Intensive Care Med. 2015;30:209–16. doi:10.1177/0885066613516411.

22. Group TPALICC. Pediatric acute respiratory distress syndrome: consensus recommendations from the pediatric acute lung injury consensus conference. Pediatr Crit Care Med. 2015;16:428–39. doi:10.4187/respcare.01515.

23. Khemani RG, Rubin S, Belani S, et al. Pulse oximetry vs. PaO_2 metrics in mechanically ventilated children: Berlin definition of ARDS and mortality risk. Intensive Care Med. 2015;41:94–102. doi:10.1007/s00134-014-3486-2.

24. Ferguson ND, Fan E, Camporota L, et al. The Berlin definition of ARDS: an expanded rationale, justification, and supplementary material. Intensive Care Med. 2012;38:1573–82. doi:10.1007/s00134-012-2682-1.

25. Villar J, Pérez-Méndez L, Kacmarek RM. Current definitions of acute lung injury and the acute respiratory distress syndrome do not reflect their true severity and outcome. Intensive Care Med. 1999;25:930–5. doi:10.1007/s001340050984.

26. Papazian L, Forel J-M, Gacouin A, et al. Neuromuscular blockers in early acute respiratory distress syndrome. N Engl J Med. 2010;363:1107–16. doi:10.1056/NEJMoa1005372.

27. Guérin C, Reignier J, Richard J-C, et al. Prone positioning in severe acute respiratory distress syndrome. N Engl J Med. 2013;368:2159–68. doi:10.1056/NEJMoa1214103

28. Mayordomo-Colunga J, Pons M, López Y, et al. Predicting non-invasive ventilation failure in children from the SpO_2/FiO_2 (SF) ratio. Intensive Care Med. 2013;39:1095–103. doi:10.1007/s00134-013-2880-5.

29. Tripathi RS, Blum JM, Rosenberg AL, Tremper KK. Pulse oximetry saturation to fraction inspired oxygen ratio as a measure of hypoxia under general anesthesia and the influence of positive end-expiratory pressure. J Crit Care. 2010;25:542.e9–13. doi:10.1016/j.jcrc.2010.04.009.

30. Sanz F, Dean N, Dickerson J, et al. Accuracy of PaO_2/FiO_2 calculated from SpO_2 for severity assessment in ED patients with pneumonia. Respirology. 2015;20:813–8. doi:10.1111/resp.12560.

31. Allardet-Servent J, Forel J-M, Roch A, et al. FiO_2 and acute respiratory distress syndrome definition during lung protective ventilation*. Crit Care Med. 2009;37:202-e6. doi:10.1097/CCM.0b013e31819261db.

32. Feiner JR, Weiskopf RB. Evaluating pulmonary function: an assessment of PaO_2/FiO_2. Crit Care Med. 2017;45:e40–8. doi:10.1097/CCM.0000000000002017.

33. Villar J, Pérez-Méndez L, Blanco J, et al. A universal definition of ARDS: the PaO_2/FiO_2 ratio under a standard ventilatory setting-a prospective, multicenter validation study. Intensive Care Med. 2013;39:583–92. doi:10.1007/s00134-012-2803-x.

34. López-Fernández Y, Azagra AM, de la Oliva P, et al. Pediatric acute lung injury epidemiology and natural history study: incidence and outcome of the acute respiratory distress syndrome in children. Crit Care Med. 2012;40:3238–45. doi:10.1097/CCM.0b013e318260caa3.

35. Bone RC, Maunder R, Slotman G, et al. An early test of survival in patients with the adult respiratory distress syndrome. The PaO_2/FiO_2 ratio and its differential response to conventional therapy. Prostaglandin E1 Study Group. Chest. 1989;96:849–51. doi:10.1378/chest.96.4.849.

36. Cooke CR, Shah CV, Gallop R, et al. A simple clinical predictive index for objective estimates of mortality in acute lung injury. Crit Care Med. 2009;37:1913–20. doi:10.1097/CCM.0b013e3181a009b4.

37. Villar J, Pérez-Méndez L, Basaldúa S, et al. A risk tertiles model for predicting mortality in patients with acute respiratory distress syndrome: age, plateau pressure, and PaO_2/FiO_2 at ARDS onset can predict mortality. Respir Care. 2011;56:420–8. doi:10.4187/respcare.00811.

38. Bersten AD, Edibam C, Hunt T, Moran J. Incidence and mortality of acute lung injury and the acute respiratory distress syndrome in three Australian States. Am J Respir Crit Care Med. 2002;165:443–8. doi:10.1164/ajrccm.165.4.2101124.

39. Luhr OR, Karlsson M, Thorsteinsson A, et al. The impact of respiratory variables on mortality in non-ARDS and ARDS patients requiring mechanical ventilation. Intensive Care Med. 2000;26:508–17. doi:10.1007/s001340051197.

40. Knaus WA, Sun X, Hakim RB, Wagner DP. Evaluation of definitions for adult respiratory distress syndrome. Am J Respir Crit Care Med. 1994;150:311–7.

41. Sloane PJ, Gee MH, Gottlieb JE, et al. A multicenter registry of patients with acute respiratory distress syndrome. Physiology and outcome. Am Rev Respir Dis. 1992;146:419–26. doi:10.1164/ajrccm/146.2.419.

42. Riviello ED, Kiviri W, Twagirumugabe T, et al. Hospital incidence and outcomes of the acute respiratory distress syndrome using the Kigali modification of the Berlin definition. Am J Respir Crit Care Med. 2016;193:52–9. doi:10.1164/rccm.201503-0584OC.

43. Villar J, Blanco J, del Campo R, et al. Assessment of PaO_2/FiO_2 for stratification of patients with moderate and severe acute respiratory distress syndrome. BMJ Open. 2015;5:e006812. doi:10.1136/bmjopen-2014-006812.

7

Tracheotomy in the intensive care unit: guidelines from a French expert panel

Jean Louis Trouillet[1], Olivier Collange[2,3], Fouad Belafia[4], François Blot[5], Gilles Capellier[6,7], Eric Cesareo[8,9], Jean-Michel Constantin[10,11], Alexandre Demoule[12], Jean-Luc Diehl[13,14], Pierre-Grégoire Guinot[15,16], Franck Jegoux[17], Erwan L'Her[18,19], Charles-Edouard Luyt[1,20], Yazine Mahjoub[21], Julien Mayaux[12], Hervé Quintard[22,23], François Ravat[24], Sebastien Vergez[25], Julien Amour[26] and Max Guillot[3,27]*

Abstract

Tracheotomy is widely used in intensive care units, albeit with great disparities between medical teams in terms of frequency and modality. Indications and techniques are, however, associated with variable levels of evidence based on inhomogeneous or even contradictory literature. Our aim was to conduct a systematic analysis of the published data in order to provide guidelines. We present herein recommendations for the use of tracheotomy in adult critically ill patients developed using the Grading of Recommendations Assessment, Development, and Evaluation (GRADE) method. These guidelines were conducted by a group of experts from the French Intensive Care Society (Société de Réanimation de Langue Française) and the French Society of Anesthesia and Intensive Care Medicine (Société Francaise d'Anesthésie Réanimation) with the participation of the French Emergency Medicine Association (Société Française de Médecine d'Urgence), the French Society of Otorhinolaryngology. Sixteen experts and two coordinators agreed to consider questions concerning tracheotomy and its practical implementation. Five topics were defined: indications and contraindications for tracheotomy in intensive care, tracheotomy techniques in intensive care, modalities of tracheotomy in intensive care, management of patients undergoing tracheotomy in intensive care, and decannulation in intensive care. The summary made by the experts and the application of GRADE methodology led to the drawing up of 8 formal guidelines, 10 recommendations, and 3 treatment protocols. Among the 8 formal guidelines, 2 have a high level of proof (Grade 1+/−) and 6 a low level of proof (Grade 2+/−). For the 10 recommendations, GRADE methodology was not applicable and instead 10 expert opinions were produced.

Background

Tracheotomy is a procedure commonly used in intensive care, albeit with great disparities between medical teams in terms of frequency (5–54%) and modality (surgical or percutaneous) [1, 2]. Although tracheotomy has a long history, its utility, indications, duration, and techniques are the subject of debate [3, 4]. Also, the real or potential advantages of tracheotomy need to be weighed against its risks, which are rare but sometimes serious. The advantages are a reduction in pharyngolaryngeal lesions, lower risk of sinusitis, reduced sedation requirements, easier buccopharyngeal hygiene, improved patient comfort with easier communication, facilitated care by nursing personnel, maintenance of swallowing, possible glottic closure, simpler reinsertion in cases of accidental decannulation, and easier weaning from mechanical ventilation [5]. In some studies, early use of tracheotomy was associated with decreased incidence of ventilator-acquired pneumonia, reduced duration of mechanical ventilation and of intensive care, and so of costs, and decreased hospital mortality [6, 7]. However, several recent randomized trials found no evidence of these benefits [8–11]. The most frequent complications can be qualified as minor (for example, minor stomal bleeding). Rare and

*Correspondence: max.guillot@chru-strasbourg.fr
[27] Hôpitaux Universitaires de Strasbourg, Hôpital de Hautepierre, Réanimation Médicale, Avenue Molière, 67200 Strasbourg, France

life-threatening complications, such as lesions of the brachiocephalic artery trunk, have been reported.

Among the controversies surrounding tracheotomy in intensive care, the greatest is probably that of its indication. Tracheotomy is most often considered in cases of failed extubation and of prolonged mechanical ventilation. Three remarks are relevant here. First, there is currently no consensus regarding the contribution of failed extubation (one, two, three attempts? in what conditions?) and of prolonged mechanical ventilation. Second, it may be worthwhile preventing failure of extubation and not adding the deleterious effects of prolonged intubation to those of tracheotomy. The intensivist should predict the failure of extubation and the duration of ventilation so as to perform tracheotomy without delay [5], but prediction of the duration of ventilation is an inexact "science" [12, 13]. Third, the duration of mechanical ventilation and the success of extubation depend on intensive care management as a whole (notably the appropriate treatment of an infection, the water–sodium balance and acid–base balance, nutrition, and sedation). In particular, a sedation protocol is essential.

The most recent SRLF guidelines concerning the surgical approach to the trachea of ventilated patients in intensive care date back to 1998 [14]. There are no recent international guidelines and national guidelines are rare [15, 16]. In the absence of clearly defined and unquestionable criteria, tracheotomy is most often decided solely by the medical team in charge of the patient. In the last ten or so years, the medical literature has been enriched by new clinical data, often compiled in the form of meta-analyses [17–19]. It was against this backdrop that the Société de Réanimation de Langue Française (SRLF) and the Société Française d'Anesthésie et de Réanimation (SFAR) decided to draw up the present guidelines entitled "Tracheotomy in the Intensive Care Unit." The aim of these guidelines is to define the indications, contraindications, modalities, and monitoring of tracheotomy in light of the current literature data.

Methods

These guidelines were prepared by a working group of experts from the SRLF and the SFAR. The organizing committee, together with the coordinators, first defined the questions to be addressed and then designated the experts in charge of each question. The questions were formulated according to the Patient Intervention Comparison Outcome (PICO) format. Grade of Recommendation Assessment, Development and Evaluation (GRADE) methodology was used to analyze the literature and formulate guidelines. A level of proof was defined for each bibliographical reference cited, as a function of the type of study. This level of proof could be reviewed in

light of the methodological quality of the study. An overall level of proof was determined for each endpoint, taking into account the level of proof of each reference, the between-study consistency of the results, the direct or indirect nature of the proof, and cost analysis. A "strong" overall level of proof enabled formulation of a "strong" guideline (must be done, must not be done... GRADE 1 + or 1 −). A "moderate," "weak," or "very weak" overall level of proof led to the writing of an "optional" guideline (should probably be done or should probably not be done... GRADE 2 + or 2 −). When the literature was inexistent, the question could be the subject of a guideline in the form of an expert opinion (the experts suggest...). The proposed guidelines were presented and discussed one by one. The aim was not necessarily to reach a single, unanimous opinion of all the experts for each proposal, but to derive points of agreement or disagreement and of indecision. Each expert then reviewed every guideline and rated it using a scale from 1 (complete disagreement) to 9 (complete agreement). The collective rating was done using a GRADE grid. To validate a guideline on a criterion, at least 50% of the experts had to be in broad agreement, while < 20% of them expressed the opposite opinion. For a guideline to be strong, at least 70% of the experts had to be in broad agreement. In the absence of strong agreement, the guidelines were reformulated and again rated, with a view to reaching a consensus.

Topics of the guidelines: summary of the results

Because of the specificity of emergency airway management (in emergency medicine or intensive care, and in particular in patients with cervicofacial trauma or burns), we did not include it in our literature analysis or in the guidelines. We shall, therefore, address tracheotomy only in the setting of planned tracheotomy in adults in intensive care.

Five topics were defined: indications and contraindications for tracheotomy in intensive care, tracheotomy techniques in intensive care, modalities of tracheotomy in intensive care, management of patients undergoing tracheotomy in intensive care, and decannulation in intensive care. An extensive search of the bibliography from recent years was performed using PubMed and the Cochrane database. To be selected for the analysis, articles had to be written in English or in French.

The summary made by the experts and the application of GRADE methodology led to the drawing up of 8 formal guidelines, 10 recommendations, and 3 treatment protocols. Among the 8 formal guidelines, 2 have a high level of proof (Grade 1+/−) and 6 a low level of proof (Grade 2+/−). For the 10 recommendations, GRADE methodology was not applicable and instead 10 expert opinions were produced. After 2 rounds of rating and various amendments, strong agreement was obtained for all the guidelines and protocols.

Indications and contraindications for tracheotomy in intensive care

R1.1 The experts suggest that tracheotomy be proposed in cases of prolonged weaning from mechanical ventilation and of acquired and potentially reversible neuromuscular disorder.

(Expert opinion)

Rationale The term neuromuscular refers to acquired and potentially reversible cerebrospinal, motor, and muscle disorders (e.g., Guillain–Barré syndrome, intensive care unit acquired muscle weakness, myasthenia, lupus myelitis). No study has provided formal evidence that tracheotomy improves the prognosis for survival of patients with these types of disorders. In this indication, no randomized study has evaluated the specific usefulness of early compared with late tracheotomy. Nevertheless, studies, often retrospective, suggest that late tracheotomy raises the risk of ventilator-associated pneumonia [20]. Tracheotomy can be proposed when weaning from mechanical ventilation is prolonged: weaning lasting more than 7 days after the first spontaneous breathing trial [21].

In the case of Guillain–Barré syndrome, tracheotomy should only be considered if weaning from invasive mechanical ventilation is not achieved after completion of immunotherapy (intravenous immunoglobulins or plasma exchange). At the end of immunotherapy, deficit in plantar flexion associated with sciatic nerve block was found to be an early predictor of prolonged (> 15 days) invasive mechanical ventilation in 100% of cases [22]. Alone, deficit in plantar flexion at the end of immunotherapy had a positive predictive value of 82% for prolonged mechanical ventilation.

R1.2 The experts suggest that the indication for tracheotomy in patients with chronic respiratory failure should be the subject of multidisciplinary discussion.

(Expert opinion)

Rationale The usefulness of intermittent mechanical ventilation in the management of patients with chronic respiratory failure is beyond the scope of these recommendations. When intermittent mechanical ventilation is indicated, a randomized study does not seem necessary before recommending first-line noninvasive ventilation rather than tracheotomy.

Life-threatening decompensation of chronic respiratory failure is generally managed in intensive care. In this setting, certain forms of chronic respiratory failure, notably those resulting from neurological disorders, can be managed using tracheotomy to enable mechanical ventilation and to simplify upper airway management. A 2016 meta-analysis including data from a randomized trial and 25 observational studies suggests that intermittent mechanical ventilation can improve the quality of life of patients with chronic respiratory failure [23]. The meta-analysis considered together patients receiving intermittent noninvasive mechanical ventilation and tracheotomized patients. More specifically, several studies have looked into the usefulness of tracheotomy in amyotrophic lateral sclerosis (ALS). In a 2011 study, an Italian team found that of 60 ALS patients who underwent tracheotomy, 44 (70%) left hospital completely dependent on mechanical ventilation, 17 (28%) were partially dependent, and a single patient was completely weaned from mechanical ventilation. At 1-year follow-up, 13 (22%) patients were still alive and had a quality of life deemed similar to that of ALS patients who did not have a tracheotomy [24].

In this type of situation, the patient and his or her family must be informed that tracheotomy does not alter the prognosis of the causal disease. The usefulness of tracheotomy in improving patient comfort and management following a stay in intensive care must be accurately evaluated, in particular with the patient and the medical team. Facilitation of upper airway management does not necessarily lead to improved comfort; tracheotomy can unduly prolong suffering associated with the underlying illness. In a context of chronic respiratory failure, these ethical considerations must be carefully thought through and discussed with the patient and his or her family before performing a tracheotomy.

R1.3 Tracheotomy in intensive care should not be performed before the fourth day of mechanical ventilation.

(GRADE 1+/STRONG agreement)

Rationale The question of the timing of tracheotomy in intensive care is hard to analyze, because: 1) it is necessary beforehand to demonstrate the usefulness of tracheotomy (independently of its timing) and 2) most studies comparing early and late tracheotomy include nontracheotomized patients in the "late" group.

Several good-quality prospective studies relate to "objective" criteria (mortality, incidence of ventilator-associated lung injury, duration of mechanical ventilation and of stay in intensive care). Early tracheotomy (in general before the fourth day of mechanical ventilation) is not associated with decreases in mortality, the incidence of ventilator-associated lung injury, or the duration of mechanical ventilation [8–11, 25, 26]. It does seem to reduce the consumption of hypnotic drugs. Improvement in comfort is not proven, and is insufficiently studied, but seems likely when tracheotomy is done early.

Lastly, early tracheotomy in burn patients with cervicofacial involvement and in patients with cervicofacial trauma more properly comes under the heading of emergency tracheotomy and is not within the scope of these guidelines.

R1.4 The experts suggest that tracheotomy (percutaneous or surgical) should not be performed in intensive care in situations at high risk of complications.

(Expert opinion)

Rationale The potentially serious complications are hemorrhage, hypoxemia, and neurological deterioration. Most studies have excluded patients at risk of these complications [6, 9, 10, 25]. Tracheotomy should not, therefore, be performed in intensive care in the following situations:

- Hemodynamic instability.
- Intracranial hypertension (intracranial pressure > 15 mmHg).
- Severe hypoxemia: $PaO_2/FiO_2 < 100$ mmHg, with positive expiratory pressure > 10 cmH_2O.
- Uncorrected bleeding disorders (platelets < 50 000/mm^3 and/or international normalized ratio > 1.5 and/or partial thromboplastin time > 2 normal).
- Refusal by the patient and/or family.
- Patient is dying or active treatment is being withdrawn.

Tracheotomy techniques in intensive care

R2.1 Percutaneous tracheotomy is the standard method in intensive care patients.

(GRADE 1+/STRONG agreement)

Rationale Several randomized studies have compared the impact of the technique of tracheotomy (percutaneous or surgical) on the incidence of complications (short-, medium-, and long-term), mortality, and cost

[27–36]. The great heterogeneity of endpoints (immediate or delayed, minor or major complications) complicates comparison of studies. To date, neither of the two techniques (percutaneous or surgical) has proven superior in terms of mortality or incidence of major complications (respiratory distress, hemorrhagic shock, tracheal stenosis) [37]. A 2014 meta-analysis including 14 randomized studies suggests that the percutaneous technique is associated with a shorter operative time and a decreased incidence of stoma infection and inflammation [37]. The incidence of other complications does not seem to differ between the two tracheotomy techniques [37]. These results, plus the spread and availability of this technique in intensive care units, mean that percutaneous tracheotomy should whenever possible be preferred to surgical technique.

Whatever the technique used, prior training is needed to perform tracheotomy, which must be done by physicians able to manage any complications or accidents quickly.

R2.2 The experts suggest that medical and surgical teams should discuss and decide upon the tracheotomy technique to be used when there is a risk of complications.

(Expert opinion)

Rationale Percutaneous tracheotomy can be made difficult, even impossible, by the patient's condition. For instance, an unstable cervical spine, an anterior cervical infection, a neck that has been treated (surgery or radiotherapy), difficulty in identifying anatomical landmarks (e.g., obesity, short neck, thyroid hypertrophy), or stiffness of the cervical spine are relative contraindications to percutaneous tracheotomy and prompt instead use of surgical tracheotomy [27]. It is nevertheless difficult to draw up formal guidelines. Indeed, at-risk situations are conventionally exclusion criteria for prospective studies. Observational studies have yielded contradictory results on which technique to prefer in cases of morbid obesity, spinal fracture, or a history of tracheotomy [35, 38–53]. A single randomized prospective study has compared surgical tracheotomy with modified percutaneous tracheotomy or so-called mini-surgical percutaneous dilatational tracheotomy (surgical tracheal access followed by a percutaneous procedure) in at-risk situations (anatomical difficulties, coagulation disorders, hypoxemia, hemodynamic instability). This study found no difference between the two techniques in terms of complications [52].

Such situations should therefore prompt discussions between the medical and surgical teams to decide on what benefit tracheotomy provides and which technique is the most suitable. Percutaneous tracheotomy in these situations can be envisioned by an experienced team with access to the technical means to improve the usual procedure: fiberoptic bronchoscopy, cervical Doppler ultrasound, surgical approach to the tracheal rings, tracheotomy equipment adapted to the anatomical problem (e.g., special tracheotomy kits for obese patients).

R2.3 Percutaneous dilatational tracheotomy should probably be preferred as the standard method in intensive care patients.

(GRADE 2+/STRONG agreement)

Rationale Several randomized studies have compared the six techniques of percutaneous tracheotomy: multiple dilator, guide wire dilating forceps, single dilator, rotating dilation, balloon dilation, and translaryngeal tracheotomy. These comparisons have in general been made two-by-two with as principal endpoints the duration of the procedure, failure rate defined by a switch to an alternative technique, the rate of major complications, and the rate of minor complications. These techniques are relatively equivalent, with the exception of translaryngeal tracheotomy, which seems to be associated with a higher rate of failure and of complications, notably major [54, 55]. The single dilator technique is associated with a lower failure rate than rotating dilation [56] and a lower rate of minor complications than balloon dilation or dilation with guide wire dilating forceps [57–59]. When the single dilator technique is compared with all the others, it seems to be associated with a higher success rate (corollary of its more widespread use) [60], but also with a higher rate of minor complications (notably minor bleeding and tracheal ring fractures) [60].

Conditions necessary for tracheotomy in intensive care

R3.1 Fiberoptic bronchoscopy should probably be performed before and during percutaneous tracheotomy.

(GRADE 2+/STRONG agreement)

Rationale Fiberoptic bronchoscopy before tracheotomy is advantageous because it helps locate the point of incision, by transillumination and palpation, and helps position the endotracheal tube correctly, below the vocal cords. Fibroscopy directly visualizes all stages of the procedure (incision, placement of the guide wire and of the dilator, dilation) and the position of the tracheotomy tube [61]. Fibroscopy must be available during the tracheotomy and the clinician must be trained.

Three nonrandomized studies seem to suggest that fiberoptic bronchoscopy could be nonsignificantly associated with more complications [62–64], but they are subject to substantial methodological bias and their results seem difficult to interpret.

A single randomized trial in 60 patients has shown that fiberoptic bronchoscopy is associated with a 47% (95% CI 23–64%) decrease in early complications of percutaneous tracheotomy in intensive care [65]. The main complications observed were accidental extubation, perforation of the cuff of the endotracheal tube, and hemorrhage. In addition, the number of incisions needed for tracheotomy was statistically smaller in the fiberoptic bronchoscopy group.

In summary, the only randomized study performed found that there are fewer complications of percutaneous tracheotomy when fiberoptic bronchoscopy is used.

R3.2 A laryngeal mask airway should probably not be used during percutaneous tracheotomy in intensive care.

(GRADE 2−/STRONG agreement)

Rationale Several randomized studies have compared two procedures for extubation of the endotracheal tube from the trachea while maintaining invasive mechanical ventilation: extubation followed by placement of a laryngeal mask airway or withdrawal of the endotracheal tube until the cuff is at the level of the vocal cords. A 2014 meta-analysis of 8 randomized controlled trials of the usefulness of placement of a laryngeal mask airway [66] showed that these trials examined four main outcomes: mortality (one study), the proportion of patients with one or more serious adverse events (seven studies), duration of the procedure (six studies), and failure of the procedure requiring a switch to any other procedure (seven studies). For each of these outcomes, the quality of the proof was considered low. Use of a laryngeal mask airway is not associated with decreases in mortality, complication rate, or failure related to the procedure, but does shorten the length of the procedure by an average of 1.46 (1.01–1.92) minutes. A single randomized controlled study conducted after this meta-analysis [67] found that more patients needed conversion to another procedure and had more clinically significant complications with a laryngeal mask airway.

R3.3 Cervical ultrasound should probably be performed with percutaneous tracheotomy in intensive care.

(GRADE 2+/Strong agreement)

Rationale Ultrasound visualizes the trachea and the tracheal rings, thus optimizing positioning of point of incision while avoiding injury to blood vessels and/or the thyroid [68]. Four open randomized studies in a total of 560 patients have tested the usefulness of Doppler ultrasound in preventing complications of percutaneous tracheotomy [69–72]. Of 275 patients who underwent ultrasound-guided localization before tracheotomy, 40 (14.5%) presented a complication during or after the procedure. In the absence of Doppler ultrasound, 74 (26%) of the 285 patients presented at least one complication during or after the procedure, i.e., a 44% (95% CI 21–60) decrease in the risk of complications. The risk of puncturing a blood vessel is reduced by localization beforehand. The success of the procedure at the first attempt is significantly greater with Doppler ultrasound: 94.9% (168/177) versus 90.4% (160/177). There is, however, great heterogeneity between these studies, as the randomization procedure is not always well described [70, 71] and the definition of complications is not uniform.

The strength of the recommendation (2 +) is related to the as-yet infrequent use of ultrasound with tracheotomy and to the quality of the randomized trials.

In conclusion, Doppler ultrasound increases the success rate of tracheotomy and reduces its immediate complications, provided the clinician masters the technique.

R3.4 The experts suggest that antibiotic prophylaxis should not be prescribed for tracheotomy.

(Expert opinion)

Rationale Because it opens the trachea, percutaneous tracheotomy can be considered as clean-contaminated surgery. The rate of infection of the operative site ranges between 0 and 33% depending on the study. Most studies comparing percutaneous tracheotomy and surgical tracheotomy indicate a higher rate of infection of the operative site for the surgical procedure. The infection rate for percutaneous tracheotomy is generally between 0 and 4%. In a retrospective study in 297 patients who underwent percutaneous tracheotomy, Hagiya et al. [73] reported a significantly lower rate of infection at the tracheotomy site in patients on antibiotic therapy: 2.36 versus 7.25% ($p = 0.002$). In contrast, there is no randomized study that has assessed the usefulness of antibiotic prophylaxis for tracheotomy. The quality of evidence is therefore very poor. The 2010 SFAR update concerning antibiotic prophylaxis in surgery and interventional medicine advises against antibiotic prophylaxis for

tracheotomy (whether surgical or percutaneous is not specified) [74].

R3.5 The experts suggest that a standardized procedure be implemented in intensive care units that perform percutaneous tracheotomy.

(Expert opinion)

Rationale Percutaneous tracheotomy in intensive care is an invasive procedure which can lead to potentially serious complications [75] and for which there are contraindications. The learning curve for percutaneous tracheotomy is on average more than 80 consecutive procedures by the same team and with the same technique [76]. In addition, rules should be observed to optimize safety [75]. Intensive care units should define a standard procedure for percutaneous tracheotomy, which could indicate the following points: medical and paramedical personnel required, necessary pre-surgery laboratory tests and radiography, equipment required for airway management, equipment needed for the procedure (notably, the role of Doppler ultrasound and fiberoptic bronchoscopy), position of the patient, method of ventilation, type of analgesia, ways of checking the position of the tracheotomy tube at the end of the procedure, and then the modalities for monitoring the intensive care patient following surgery (Figs. 1, 2).

Tracheotomy monitoring and maintenance in intensive care

R4.1 The experts suggest that intensive care units should have a tracheotomy management protocol.

(Expert opinion)

Rationale The numerous secondary complications of tracheotomy include skin infection, granuloma, secondary bleeding from the stoma, tracheal stenosis, tracheomalacia, and erosion of blood vessels (brachiocephalic vein, brachiocephalic artery) [15, 77, 78]. There is no prospective study comparing different kinds of local care, such as antisepsis, type of dressing, or way of securing. Prospective randomized studies comparing surgical and percutaneous techniques, and different types of percutaneous techniques, do not specify the protocol. Studies evaluating practices for tracheotomy follow-up in intensive care reveal large disparities, absence of formalization, and lack of guidelines for follow-up during or after intensive care [79, 80]. Use of a standard care protocol reduced local lesions [81]. Based on limited data or expert opinions, monitoring is recommended to ensure

Equipment and supplies required:

- o Bronchial endoscope (with video if possible).
- o Percutaneous tracheotomy kit.
- o Reintubation equipment.
- o Ultrasound machine (for departments with the expertise).
- o Monitoring (hemodynamic and ventilatory).
- o Coagulation tests (if findings abnormal, correction made).

- Personnel required:
  - o 2 physicians (1 for surgery + 1 for fiberoptic bronchoscopy).
  - o A least 1 paramedic to help perform the procedure.

- Preparation:
  - o Patient intubated and ventilated in volume controlled mode, with $FiO_2 = 1$.
  - o General anesthesia with neuromuscular block.
  - o Hyperextension of the head, using a pillow under the shoulders to extend the neck.
  - o Skin preparation of the surgical field.

- Conditions (key points):
  - o Location of the planned point of incision by palpation and transillumination (ultrasound can be an additional aid in departments with the expertise). The point of incision should ideally be between the 1st and 2nd tracheal rings.
  - o Visually guided withdrawal of the endotracheal tube and its immobilization below the glottis, with the cuff inflated.
  - o Compensation for loss of ventilation when needed, throughout the procedure if necessary.
  - o Direct visualization of tracheal puncture.
  - o Continuation of the procedure using the chosen technique under direct visualization.
  - o Placement of the tracheotomy tube under direct visualization.

- After cannulation:
  - o Connection of the tracheotomy tube to the ventilator and adjustment of ventilation.
  - o Maintenance and securing of the tracheotomy tube by a device adapted to the condition of the patient's skin.
  - o Endoscopic check that the tracheotomy tube is in the right position. Bronchial hygiene therapy if necessary.

Writing of a tracheotomy report.

Fig. 1 Proposal for a protocol associated with guideline 3.5 (Expert opinion)

that cuff pressure does not exceed 30 cmH$_2$O [77, 78, 82]. Too low a pressure could lead to inhalation of oropharyngeal secretions [15]. Increased cuff pressure favors ischemia of the tracheal mucosa, which is a source of tracheal stenosis. A check every 8 h is proposed.

Local infection and gastroesophageal reflux damage the cartilage of the tracheal rings, potentially leading to chondritis, tracheal stenosis, and tracheomalacia

[83]. By analogy with work done on endotracheal intubation, it is recommended to use tubes fitted with a suction catheter that opens above the cuff, for regular aspiration of retained secretions from the subglottic space.

Special attention should be paid to securing the tracheotomy tube, maintenance of a corrugated tube, and prevention of repeated local trauma caused by the moving and weight of the tubes (avoid pulling the tracheotomy

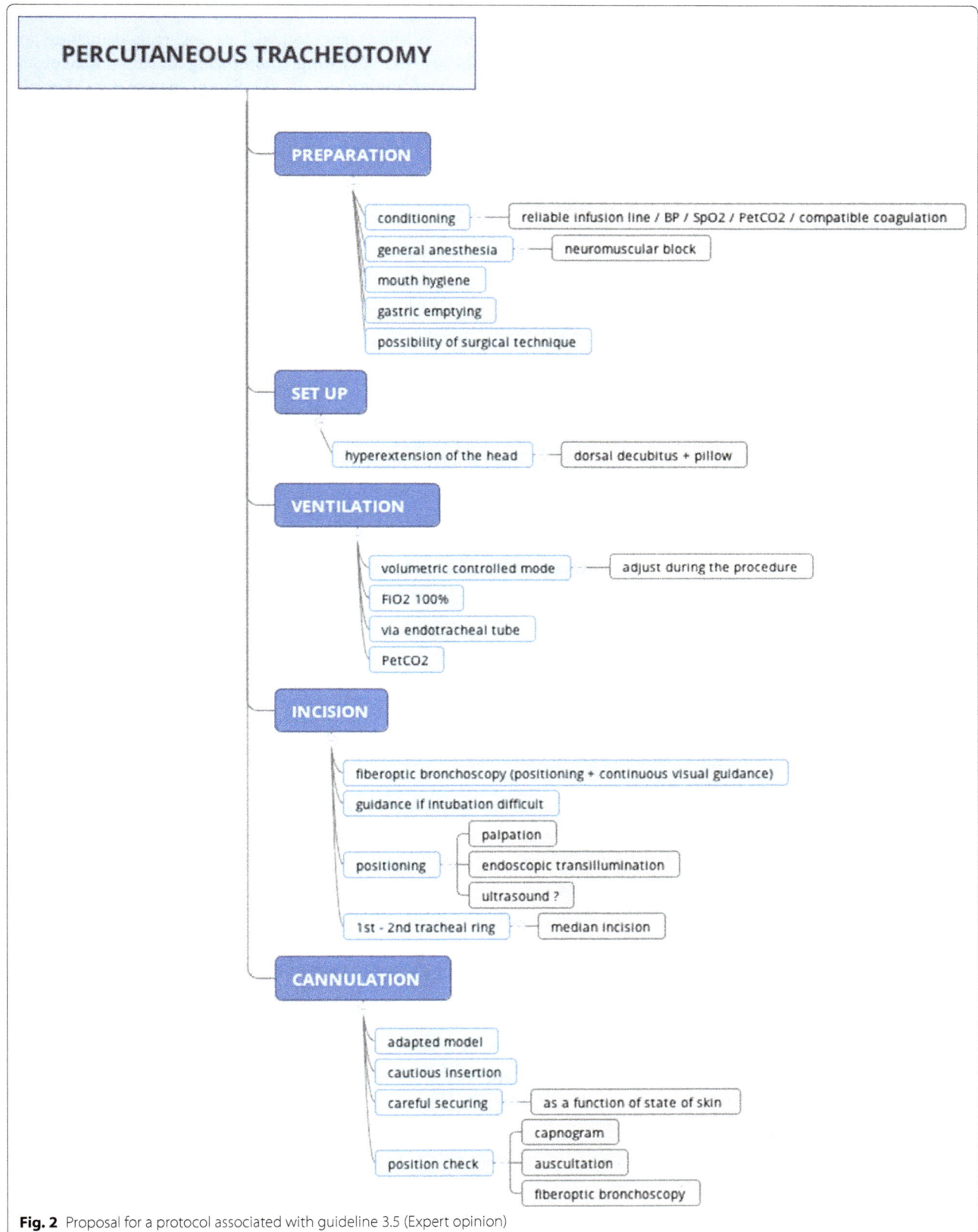

PERCUTANEOUS TRACHEOTOMY

PREPARATION
- conditioning — reliable infusion line / BP / SpO2 / PetCO2 / compatible coagulation
- general anesthesia — neuromuscular block
- mouth hygiene
- gastric emptying
- possibility of surgical technique

SET UP
- hyperextension of the head — dorsal decubitus + pillow

VENTILATION
- volumetric controlled mode — adjust during the procedure
- FIO2 100%
- via endotracheal tube
- PetCO2

INCISION
- fiberoptic bronchoscopy (positioning + continuous visual guidance)
- guidance if intubation difficult
- positioning
  - palpation
  - endoscopic transillumination
  - ultrasound ?
- 1st - 2nd tracheal ring — median incision

CANNULATION
- adapted model
- cautious insertion
- careful securing — as a function of state of skin
- position check
  - capnogram
  - auscultation
  - fiberoptic bronchoscopy

Fig. 2 Proposal for a protocol associated with guideline 3.5 (Expert opinion)

tube). There are no specific data on local care (antisepsis, products, frequency). A single study found no difference in bacterial contamination or local infection between the application of compresses or soft dressings [84]. Few studies specify the performance and type of local care (4–6 applications of isotonic saline, for example, in Lagambina et al.) [77, 85].

The experts consider it useful to check the position of the tracheotomy tube (chest X-ray, ease of tracheal suction, absence of dyspnea) and, if necessary, to use fiberoptic bronchoscopy to look for injury or stenosis, without specifying the frequency or timing.

To meet intensive care safety requirements, management of the tracheotomized patient should include and specify the following: monitoring of the tracheotomy stoma, monitoring of ventilation parameters, specific local care, care of the tracheotomy tube, nature and frequency of the care provided (Fig. 3).

R4.2 The experts recommend airway humidification in patients with a tracheotomy in intensive care.

Immediate post-tracheotomy care:

- Personnel trained in management of tracheotomy.
- Verification of the position (landmarks), with one end of the tracheotomy tube 4 to 6 cm from the carina in the tracheal lumen, securing of tube (skin sutures, ties, or Velcro), avoiding overly tight or loose fitting (movement limited to 1 finger width).
- Check airway access: easy trachea suction, monitoring of $PetCO_2$, peak pressure (comparison with pre-tracheotomy values), absence of subcutaneous emphysema in the cervical or thoracic region, verification of hemodynamic stability and of the absence of heart rhythm disorders, check the position of the tube (chest X-ray).
- Check the cuff pressure according to the guidelines applicable to airway access (P<30 cmH_2O ; 25-35 depending on the team).
- Have in the room or close at hand equipment for reintubation and tracheotomy, in case of early accidental dislodgement.

Care on days 0-4:

- Monitoring for hemorrhagic signs (apparent at scar site or on tracheal suction) every 3 hours postoperatively.
- Examination of the scar and checking for signs of local infection.
- Dressing changed with physiological saline 3 times every 24 hours (to avoid accumulation of secretions and moisture at the stoma).
- Tracheal suction according to usual practice (defined frequency or on request), but measuring the maximum depth (down to the carina, up one centimeter and note the distance).
- Airway humidification (heated humidifier, if necessary). Care of the inner cannula with cuffed tube.
- Raise the head by 30°, in the median position, and be careful to preserve the axis of the head and trunk during mobilization and changes of position.
- Check that the respirator tube is not pressing on the tracheotomy stoma.

Subsequent care:

- Change the fixation every day or more often if oozing (hemorrhage or pus).
- Check the scar every day.
- Cleansing with isotonic saline.

Fig. 3 Proposed care protocol associated with guideline 4.1 (Expert opinion)

(Expert opinion)

Rationale There are no data on airway humidification in patients with a tracheotomy in intensive care. Lack of airway humidification can lead to obstruction of the tracheotomy tube in patients who need oxygen therapy in intensive care [86]. The UK 2014 guidelines suggest that humidification be envisioned for all patients undergoing tracheotomy. Airway humidification should be adapted in particular to the ventilatory support and to the amount of bronchial secretion [86].

No study has determined which airway humidification technique should be preferred in mechanically ventilated patients undergoing tracheotomy in intensive care. Only two studies have evaluated the effect on the incidence of ventilator-associated lung injury of different humidification systems (heated humidifiers or heat and moisture exchangers) in patients undergoing tracheotomy. Their results are discordant. The first study of 185 patients in each group and only 11 tracheotomized patients [87] found no benefit of airway humidification with any particular system. The second study, in a comparison of only 15 and 16 tracheotomized patients, showed a significant decrease in the incidence of ventilator-associated lung injury in the group with a heated humidifier [88].

R4.3 The experts suggest that tracheotomy tubes should not be routinely changed in intensive care.

(Expert opinion)

Rationale No literature study has examined the frequency of tracheotomy tube changes and the incidence of lung disease. A single prospective study in a long-stay hospital for ventilated patients with a tracheotomy showed a reduction in the incidence of granulation tissue when tubes were changed every two weeks [89]. A non-randomized prospective study in a center for mechanical ventilation weaning showed that a change of tracheotomy tubes before the seventh day after tracheotomy was associated with faster resumption of nutrition and speech. The authors ascribed this effect to a reduction in tracheotomy tube size [90]. They reported no complication associated with the change of tracheotomy tube.

In intensive care, in a practice survey in the USA, 80% of tracheotomy tubes were changed routinely, but with substantial variability [91]. A Dutch practice survey observed that 60% of departments never change the tracheotomy tube [92].

The guidelines of the Belgian Society of Pneumology and the Belgian Association for Cardiothoracic Surgery [15] propose tracheotomy tube changes only if there is a specific indication. The British Intensive Care Society [86] advocates changing a tracheotomy tube without an inner cannula every 7–14 days and a tracheotomy tube with an inner cannula every 30 days. Tube change should be performed no less than 4 days after surgical tracheotomy, and 7–10 days after percutaneous tracheotomy. Subsequently, the frequency of tube change must be adapted to the individual patient's condition [86].

The European Directive [93] advocates changing medical devices every 30 days. One study shows a structural alteration of the wall of 58% of tracheotomy tubes after 30 days of use [94]. A tracheotomy tube change early in intensive care is associated with risks (tube displacement and respiratory arrest) [15].

In summary, tracheotomy tube change must be guided by clinical considerations and should be envisaged, in particular, in cases of suspected local infection, bleeding, or to reduce the caliber of the tracheotomy tube and to facilitate the patient's speech.

Tracheotomy decannulation

R5.1 The experts suggest that a multidisciplinary decannulation protocol should be available in intensive care units.

(Expert opinion)

R5.2 The tracheotomy tube cuff should probably be deflated when the patient is breathing spontaneously.

(GRADE 2+/STRONG agreement)

Rationale Numerous observational and before/after studies conclude that use of a weaning protocol shortens weaning time and reduces the decannulation failure rate and the complication rate [95–104]. In a controlled, randomized, single-center trial in 195 patients, cuff deflation once the patient was disconnected from the ventilator reduced failure of decannulation, shortened weaning from mechanical ventilation, and decreased tracheostomy-related complications [105].

This consensual multidisciplinary protocol, which was written and is applied routinely by all members of the intensive care team who use tracheotomy, should at least define the following (Fig. 4): prior neurological

Prerequisite:

Weaning from mechanical ventilation 24/24 hours in cases of previous neurological disease.

Conditions of examination:

- Cuff deflated.
- Prior aspiration of secretions.
- Seated position >70°.
- No anesthesia so as not to generate swallowing difficulties.
- Nasal endoscopy to the cuff.

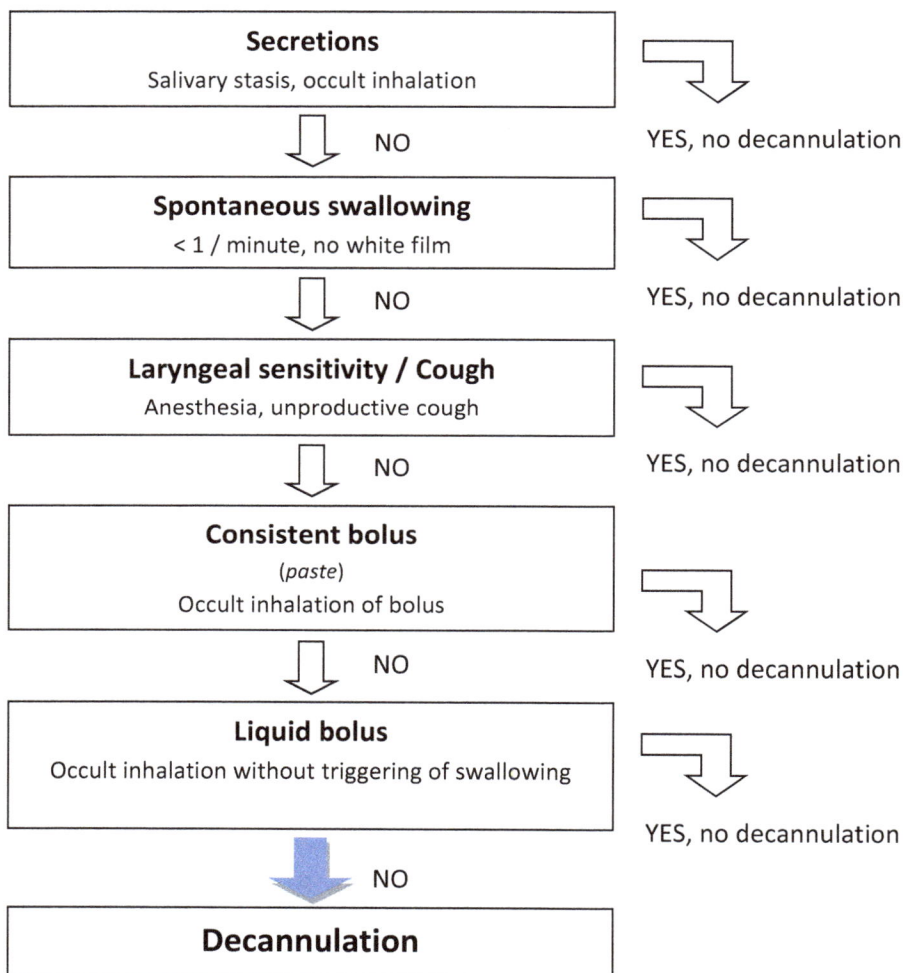

Secretions Salivary stasis, occult inhalation

⬇ NO → YES, no decannulation

Spontaneous swallowing < 1 / minute, no white film

⬇ NO → YES, no decannulation

Laryngeal sensitivity / Cough Anesthesia, unproductive cough

⬇ NO → YES, no decannulation

Consistent bolus (*paste*) Occult inhalation of bolus

⬇ NO → YES, no decannulation

Liquid bolus Occult inhalation without triggering of swallowing

⬇ NO → YES, no decannulation

Decannulation

Fig. 4 Proposed endoscopic protocol associated with guideline 5.1 (Expert opinion): *(according to Warnecke et al. Crit Care Med 2013 (106))*

examination and pharyngolaryngeal examinations, medical and paramedical personnel involved in decannulation, equipment needed for decannulation, immediate and subsequent monitoring of decannulation, and type and location of equipment required in cases of respiratory distress following decannulation.

R5.3 A pharyngolaryngeal examination should probably be performed at or following decannulation.

(GRADE 2+/STRONG agreement)

Rationale Few prospective controlled studies consider the pharyngolaryngeal examination required during or following decannulation of intensive care patients or whether or not routine fiberoptic bronchoscopy is needed. A prospective observational study by practitioners blinded to each other's decisions [106] shows the benefit of routine laryngotracheal endoscopy by the intensivist at decannulation, in comparison with routine clinical assessment of swallowing, possibly completed by the Evans blue dye test. Among the 100 neurological patients in the cohort, endoscopic evaluation allowed successful decannulation in 27 patients for whom clinical assessment had predicted failure of weaning. The recannulation rate was 1.9%. Pharyngolaryngeal examination on decannulation comprises sequential assessments of salivary stasis and silent inhalation, spontaneous swallowing, and laryngeal sensitivity, before considering a swallowing test using paste and then liquid. No patient who passed these three assessments had difficulty swallowing in the tests with paste and liquid.

Other prospective, observational, but noncomparative studies confirm [107, 108]: 1) a higher incidence of swallowing dysfunction in tracheotomized patients ventilated for a prolonged period; 2) a longer intensive care stay and increased risk of inhalation and of pharyngolaryngeal lesions when tracheotomy is prolonged or decannulation is delayed.

This article is being published jointly in Anaesthesia Critical Care & Pain Medicine and Annals of Intensive Care. The manuscript validated by the board of the SRLF (12/13/2016) and the SFAR (12/15/2016).

Abbreviations
ALS: amyotrophic lateral sclerosis; GRADE: Grading of Recommendations Assessment, Development, and Evaluation; PICO: Patient Intervention Comparison Outcome; SFAR: Société Francaise d'Anesthésie Réanimation; SFMU: Société Française de Médecine d'Urgence; SFORL: Société Française d'Otorhinolaryngologie; SRLF: Société de Réanimation de Langue Française.

Authors' contributions
JLT and OC proposed the elaboration of this recommendation and manuscript in agreement with the "Société de Réanimation de Langue Française" and "Société Française d'Anesthésie et de Réanimation"; JA and MG wrote the methodology section and gave the final version with the final presentation. FB, FB, EC, J-L D, FJ contributed to elaborate recommendations and write the rationale of "Indications and contraindications for tracheotomy in intensive care." AD and FJ contributed to elaborate recommendations and to write the rationale of "Tracheotomy techniques in intensive care." CEL, YM, P-GG, FR contributed to elaborate recommendations and to write the rationale of Conditions necessary for tracheotomy in intensive care. GC, HQ, JM contributed to elaborate recommendations and to write the rationale of "Tracheotomy monitoring and maintenance in intensive care." J-MC, EL, SV contributed to elaborate recommendations and to write the rationale of "Tracheotomy decannulation." All authors provide references. JLT, OC, JA and MG drafted the manuscript. All authors read and approved the final manuscript.

Author details
[1] Service de Réanimation, Groupe Hospitalier Pitié-Salpêtrière, Assistance Publique-Hôpitaux de Paris, Paris, France. [2] Hôpitaux Universitaires de Strasbourg, Nouvel Hôpital Civil, Pôle d'Anesthésie-Réanimation Chirurgicale, SAMU, SMUR, NHC, 1 Place de l'Hôpital, 67000 Strasbourg, France. [3] EA 3072, FMTS, Université de Strasbourg, Strasbourg, France. [4] Intensive Care Unit and Department of Anesthesiology, Research Unit INSERM U1046, University of Montpellier Saint Eloi Hospital and Montpellier School of Medicine, Montpellier, France. [5] Medical-Surgical Intensive Care Unit, Gustave Roussy Cancer Campus, Villejuif, France. [6] CHRU Besançon 25000, EA3920 Université de Franche-Comté, Besançon, France. [7] Australian and New Zealand Intensive Care Research Centre, Department of Epidemiology and Preventive Medicine, Monash University, Clayton, Australia. [8] SAMU de Lyon and Department of Emergency Medicine, Hospices Civils de Lyon, Edouard Herriot Hospital, Lyon, France. [9] Lyon Sud School of Medicine, University Lyon 1, Oullins, France. [10] Department of Preoperative Medicine, University Hospital of Clermont-Ferrand, Clermont-Ferrand, France. [11] R2D2, EA-7281, Auvergne University, Clermont-Ferrand, France. [12] INSERM, UMRS1158 Neurophysiologie Respiratoire Expérimentale et Clinique; AP-HP, Groupe Hospitalier Pitié-Salpêtrière Charles Foix, Service de Pneumologie et Réanimation Médicale du Département R3S, Sorbonne Université, Paris, France. [13] Medical ICU, AP-HP, Georges Pompidou European Hospital, Paris, France. [14] INSERM UMR-S1140, Paris Descartes University and Sorbonne Paris Cité, Paris, France. [15] Anaesthesiology and Critical Care Department, Amiens University Hospital, Place Victor Pauchet, 80054 Amiens, France. [16] INSERM U1088, Jules Verne University of Picardy, 80054 Amiens, France. [17] Service ORL et Chirurgie Cervico-maxillo-Faciale, CHU PONTCHAILLOU, Rue H. Le Guilloux, 35033 Rennes Cedex 9, France. [18] CeSim/LaTIM INSERM UMR 1101, Université de Bretagne Occidentale, Rue Camille Desmoulins, 29200 Brest Cedex, France. [19] Médecine Intensive et Réanimation, CHRU de Brest, Boulevard Tanguy Prigent, 29200 Brest Cedex, France. [20] UPMC Université Paris 06, INSERM, UMRS-1166, ICAN Institute of Cardiometabolism and Nutrition, Sorbonne Universités, Paris, France. [21] Department of Anesthesia and Intensive Care, Amiens-Picardie University Hospital, Amiens, France. [22] Réanimation médico chirurgicale Hôpital Pasteur 2 CHU de Nice, 30 voie romaine, 06000 Nice, France. [23] CNRS UMR 7275, IPMC Sophia Antipolis, Valbonne, France. [24] Centre des brûlés, Centre Hospitalier St Joseph et St Luc, 20 quai Claude Bernard, 69007 Lyon, France. [25] ORL Chirurgie Cervicofaciale, CHU Toulouse Rangueil-Larrey, 24 chemin de Pouvourville, 31059 Toulouse Cedex 9, France. [26] Département d'Anesthésie et de Réanimation Chirurgicale, Institut de Cardiologie, Groupe Hospitalier Pitié-Salpêtrière, 47-83 Boulevard de l'Hôpital, 75013 Paris, France. [27] Hôpitaux Universitaires de Strasbourg, Hôpital de Hautepierre, Réanimation Médicale, Avenue Molière, 67200 Strasbourg, France.

Acknowledgements
Not applicable.

Competing interests
The authors declare that they have no competing interests.

Funding
This work was financially supported by the Société de Réanimation de Langue Française (SRLF) and the Société Française d'Anesthésie et de Réanimation (SFAR).

References
 1. Blot F, Melot C. Commission d'Epidémiologie et de Recherche Clinique. Indications, timing, and techniques of tracheostomy in 152 French ICUs. Chest. 2005;127(4):1347–52.
 2. Freeman BD, Kennedy C, Coopersmith CM, Buchman TG. Examination of non-clinical factors affecting tracheostomy practice in an academic surgical intensive care unit. Crit Care Med. 2009;37(12):3070–8.
 3. Freeman BD, Morris PE. Tracheostomy practice in adults with acute respiratory failure. Crit Care Med. 2012;40(10):2890–6.
 4. Banfi P, Robert D. Early tracheostomy or prolonged translaryngeal intubation in the ICU: a long running story. Respir Care. 2013;58(11):1995–6.
 5. Durbin CG. Tracheostomy: why, when, and how? Respir Care. 2010;55(8):1056–68.
 6. Rumbak MJ, Newton M, Truncale T, Schwartz SW, Adams JW, Hazard PB. A prospective, randomized, study comparing early percutaneous dilational tracheotomy to prolonged translaryngeal intubation (delayed tracheotomy) in critically ill medical patients. Crit Care Med. 2004;32(8):1689–94.
 7. Hyde GA, Savage SA, Zarzaur BL, Hart-Hyde JE, Schaefer CB, Croce MA, et al. Early tracheostomy in trauma patients saves time and money. Injury. 2015;46(1):110–4.
 8. Blot F, Similowski T, Trouillet J-L, Chardon P, Korach J-M, Costa M-A, et al. Early tracheotomy versus prolonged endotracheal intubation in unselected severely ill ICU patients. Intensive Care Med. 2008;34(10):1779–87.
 9. Terragni PP, Antonelli M, Fumagalli R, Faggiano C, Berardino M, Pallavicini FB, et al. Early vs late tracheotomy for prevention of pneumonia in mechanically ventilated adult ICU patients: a randomized controlled trial. JAMA. 2010;303(15):1483–9.
10. Trouillet J-L, Luyt C-E, Guiguet M, Ouattara A, Vaissier E, Makri R, et al. Early percutaneous tracheotomy versus prolonged intubation of mechanically ventilated patients after cardiac surgery: a randomized trial. Ann Intern Med. 2011;154(6):373–83.
11. Young D, Harrison DA, Cuthbertson BH, Rowan K, TracMan Collaborators. Effect of early vs late tracheostomy placement on survival in patients receiving mechanical ventilation: the TracMan randomized trial. JAMA. 2013;309(20):2121–9.
12. Figueroa-Casas JB, Connery SM, Montoya R, Dwivedi AK, Lee S. Accuracy of early prediction of duration of mechanical ventilation by intensivists. Ann Am Thorac Soc. 2014;11(2):182–5.
13. Thille AW, Boissier F, Ben Ghezala H, Razazi K, Mekontso-Dessap A, Brun-Buisson C. Risk factors for and prediction by caregivers of extubation failure in ICU patients: a prospective study. Crit Care Med. 2015;43(3):613–20.
14. Chastre J, Bedock B, Clair B, Gehanno P, Lacaze T, Lesieur O, et al. Quel abord trachéal pour la ventilation mécanique des malades de réanimation? (à l'exclusion du nouveau-né) 18e Conférence de Consensus en Réanimation et Médecine d'Urgence. Réanim Urgences. 1998;7:435–42.
15. De Leyn P, Bedert L, Delcroix M, Depuydt P, Lauwers G, Sokolov Y, et al. Tracheotomy: clinical review and guidelines. Eur J Cardio-Thorac Surg Off J Eur Assoc Cardio-Thorac Surg. 2007;32(3):412–21.
16. Madsen KR, Guldager H, Rewers M, Weber S-O, Købke-Jacobsen K, Jensen R, et al. Guidelines for Percutaneous Dilatational Tracheostomy (PDT) from the Danish Society of Intensive Care Medicine (DSIT) and the Danish Society of Anesthesiology and Intensive Care Medicine (DASAIM). Dan Med Bull. 2011;58(12):C4358.
17. Siempos II, Ntaidou TK, Filippidis FT, Choi AMK. Effect of early versus late or no tracheostomy on mortality and pneumonia of critically ill patients receiving mechanical ventilation: a systematic review and meta-analysis. Lancet Respir Med. 2015;3(2):150–8.
18. Brass P, Hellmich M, Ladra A, Ladra J, Wrzosek A. Percutaneous techniques versus surgical techniques for tracheostomy. Cochrane Database Syst Rev. 2016;7:CD008045.
19. Andriolo BNG, Andriolo RB, Saconato H, Atallah ÁN, Valente O. Early versus late tracheostomy for critically ill patients. Cochrane Database Syst Rev. 2015;1:CD007271.
20. Ali MI, Fernández-Pérez ER, Pendem S, Brown DR, Wijdicks EFM, Gajic O. Mechanical ventilation in patients with Guillain-Barré syndrome. Respir Care. 2006;51(12):1403–7.
21. Béduneau G, Pham T, Schortgen F, Piquilloud L, Zogheib E, Jonas M, et al. Epidemiology of weaning outcome according to a new definition. the WIND study. Am J Respir Crit Care Med. 2017;195(6):772–83.
22. Fourrier F, Robriquet L, Hurtevent J-F, Spagnolo S. A simple functional marker to predict the need for prolonged mechanical ventilation in patients with Guillain-Barré syndrome. Crit Care. 2011;15(1):R65.
23. MacIntyre EJ, Asadi L, Mckim DA, Bagshaw SM. Clinical outcomes associated with home mechanical ventilation: a systematic review. Can Respir J. 2016;2016:6547180.
24. Vianello A, Arcaro G, Palmieri A, Ermani M, Braccioni F, Gallan F, et al. Survival and quality of life after tracheostomy for acute respiratory failure in patients with amyotrophic lateral sclerosis. J Crit Care. 2011;26(3):329.e7-14.
25. Diaz-Prieto A, Mateu A, Gorriz M, Ortiga B, Truchero C, Sampietro N, et al. A randomized clinical trial for the timing of tracheotomy in critically ill patients: factors precluding inclusion in a single center study. Crit Care. 2014;18(5):585.
26. Rodriguez JL, Steinberg SM, Luchetti FA, Gibbons KJ, Taheri PA, Flint LM. Early tracheostomy for primary airway management in the surgical critical care setting. Surgery. 1990;108(4):655–9.
27. Antonelli M, Michetti V, Di Palma A, Conti G, Pennisi MA, Arcangeli A, et al. Percutaneous translaryngeal versus surgical tracheostomy: a randomized trial with 1-yr double-blind follow-up. Crit Care Med. 2005;33(5):1015–20.
28. Freeman BD, Isabella K, Cobb JP, Boyle WA, Schmieg RE, Kolleff MH, et al. A prospective, randomized study comparing percutaneous with surgical tracheostomy in critically ill patients. Crit Care Med. 2001;29(5):926–30.
29. Friedman Y, Fildes J, Mizock B, Samuel J, Patel S, Appavu S, et al. Comparison of percutaneous and surgical tracheostomies. Chest. 1996;110(2):480–5.
30. Gysin C, Dulguerov P, Guyot JP, Perneger TV, Abajo B, Chevrolet JC. Percutaneous versus surgical tracheostomy: a double-blind randomized trial. Ann Surg. 1999;230(5):708–14.
31. Heikkinen M, Aarnio P, Hannukainen J. Percutaneous dilational tracheostomy or conventional surgical tracheostomy? Crit Care Med. 2000;28(5):1399–402.
32. Holdgaard HO, Pedersen J, Jensen RH, Outzen KE, Midtgaard T, Johansen LV, et al. Percutaneous dilatational tracheostomy versus conventional surgical tracheostomy. A clinical randomised study. Acta Anaesthesiol Scand. 1998;42(5):545–50.
33. Melloni G, Muttini S, Gallioli G, Carretta A, Cozzi S, Gemma M, et al. Surgical tracheostomy versus percutaneous dilatational tracheostomy. A prospective-randomized study with long-term follow-up. J Cardiovasc Surg (Torino). 2002;43(1):113–21.
34. Silvester W, Goldsmith D, Uchino S, Bellomo R, Knight S, Seevanayagam S, et al. Percutaneous versus surgical tracheostomy: a randomized controlled study with long-term follow-up. Crit Care Med. 2006;34(8):2145–52.
35. Tabaee A, Geng E, Lin J, Kakoullis S, McDonald B, Rodriguez H, et al. Impact of neck length on the safety of percutaneous and surgical tracheotomy: a prospective, randomized study. The Laryngoscope. 2005;115(9):1685–90.
36. Sustić A, Krstulović B, Eskinja N, Zelić M, Ledić D, Turina D. Surgical tracheostomy versus percutaneous dilational tracheostomy in

patients with anterior cervical spine fixation: preliminary report. Spine. 2002;27(17):1942–5 **(discussion 1945)**.

37. Putensen C, Theuerkauf N, Guenther U, Vargas M, Pelosi P. Percutaneous and surgical tracheostomy in critically ill adult patients: a meta-analysis. Crit Care Lond Engl. 2014;18(6):544.

38. Blankenship DR, Gourin CG, Davis WB, Blanchard AR, Seybt MW, Terris DJ. Percutaneous tracheostomy: don't beat them, join them. The Laryngoscope. 2004;114(9):1517–21.

39. Blankenship DR, Kulbersh BD, Gourin CG, Blanchard AR, Terris DJ. High-risk tracheostomy: exploring the limits of the percutaneous tracheostomy. The Laryngoscope. 2005;115(6):987–9.

40. Deppe A-C, Kuhn E, Scherner M, Slottosch I, Liakopoulos O, Langebartels G, et al. Coagulation disorders do not increase the risk for bleeding during percutaneous dilatational tracheotomy. Thorac Cardiovasc Surg. 2013;61(3):234–9.

41. Kluge S, Baumann HJ, Nierhaus A, Kröger N, Meyer A, Kreymann G. Safety of percutaneous dilational tracheotomy in hematopoietic stem cell transplantation recipients requiring long-term mechanical ventilation. J Crit Care. 2008;23(3):394–8.

42. Kluge S, Meyer A, Kühnelt P, Baumann HJ, Kreymann G. Percutaneous tracheostomy is safe in patients with severe thrombocytopenia. Chest. 2004;126(2):547–51.

43. Pandian V, Gilstrap DL, Mirski MA, Haut ER, Haider AH, Efron DT, et al. Predictors of short-term mortality in patients undergoing percutaneous dilatational tracheostomy. J Crit Care. 2012;27(4):420.e9-15.

44. Pandian V, Vaswani RS, Mirski MA, Haut E, Gupta S, Bhatti NI. Safety of percutaneous dilational tracheostomy in coagulopathic patients. Ear Nose Throat J. 2010;89(8):387–95.

45. Byhahn C, Lischke V, Meininger D, Halbig S, Westphal K. Peri-operative complications during percutaneous tracheostomy in obese patients. Anaesthesia. 2005;60(1):12–5.

46. Kost KM. Endoscopic percutaneous dilatational tracheotomy: a prospective evaluation of 500 consecutive cases. The Laryngoscope. 2005;115(10 Pt 2):1–30.

47. Ben Nun A, Altman E, Best LA. Extended indications for percutaneous tracheostomy. Ann Thorac Surg. 2005;80(4):1276–9.

48. Ben Nun A, Orlovsky M, Best LA. Percutaneous tracheostomy in patients with cervical spine fractures–feasible and safe. Interact CardioVasc Thorac Surg. 2006;5(4):427–9.

49. Muhammad JK, Major E, Patton DW. Evaluating the neck for percutaneous dilatational tracheostomy. J Cranio-Maxillofac Surg. 2000;28(6):336–42.

50. Muhammad JK, Major E, Wood A, Patton DW. Percutaneous dilatational tracheostomy: haemorrhagic complications and the vascular anatomy of the anterior neck. A review based on 497 cases. Int J Oral Maxillofac Surg. 2000;29(3):217–22.

51. Mayberry JC, Wu IC, Goldman RK, Chesnut RM. Cervical spine clearance and neck extension during percutaneous tracheostomy in trauma patients. Crit Care Med. 2000;28(10):3436–40.

52. Hashemian SM-R, Digaleh H, Massih Daneshvari Hospital Group. A prospective randomized study comparing mini-surgical percutaneous dilatational tracheostomy with surgical and classical percutaneous tracheostomy: a new method beyond contraindications. Medicine (Baltimore). 2015;94(47):e2015.

53. Higgins KM, Punthakee X. Meta-analysis comparison of open versus percutaneous tracheostomy. The Laryngoscope. 2007;117(3):447–54.

54. Cabrini L, Landoni G, Greco M, Costagliola R, Monti G, Colombo S, et al. Single dilator vs. guide wire dilating forceps tracheostomy: a meta-analysis of randomised trials. Acta Anaesthesiol Scand. 2014;58(2):135–42.

55. Cantais E, Kaiser E, Le-Goff Y, Palmier B. Percutaneous tracheostomy: prospective comparison of the translaryngeal technique versus the forceps-dilational technique in 100 critically ill adults. Crit Care Med. 2002;30(4):815–9.

56. Byhahn C, Westphal K, Meininger D, Gürke B, Kessler P, Lischke V. Single-dilator percutaneous tracheostomy: a comparison of PercuTwist and Ciaglia Blue Rhino techniques. Intensive Care Med. 2002;28(9):1262–6.

57. Cianchi G, Zagli G, Bonizzoli M, Batacchi S, Cammelli R, Biondi S, et al. Comparison between single-step and balloon dilatational

tracheostomy in intensive care unit: a single-centre, randomized controlled study. Br J Anaesth. 2010;104(6):728–32.

58. Ambesh SP, Pandey CK, Srivastava S, Agarwal A, Singh DK. Percutaneous tracheostomy with single dilatation technique: a prospective, randomized comparison of Ciaglia Blue Rhino versus Griggs' guidewire dilating forceps. Anesth Analg. 2002;95(6):1739–45.

59. Añón JM, Escuela MP, Gómez V, Moreno A, López J, Díaz R, et al. Percutaneous tracheostomy: Ciaglia Blue Rhino versus Griggs' guide wire dilating forceps. A prospective randomized trial. Acta Anaesthesiol Scand. 2004;48(4):451–6.

60. Sanabria A. Which percutaneous tracheostomy method is better? A systematic review. Respir Care. 2014;59(11):1660–70.

61. Terragni P, Faggiano C, Martin EL, Ranieri VM. Tracheostomy in mechanical ventilation. Semin Respir Crit Care Med. 2014;35(4):482–91.

62. Abdulla S, Conrad A, Vielhaber S, Eckhardt R, Abdulla W. Should a percutaneous dilational tracheostomy be guided with a bronchoscope? B-ENT. 2013;9(3):227–34.

63. Jackson LSM, Davis JW, Kaups KL, Sue LP, Wolfe MM, Bilello JF, et al. Percutaneous tracheostomy: to bronch or not to bronch—that is the question. J Trauma. 2011;71(6):1553–6.

64. Berrouschot J, Oeken J, Steiniger L, Schneider D. Perioperative complications of percutaneous dilational tracheostomy. The Laryngoscope. 1997;107(11 Pt 1):1538–44.

65. Saritas A, Saritas PU, Kurnaz MM, Beyaz SG, Ergonenc T. The role of fiberoptic bronchoscopy monitoring during percutaneous dilatational tracheostomy and its routine use into tracheotomy practice. JPMA J Pak Med Assoc. 2016;66(1):83–9.

66. Strametz R, Pachler C, Kramer JF, Byhahn C, Siebenhofer A, Weberschock T. Laryngeal mask airway versus endotracheal tube for percutaneous dilatational tracheostomy in critically ill adult patients. Cochrane Database Syst Rev. 2014;(6):CD009901. https://doi.org/10.1002/14651858. CD009901.pub2.

67. Price GC, McLellan S, Paterson RL, Hay A. A prospective randomised controlled trial of the LMA Supreme vs cuffed tracheal tube as the airway device during percutaneous tracheostomy. Anaesthesia. 2014;69(7):757–63.

68. Alansari M, Alotair H, Al Aseri Z, Elhoseny MA. Use of ultrasound guidance to improve the safety of percutaneous dilatational tracheostomy: a literature review. Crit Care. 2015;19:229.

69. Rudas M, Seppelt I, Herkes R, Hislop R, Rajbhandari D, Weisbrodt L. Traditional landmark versus ultrasound guided tracheal puncture during percutaneous dilatational tracheostomy in adult intensive care patients: a randomised controlled trial. Crit Care. 2014;18(5):514.

70. Yavuz A, Yılmaz M, Göya C, Alimoglu E, Kabaalioglu A. Advantages of US in percutaneous dilatational tracheostomy: randomized controlled trial and review of the literature. Radiology. 2014;273(3):927–36.

71. Ravi PR, Vijay MN. Real time ultrasound-guided percutaneous tracheostomy: is it a better option than bronchoscopic guided percutaneous tracheostomy? Med J Armed Forces India. 2015;71(2):158–64.

72. Gobatto ALN, Besen BAMP, Tierno PFGMM, Mendes PV, Cadamuro F, Joelsons D, et al. Ultrasound-guided percutaneous dilational tracheostomy versus bronchoscopy-guided percutaneous dilational tracheostomy in critically ill patients (TRACHUS): a randomized noninferiority controlled trial. Intensive Care Med. 2016;42(3):342–51.

73. Hagiya H, Naito H, Hagioka S, Okahara S, Morimoto N, Kusano N, et al. Effects of antibiotics administration on the incidence of wound infection in percutaneous dilatational tracheostomy. Acta Med Okayama. 2014;68(2):57–62.

74. Société française d'anesthésie et de réanimation. Antibioprophylaxie en chirurgie et médecine interventionnelle (patients adultes). Actualisation 2010. Ann Fr Anesth Réanim. 2011;30(2):168–90.

75. Ravat F, Pommier C, Dorne R. Percutaneous tracheostomy. Ann Francaises Anesth Réanim. 2001;20(3):260–81.

76. Massick DD, Powell DM, Price PD, Chang SL, Squires G, Forrest LA, et al. Quantification of the learning curve for percutaneous dilatational tracheotomy. The Laryngoscope. 2000;110(2 Pt 1):222–8.

77. Lagambina S, Nuccio P, Weinhouse GL. Tracheostomy care: a clinician's guide. Hosp Pract. 2011;39(3):161–7.

78. Cipriano A, Mao ML, Hon HH, Vazquez D, Stawicki SP, Sharpe RP, et al. An overview of complications associated with open and percutaneous tracheostomy procedures. Int J Crit Illn Inj Sci. 2015;5(3):179–88.

79. Mondrup F, Skjelsager K, Madsen KR. Inadequate follow-up after tracheostomy and intensive care. Dan Med J. 2012;59(8):A4481.

80. Vargas M, Sutherasan Y, Antonelli M, Brunetti I, Corcione A, Laffey JG, et al. Tracheostomy procedures in the intensive care unit: an international survey. Crit Care. 2015;19:291.

81. Lippert D, Hoffman MR, Dang P, McMurray JS, Heatley D, Kille T. Care of pediatric tracheostomy in the immediate postoperative period and timing of first tube change. Int J Pediatr Otorhinolaryngol. 2014;78(12):2281–5.

82. Leigh JM, Maynard JP. Pressure on the tracheal mucosa from cuffed tubes. Br Med J. 1979;1(6172):1173–4.

83. Sasaki CT, Horiuchi M, Koss N. Tracheostomy-related subglottic stenosis: bacteriologic pathogenesis. The Laryngoscope. 1979;89(6 Pt 1):857–65.

84. Ahmadinegad M, Lashkarizadeh MR, Ghahreman M, Shabani M, Mokhtare M, Ahmadipour M. Efficacy of dressing with absorbent foam versus dressing with gauze in prevention of tracheostomy site infection. Tanaffos. 2014;13(2):13–9.

85. Morris LL, Whitmer A, McIntosh E. Tracheostomy care and complications in the intensive care unit. Crit Care Nurse. 2013;33(5):18–30.

86. Bodenham A, Bell D, Bonner S, Branch F, Dawson D, Morgan P, et al. Standards for the care of adult patients with a temporary tracheostomy; Standards and Guidelines. Intensive Care Society; 2014.

87. Lacherade J-C, Auburtin M, Cerf C, Van de Louw A, Soufir L, Rebufat Y, et al. Impact of humidification systems on ventilator-associated pneumonia: a randomized multicenter trial. Am J Respir Crit Care Med. 2005;172(10):1276–82.

88. Lorente L, Lecuona M, Jiménez A, Mora ML, Sierra A. Ventilator-associated pneumonia using a heated humidifier or a heat and moisture exchanger: a randomized controlled trial [ISRCTN88724583]. Crit Care Lond Engl. 2006;10(4):R116.

89. Yaremchuk K. Regular tracheostomy tube changes to prevent formation of granulation tissue. The Laryngoscope. 2003;113(1):1–10.

90. Fisher DF, Kondili D, Williams J, Hess DR, Bittner EA, Schmidt UH. Tracheostomy tube change before day 7 is associated with earlier use of speaking valve and earlier oral intake. Respir Care. 2013;58(2):257–63.

91. Tabaee A, Lando T, Rickert S, Stewart MG, Kuhel WI. Practice patterns, safety, and rationale for tracheostomy tube changes: a survey of otolaryngology training programs. The Laryngoscope. 2007;117(4):573–6.

92. Veelo DP, Schultz MJ, Phoa KYN, Dongelmans DA, Binnekade JM, Spronk PE. Management of tracheostomy: a survey of Dutch intensive care units. Respir Care. 2008;53(12):1709–15.

93. Conseil Des Communautés Européennes. Directive 93/42/CEE du Conseil, du 14 juin 1993, relative aux dispositifs médicaux. 1993.

94. Backman S, Björling G, Johansson U-B, Lysdahl M, Markström A, Schedin U, et al. Material wear of polymeric tracheostomy tubes: a six-month study. The Laryngoscope. 2009;119(4):657–64.

95. Choate K, Barbetti J, Currey J. Tracheostomy decannulation failure rate following critical illness: a prospective descriptive study. Aust Crit Care. 2009;22(1):8–15.

96. Frank U, Mäder M, Sticher H. Dysphagic patients with tracheotomies: a multidisciplinary approach to treatment and decannulation management. Dysphagia. 2007;22(1):20–9.

97. Cohen O, Tzelnick S, Lahav Y, Stavi D, Shoffel-Havakuk H, Hain M, et al. Feasibility of a single-stage tracheostomy decannulation protocol with endoscopy in adult patients. The Laryngoscope. 2016;126(9):2057–62.

98. Pandian V, Miller CR, Schiavi AJ, Yarmus L, Contractor A, Haut ER, et al. Utilization of a standardized tracheostomy capping and decannulation protocol to improve patient safety. The Laryngoscope. 2014;124(8):1794–800.

99. Ceriana P, Carlucci A, Navalesi P, Rampulla C, Delmastro M, Piaggi G, et al. Weaning from tracheotomy in long-term mechanically ventilated patients: feasibility of a decisional flowchart and clinical outcome. Intensive Care Med. 2003;29(5):845–8.

100. Suiter DM, McCullough GH, Powell PW. Effects of cuff deflation and one-way tracheostomy speaking valve placement on swallow physiology. Dysphagia. 2003;18(4):284–92.

101. Pryor LN, Ward EC, Cornwell PL, O'Connor SN, Chapman MJ. Clinical indicators associated with successful tracheostomy cuff deflation. Aust Crit Care. 2016;29(3):132–7.

102. Santus P, Gramegna A, Radovanovic D, Raccanelli R, Valenti V, Rabbiosi D, et al. A systematic review on tracheostomy decannulation: a proposal of a quantitative semiquantitative clinical score. BMC Pulm Med. 2014;14:201.

103. Rumbak MJ, Graves AE, Scott MP, Sporn GK, Walsh FW, Anderson WM, et al. Tracheostomy tube occlusion protocol predicts significant tracheal obstruction to air flow in patients requiring prolonged mechanical ventilation. Crit Care Med. 1997;25(3):413–7.

104. de Zanata I. L, Santos RS, Hirata GC. Tracheal decannulation protocol in patients affected by traumatic brain injury. Int. Arch Otorhinolaryngol. 2014;18(2):108–14.

105. Hernandez G, Pedrosa A, Ortiz R, Accuaroni MDMC, Cuena R, Collado CV, et al. The effects of increasing effective airway diameter on weaning from mechanical ventilation in tracheostomized patients: a randomized controlled trial. Intensive Care Med. 2013;39(6):1063–70.

106. Warnecke T, Suntrup S, Teismann IK, Hamacher C, Oelenberg S, Dziewas R. Standardized endoscopic swallowing evaluation for tracheostomy decannulation in critically ill neurologic patients. Crit Care Med. 2013;41(7):1728–32.

107. Romero CM, Marambio A, Larrondo J, Walker K, Lira M-T, Tobar E, et al. Swallowing dysfunction in nonneurologic critically ill patients who require percutaneous dilatational tracheostomy. Chest. 2010;137(6):1278–82.

108. Rodrigues LB, Nunes TA. Importance of flexible bronchoscopy in decannulation of tracheostomy patients. Rev Col Bras Cir. 2015;42(2):75–80.

8

Assessment of fluid responsiveness in spontaneously breathing patients

Renato Carneiro de Freitas Chaves[1*], Thiago Domingos Corrêa[1,2], Ary Serpa Neto[1,3], Bruno de Arruda Bravim[1], Ricardo Luiz Cordioli[1], Fabio Tanzillo Moreira[1], Karina Tavares Timenetsky[1] and Murillo Santucci Cesar de Assunção[1]

Abstract

Patients who increase stoke volume or cardiac index more than 10 or 15% after a fluid challenge are usually considered fluid responders. Assessment of fluid responsiveness prior to volume expansion is critical to avoid fluid overload, which has been associated with poor outcomes. Maneuvers to assess fluid responsiveness are well established in mechanically ventilated patients; however, few studies evaluated maneuvers to predict fluid responsiveness in spontaneously breathing patients. Our objective was to perform a systematic review of literature addressing the available methods to assess fluid responsiveness in spontaneously breathing patients. Studies were identified through electronic literature search of PubMed from 01/08/2009 to 01/08/2016 by two independent authors. No restrictions on language were adopted. Quality of included studies was evaluated with Quality Assessment of Diagnostic Accuracy Studies tool. Our search strategy identified 537 studies, and 9 studies were added through manual search. Of those, 15 studies (12 intensive care unit patients; 1 emergency department patients; 1 intensive care unit and emergency department patients; 1 operating room) were included in this analysis. In total, 649 spontaneously breathing patients were assessed for fluid responsiveness. Of those, 340 (52%) were deemed fluid responsive. Pulse pressure variation during the Valsalva maneuver (ΔPPV) of 52% (AUC $\pm$ SD: 0.98 $\pm$ 0.03) and passive leg raising-induced change in stroke volume (ΔSV-PLR) > 13% (AUC $\pm$ SD: 0.96 $\pm$ 0.03) showed the highest accuracy to predict fluid responsiveness in spontaneously breathing patients. Our systematic review indicates that regardless of the limitations of each maneuver, fluid responsiveness can be assessed in spontaneously breathing patients. Further well-designed studies, with adequate simple size and power, are necessary to confirm the real accuracy of the different methods used to assess fluid responsiveness in this population of patients.

Keywords: Fluid responsiveness, Spontaneously breathing, Echocardiography, Stroke volume, Pulse pressure, Intensive care, Critical care

Background

Intravascular volume expansion is a common intervention in critically ill patients [1]. Patients who will benefit from intravascular volume expansion, i.e., will boost stroke volume (SV) after a volume expansion, have both ventricles in the ascending portion of the Frank–Starling curve, characterizing a preload dependency [1, 2]. Nevertheless, nearly 50% of critically ill patients will not benefit from an intravascular volume expansion [2, 3]. Conversely, an accurate assessment of fluid responsiveness prior to volume expansion is critical to avoid fluid overload, which has been associated with increased morbidity and mortality in critically ill patients [4–6].

The concept of predicting fluid responsiveness was initially reported in deeply sedated patients under volume-controlled mechanical ventilation with tidal volume

*Correspondence: chavesrcf@hotmail.com
[1] Intensive Care Unit, Hospital Israelita Albert Einstein, Av. Albert Einstein, 627/701, 5th Floor, São Paulo, SP 05651-901, Brazil

(VT) of at least 8 ml/Kg and positive end-expiratory pressure (PEEP) lower than 10 cm H_2O [7]. Nonetheless, since many patients in the intensive care unit (ICU) are not under such conditions, for many years the presence of spontaneous breathing or inspiratory efforts, with or without an endotracheal tube, was considered a major limitation to assess fluid responsiveness in critically ill patients [8].

Knowledge on the interaction between heart, lung and abdominal compartment is critical to understanding the concept of fluid responsiveness [9, 10]. In spontaneous breathing patients without mechanical ventilation, intrathoracic pressure decreases, while venous return and stroke volume increases during inspiration [10]. On the other hand, at expiration, intrathoracic pressure increases, while venous return and stroke volume decreases [10]. Thus, quantifying stroke volume variation, between respiratory cycles could be used to assess fluid responsiveness [1].

Static [11, 12] and dynamic [8, 13] parameters have been proposed to assess fluid responsiveness in critically ill patients. The available evidence clearly shows that dynamic parameters exhibited a higher accuracy than static parameters to predict fluid responsiveness [13, 14]. Pulse pressure variation, [15–20] echocardiography maneuvers [21–28] and passive leg raising [18, 21–23, 25, 27, 29] are tools that could be used to assess fluid responsiveness in spontaneously breathing patients.

Thus, our primary objective was to perform a systematic review addressing the available methods for fluid responsiveness assessment in spontaneously breathing patients. A secondary objective was to summarize the performance of available methods to assess fluid responsiveness in spontaneously breathing patients.

Methods

This systematic review was reported following the PRISMA (Preferred Reporting Items for Systematic Reviews and Meta-Analyses) guidelines [30].

Eligibility criteria

Articles were selected for inclusion if they evaluated fluid responsiveness in spontaneous breathing adult patients. Articles were assessed for eligibility if one of the following standard definitions of fluid responsiveness and fluid challenge was adopted: increase in stroke volume (SV) $\geq$ 10% and/or cardiac output (CO) $\geq$ 10% and/ or cardiac index (CI) [31] $\geq$ 10% and/or aortic velocity–time integral (VTI) $\geq$ 10% after a fluid challenge [2, 32]. Fluid challenge was considered adequate if at least 250 ml over 30 min of intravenous (I.V.) fluid was infused [2, 33]. Spontaneously breathing was defined as patients without any ventilatory support, patients on noninvasive mechanical ventilation or patients on invasive mechanical ventilation in a spontaneous mode. Patients in the following clinical scenarios were included: ICU, emergency department (ED) and operating room.

Identifying studies

An electronic literature search was carried out by two authors through a computerized blinded search on PubMed. The following search strategy was applied: (((("hemodynamics"[MeSH Terms] OR "hemodynamics"[All Fields]) AND ("respiration"[MeSH Terms] OR "respiration"[All Fields] OR "cell respiration"[MeSH Terms] OR ("cell"[All Fields] AND "respiration"[All Fields]) OR "cell respiration"[All Fields]) AND ("cardiac output"[MeSH Terms] OR ("cardiac"[All Fields] AND "output"[All Fields]) OR "cardiac output"[All Fields]))). Literature search was limited to a period of time (01/08/2009 to 01/08/2016) and to "human." No restrictions on language were adopted. Additionally, we hand-searched the reference lists of the included studies to identify other relevant studies.

Study selection

Prospective studies that reported sensitivity, specificity, cutoff value of each maneuver to assess fluid responsiveness, number of patients included and frequency of fluid responsiveness and non-fluid responsiveness patients were included in this systematic review. Review articles, editorials, studies assessing fluid responsiveness during mechanical ventilation and studies that did not report outcomes of interest were excluded.

Data extraction

Two authors independently screened all retrieved citations by reviewing their titles and abstracts (RCFC and FTM). Then, the reviewers independently evaluated the full-text manuscripts for eligibility using a standardized form. Reviewers independently extracted the relevant data from the full-text manuscripts and assessed the risk of bias using a standardized form. Any disagreement between the authors was resolved by a third author (ASN).

Quality assessment

The quality of each study was evaluated by the Quality Assessment of Diagnostic Accuracy Studies tool (QUADAS) [34]. Details of the quality assessment are reported in Additional file 1.

Primary objective

The primary objective was to report the available methods to assess fluid responsiveness in spontaneously breathing patients.

Secondary objectives

Secondary objectives were to assess diagnostic performance and build a receiver operating characteristics curve (ROC curve) of methods available to assess fluid responsiveness in spontaneously breathing patients.

Methods for fluid responsiveness assessment

Assessed methods to predict fluid responsiveness were pulse pressure variation (ΔPP); [15, 17, 19] systolic pressure variation (ΔSP); [15] ΔPP during forced inspiratory effort (ΔPPf); [15] ΔSP during forced inspiratory effort (ΔSPf); [15] ΔPP during the Valsalva maneuver (ΔPPV); [16] ΔSP during the Valsalva maneuver (ΔVSP); [16] lowest pulse pressure (PPmin); [16] stroke volume variation (ΔSV); [17, 21, 26] passive leg raising (PLR)-induced change in stroke volume (ΔSV-PLR); [18, 23, 29] PLR-induced change in radial pulse pressure (ΔPP-PLR); [18] PLR-induced change in the velocity peak of femoral artery flow (ΔVF-PLR); [18] deep inspiration maneuver-induced change in pulse pressure (ΔPPdim); [19] respiratory change in velocity peak of femoral artery flow (ΔVF); [19] deep inspiration maneuver-induced change in velocity peak of femoral artery flow (ΔVFdim); [19] ΔPP during forced inspiratory breathing (ΔPP$_{FB}$); [20] PLR-induced change in stroke volume index (SVi-PLR); [21] change in cardiac output (ΔCO); [22] inferior vena cava collapsibility index (cIVC); [24, 26–28] E wave velocity; [24] aortic velocity time index (VTI) variations during PLR (ΔVTI-PLR); [25] VTI $\le$ 21 cm; [25] aortic velocity variation (AoVV); [26] inferior vena cava maximum diameter (IVCmax); [27] ΔCO between baseline and after PLR (ΔCO-PLR) [27].

Pulse pressure variation was calculated as the difference in pulse pressure maximal (PPmax) and pulse pressure minimal (PPmin) over the respiratory cycle divided by the mean between PPmax and PPmin [ΔPP = (PPmax − PPmin)/(PPmax + PPmin)/2] [16, 19, 20]. Passive leg raising consists in moving the patient from the 45° semirecumbent position to a horizontal position with the lower limbs lifted 30°–45° relative to the trunk [1, 18]. PLR was determined as the difference between baseline and the highest value induced during the PLR or after the PLR [21, 23, 27]. Inferior vena cava collapsibility index represents the difference in the vena cava maximum diameter (IVCmax) and vena cava minimum diameter (IVCmin) divided by the vena cava maximum diameter over the respiratory cycle [cIVC = (IVCmax − IVCmin)/(IVCmax)] [26, 27]. Valsalva maneuver consists of sustaining a forced expiration effort against a closed mouth [16]. Forced inspiratory breaths consist of three respiratory cycles of deep inspiration immediately followed by slow passive expiration [20]. Deep inspiration maneuver consists of slow continuous inspiration strain (5–8 s) followed by slow passive exhalation [19].

Statistical analysis

The number of patients included, study design, setting, inclusion and exclusion criteria, time and type of fluid infused, the best cutoff value of each maneuver and definition of fluid responders were extracted from published studies. The accuracy of each diagnostic test was assessed with sensitivity (Sens), specificity (Spec), positive predictive value (PPV), negative predictive value (NPV), positive likelihood ratio (LR +), negative likelihood ratio (LR −), AUC along with its standard deviation (SD) or 95% confidence interval (95% CI). Whenever not reported, accuracy, PPV, NPV, LR + and LR − were calculated using the Review Manager (RevMan) [computer program]—version 5.3—Copenhagen: The Nordic Cochrane Centre, The Cochrane Collaboration, 2014.

A receiver operator characteristics curve (ROC curve) was constructed using the sensitivity and specificity of each maneuver extracted from included study using Meta-DiSc version 1.4 (Universidad Complutense, Madrid, Spain) [35]. Methods for fluid responsiveness assessment were classified according to their accuracy [area under the receiver operating characteristics curve (AUC)]. AUC from 0.90 to 1.00 was considered excellent, from 0.80 to 0.89 adequate, from 0.70 to 0.79 fair, from 0.60 to 0.69 poor and from 0.50 to 0.59 failure [36].

Results

Search results

The initial search strategy identified 537 studies (Fig. 1). After screening the reference lists of the included studies, 9 potentially relevant articles were included and 546 potentially relevant articles were selected. Fifteen prospective studies (649 patients in total) were included in this systematic review after the exclusion of 531 studies

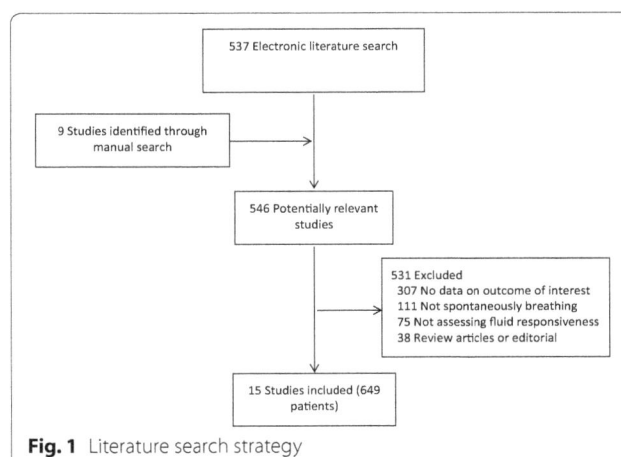

Fig. 1 Literature search strategy

(307 studies had no data on outcome of interest, 111 studies did not regard spontaneously breathing patients, 75 studies did not access fluid responsiveness, and 38 were review articles or editorials) (Fig. 1).

Characteristics of included studies

Characteristics of included studies are presented in Tables 1 [15–20] and 2 [21–29]. Out of fifteen studies included, twelve evaluated fluid responsiveness in ICU patients, [15–19, 21–27] one included ED patients, [29] one included ICU and ED patients [28] and one included operating room patients (elective thoracic surgery) [20] (Tables 1 and 2).

Out of 649 spontaneously breathing patients assessed for fluid responsiveness, 340 patients (52%) were responders. In 12 studies [12/15 (80%)], only spontaneous breathing patients without any type of ventilatory support were included (572 patients) [15, 16, 18–20, 22, 24–29]. Out of those, 51% (291/572) of patients without ventilatory support were considered fluid responsive (Tables 1 and 2). In 3 studies [3/15 (20%)], spontaneous breathing patient without any ventilatory support and patients under mechanical ventilation in a spontaneous mode were included (77 patients) [17, 21, 23]. Of those, 63% (49/77) patients were deemed responsive to a fluid challenge (Tables 1 and 2).

Table 1 Characteristics of included studies addressing pulse pressure variation for fluid responsiveness in spontaneously breathing patients

Author, year	N	Setting	Inclusion criteria	Exclusion criteria	Ventilation	Fluid challenge	Definition of responders	Maneuvers
Soubrier, 2007 [15]	32	ICU	1. Low blood pressure 2. Tachycardia 3. Oliguria 4. Mottled skin	1. Arrhythmia 2. Lack of cooperation	SB	500 ml I.V. 6% HES over 20 min	↑CI ≥ 15%	1. ΔPP 2. ΔSP 3. ΔPPf 4. ΔSPf
M. García, 2009 [16]	30	ICU	1. Hypotension 2. Tachycardia 3. Oliguria	1. Arrhythmia 2. History of syncope 3. Lack of cooperation	SB	500 ml I.V. 6% HES over 30 min	↑SVi > 15%	1. ΔPPV by PCA 2. ΔVSP by PCA 3. PPmin
Monnet, 2009 [17]	23	ICU	1. SBP < 90 mmHg 2. Tachycardia 3. UO < 0.5 ml/kg/h 4. Mottled skin	1. Not sustain an inspiration for over 15 seconds	SB and SBmv	500 ml I.V. saline over 10 min	↑CI > 15%	1. ΔPP by PCA 2. ΔSV by PCA
Préau, 2010 [18]	34	ICU	1. SBP < 90 mmHg 2. Tachycardia 3. UO < 0.5 mL/kg/h 4. Mottled skin	1. Arrhythmia 2. Aortic insufficiency 3. VNI was warranted	SB	500 mL I.V. 6% HES over 30 min	↑SV ≥ 15%	1. ΔSV-PLR by TE 2. ΔPP-PLR 3. ΔVF-PLR by Doppler
Préau, 2012 [19]	23	ICU	1. SBP < 90 mmHg 2. Tachycardia 3. Regular cardiac rhythm 4. UO < 0.5 mL/kg/h	1. RR > 30 2 Not sustain an inspiration for over 5 s 3. Aortic insufficiency 4. MV was warranted	SB	500 mL I.V. 6% HES over 30 min	↑SV > 15%	1. ΔPP 2 ΔPPdim 3. ΔVF by Doppler 4. ΔVFdim by Doppler
Hong, 2014 [20]	59	OP	1. Age 18–80 years 2. Elective thoracic surgery	1. Arrhythmia 2. Intracardiac shunt 3. Valvulopathy 4 Cardiac or pulmonary dysfunction	SB	6 ml/kg of I.V. HES for 10 min	↑CI ≥ 15%	1. ΔPP$_{FB}$ by PCA

ICU intensive care unit, *OP* operating room, *SBP* systolic blood pressure, *UO* urine output, *VNI* ventilation noninvasive, *RR* respiratory rate, *MV* mechanical ventilation, *COPD* chronic obstructive pulmonary disease, *SB* spontaneous breathing without any ventilatory support, *SBmv* mechanical ventilation during spontaneous mode, *I.V.* intravenous, *HES* hydroxyethyl starch, ↑ = increase, *CI* cardiac index, *SV* stroke volume, *ΔPP* pulse pressure variation, *ΔSP* systolic pressure variation, *ΔPPf* ΔPP during forced inspiratory effort, *ΔSPf* ΔSP during forced inspiratory effort, *ΔPPV* ΔPP during the Valsalva maneuver, *PCA* pulse contour analysis, *ΔVSP* ΔSP during the Valsalva maneuver, *PPmin* lowest pulse pressure, *ΔSV* stroke volume variation, *PLR* passive leg raising, *ΔSV-PLR* PLR-induced change in stroke volume, *ΔPP-PLR* PLR-induced change in radial pulse pressure, *ΔVF-PLR* PLR-induced change in the velocity peak of femoral artery flow, *ΔPPdim* deep inspiration maneuver-induced change in pulse pressure, *ΔVF* respiratory change in velocity peak of femoral artery flow, *ΔVFdim* deep inspiration maneuver-induced change in velocity peak of femoral artery flow, *ΔPP$_{FB}$* ΔPP during forced inspiratory breathing

Table 2 Characteristics of included studies addressing echocardiography maneuvers, pulse contour analysis or noninvasive cardiac output monitor (NICOM®) for fluid responsiveness in spontaneously breathing patients

Author, year	N	Setting	Inclusion criteria	Exclusion criteria	Ventilation	Fluid challenge	Definition of responders	Maneuvers
Lamia, 2007 [21]	24	ICU	1. MAP < 60 mmHg 2. Tachycardia 3. UO < 0.5 ml/kg/h 4. Delayed CRT	1. Aortic valvu-lopathy 2. Mitral insuf-ficiency or stenosis	SB and SBmv	500 ml I.V. saline for 15 min	↑SVi ≥ 15%	1. SVi-PLR by TE
Maizel, 2007 [22]	34	ICU	1. Hypotension 2. Acute renal failure 3. Dehydration	1. Hemorrhage 2. PLR contrain-dications 3. Arrhythmia	SB	500 ml I.V. saline over 15 min	↑CO ≥ 12%	1. ΔCO-PLR by TE 2. ΔSV-PLR by TE
Biais, 2009 [23]	30	ICU	1. SBP < 90 mmHg 2. Tachycardia 3. Acute renal failure 4 Mottled skin	1. ↑ intra-abdominal pressure 2. BMI < 15 or > 40 kg/m2 3. Valvulopathy 4 Intracardiac shunt	SB and SBmv	500 ml I.V. saline for 15 min	↑SV > 15%	1. ΔSV-PLR$_{TE}$ by TE 2. ΔSV-PLR$_{FloT}$ by PCA
Muller, 2012 [24]	40	ICU	1. MAP < 65 mmHg 2. Tachycardia 3. UO < 0.5 mL/Kg/h 4. Mottled skin	1. Pulmonary edema 2. Right ventricu-lar failure 3. Elevated left atrial pressure	SB	500 mL I.V. 6% HES over 15 min	↑VTI ≥ 15%	1. cIVC by TE 2. E wave velocity by TE
Brun, 2013 [25]	23	ICU	1. Severe preec-lampsia	1. Cardiac or renal disorders prior to preg-nancy	SB	500 ml I.V. saline over 15 min	↑SVi ≥ 15%	1. ΔVTI-PLR 2. VTI
Lanspa, 2013 [26]	14	ICU	1. Age ≥ 14 years 2. Infection and SIRS 3. Refractory hypo-tension	1. Pregnancy 2. Aortic stenosis 3. Arrhythmia 4. COPD and asthma	SB	10 mL/kg of I.V. crystalloids over 20 min	↑CI ≥ 15%	1. cIVC by TE 2. ΔSV by PCA 3. AoVV by TE
Airapetian, 2015 [27]	59	ICU	1. Physician decided to perform fluid expansion	1. Hemorrhage 2. Arrhythmia 3. Compression stockings 4. PLR contrain-dications	SB	PLR and 500 ml I.V. saline over 15 min	↑CO ≥ 10%	1. cIVC by TE 2. IVCmax by TE 3. ΔCO-PLR by TE
Duus, 2015 [29]	100	ED	1. Age ≥ 18 years 2. Clinical team intended to administer IV fluid	1. Acuity precluding participation in research 2 PLR contraindi-cations	SB	5 ml/kg I.V. saline	↑SV > 10%	1. ΔSV-PLR using NICOM®
Corl, 2017 [28]	124	ED and ICU	1. PAS < 90 mmHg 2. Tachycardia 3. UO < 0.5 ml/kg/h 4. Hypoperfusion	1. Cardiogenic, obstructive or neurogenic shock 2. Age < 18 years 3. Hospitalization for > 36 h	SB	500 ml I.V. saline	↑CI ≥ 10%	1. cIVC by TE

ICU intensive care unit, *ED* emergency department, *MAP* mean arterial pressure, *UO* urine output, *CRT* capillary refill time, *SBP* systolic blood pressure, *PLR* passive leg raising, ↑ = increase, *BMI* body mass index, *COPD* chronic obstructive pulmonary disease, *SB* spontaneous breathing without any ventilatory support, *SBmv* mechanical ventilation during spontaneous mode, *I.V.* intravenous, *HES* hydroxyethyl starch, *SV* stroke volume, *CO* cardiac output, *VTI* aortic velocity–time integral, *SVi* stroke volume index, *CI* cardiac index, *PLR* passive leg raising, *SVi-PLR* PLR-induced change in stroke volume index, *TE* transthoracic echocardiography, *ΔCO* change in cardiac output, *ΔCO-PLR* ΔCO between baseline and after PLR, *ΔSV* stroke volume variation, *ΔSV-PLR* PLR-induced change in stroke volume, *FloT* FloTrac™, *PCA* pulse contour analysis, *cIVC* inferior vena cava collapsibility index, *VTI* aortic velocity–time integral, *ΔVTI-PLR* VTI variations during PLR, *AoVV* aortic velocity variation, *NICOM®* noninvasive cardiac output monitor, *IVCmax* inferior vena cava maximum diameter

Fluid challenge characteristics

Fluid challenge was performed in seven (46.6%) studies through an I.V. infusion of 500 ml of saline; [17, 21–23, 25, 27, 28] five studies (33.3%) with 500 ml of hydroxyethyl starch (HES); [15, 16, 18, 19, 24] one (6.7%) study with 6 ml/kg of HES; [20] one (6.7%) study applied 10 mL/kg of crystalloid; [26] and one (6.7%) study used 5 ml/kg saline [29] (Tables 1 and 2).

Adopted definitions of fluid responsiveness were an increase in SV > 10% [29] or > 15%; [18, 19, 23] an increase in stroke volume index (SVi) $\geq$ 15%; [16, 21, 25] an increase in CI $\geq$ 10% [28] or $\geq$ 15%; [15, 17, 20, 26] an increase in CO $\geq$ 10% [27] or 12% [22] or an VTI $\geq$ 15% [24] (Tables 1 and 2). The triggers for intravascular volume expansion varied across the studies and are presented in Tables 1 and 2.

Methods for fluid responsiveness assessment

Thirty-four maneuvers for predicting fluid responsiveness in spontaneously breathing patients were reported (Tables 1 and 2). Studies that adopted pulse pressure variation to assess fluid responsiveness are summarized in Table 1. Studies that adopted echocardiography maneuvers, pulse contour analysis or noninvasive cardiac output monitor (NICOM®) are summarized in Table 2.

Performance of maneuvers for predicting fluid responsiveness

Pooled analysis (15 studies; 649 patients)

Out of 34 reported maneuvers for predicting fluid responsiveness in spontaneously breathing patients, 13 (38%) maneuvers had excellent accuracy (AUC from 0.9 to 1), 9 (26%) had adequate accuracy (AUC from 0.8 to 0.89), 6 (18%) had fair accuracy (AUC from 0.7 to 0.79), 5 (15%) had poor accuracy (AUC from 0.6 to 0.69) and 1 maneuver (3%) was classified as failure (AUC from 0.5 to 0.59) (Fig. 2) (Tables 3 and 4).

ΔPPV of 52% (AUC $\pm$ SD: 0.98 $\pm$ 0.03), [16] ΔSV-PLR > 13% (AUC $\pm$ SD: 0.96 $\pm$ 0.03), [23] ΔPPdim $\geq$ 12% (AUC $\pm$ SD: 0.95 $\pm$ 0.05), [19] ΔVFdim $\geq$ 12% (AUC $\pm$ SD: 0.95 $\pm$ 0.05) [19] and ΔSV-PLR $\geq$ 10% (AUC $\pm$ SD: 0.94 $\pm$ 0.04) [18] showed the highest accuracy to predict fluid responsiveness in spontaneously breathing patients (Fig. 2) (Tables 3 and 4). AoVV $\geq$ 25% [AUC (95% CI): 0.67 (0.32–1.00)], [26] cIVC > 42% [AUC (95% CI): 0.62 (0.66–0.88)], [27] IVCmax at baseline < 2.1 cm [AUC (95% CI): 0.07 (0.49–0.75)] [27] and ΔSV $\geq$ 10% [AUC (95% CI): 0.57(0.34-0.78)] [17] showed the worst values of accuracy to predict fluid responsiveness (Fig. 2) (Tables 3 and 4).

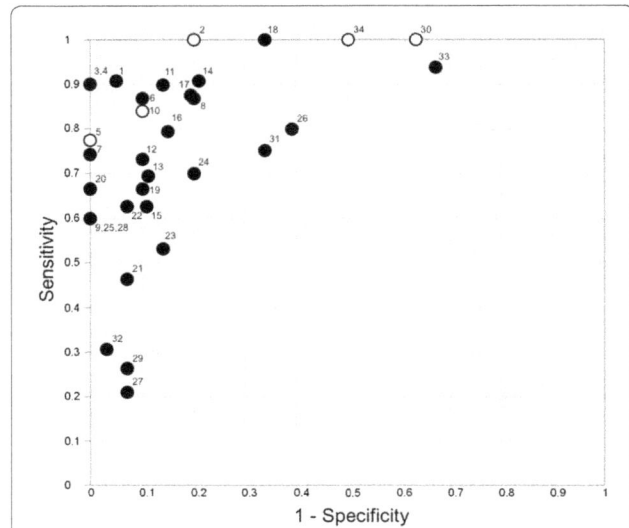

Fig. 2 Receiver operating characteristics curve with all methods found in the literature search of assessment volume responsiveness in spontaneous breathing patients. Closed circles represent studies including spontaneous breathing patients without ventilator support; open circles represent studies including patients under mechanical ventilation during spontaneous mode and spontaneous breathing without ventilator support. 1 = ΔPPV of 52%; 2 = ΔSV-PLR$_{TTE}$ >13%; 3 = ΔPPdim $\geq$12%; 4 = ΔVFdim $\geq$12%; 5 = SVi-PLR $\geq$12.5%; 6 = ΔSV-PLR $\geq$10%; 7 = ΔVTI-PLR >12%; 8 = ΔVF-PLR $\geq$8%; 9 = ΔSV $\geq$17%; 10 = ΔSV-PLR$_{FloT}$ >16%; 11 = ΔPP$_{FB}$ = 13.7%; 12 = ΔVSP of 30%; 13 = ΔSV >12%; 14 = PPmin of 45mmHg; 15 = ΔCO >12%; 16 = ΔPP-PLR $\geq$9%; 17 = cIVC of 25%; 18 = cIVC $\geq$15%; 19 = E wave velocity of 0.7; 20 = VTI $\leq$21cm; 21 = ΔSP of 9%; 22 = ΔPP of 12%; 23 = ΔCO-PLR >10%; 24 = cIVC =40%; 25 = ΔVF $\geq$10%; 26 = ΔSV-PLR; 27 = ΔPPf of 33%; 28 = ΔPP $\geq$10%; 29 = ΔSPf of 30%; 30 = ΔPP $\geq$11%; 31 = AoVV $\geq$25%; 32 = cIVC >42%, 33 = IVCmax <2.1cm, 34 = ΔSV$\geq$10%

Spontaneous breathing patients without ventilatory support

ΔVSP of 52% [AUC $\pm$ SD: 0.98 $\pm$ 0.03] [16] had the highest accuracy and cIVC > 42% [AUC (95% CI): 0.62 (0.66–0.88)] and IVCmax < 2.1 cm [AUC (95% CI) 0.62 (0.49–0.75)] the worst accuracy to predict fluid responsiveness in spontaneous breathing patients without ventilatory support (12 studies totaling 572 patients) (Additional file 1: Figure S1).

Spontaneous breathing with ventilatory support

ΔSV-PLR$_{TE}$ > 13% [AUC $\pm$ SD: 0.96 $\pm$ 0.03] had the highest accuracy, while ΔSV $\geq$ 10% [AUC (95% CI) 0.57(0.34–0.78)] had the worst accuracy to predict fluid responsiveness in mechanically ventilated patients in a spontaneous mode (3 studies totaling 77 patients) (Additional file 1: Figure S2).

Table 3 Performance of included studies that addressed pulse pressure variation to predict fluid responsiveness in spontaneously breathing patients

Author, Year	Maneuver	Sens (%)	Spec (%)	PPV (%)	NPV (%)	LR +	LR−	AUC ± SD or (95% CI)
Soubrier, 2007 [15]	ΔPP of 12%	63	92	92	63	8.20	0.39	0.81. ± 0.08
	ΔSP of 9%	47	92	90	54	6.15	0.57	0.82 ± 0.08
	ΔPPf of 33%	21	92	80	44	3.01	0.85	0.72 ± 0.09
	ΔSPf of 30%	26	92	83	46	3.75	0.80	0.69 ± 0.10
M. García, 2009 [16]	ΔPPV of 52%	91	95	91	95	17,3	0.01	0.98 ± 0.03
	ΔVSP of 30%	73	90	80	85	6.91	0.30	0.90 ± 0.07
	PPmin of 45 mmHg	91	79	71	94	4.32	0.12	0.89 ± 0.06
Monnet, 2009 [17]	ΔPP ≥ 11%	100	37	80	100	1.75		0.68 (0.45–0.88)
	ΔSV ≥ 10%	100	50	84	100	2.00		0.57 (0.34–0.78)
Préau, 2010 [18]	ΔSV-PLR ≥ 10%	86	90	86	90	8.57	0.16	0.94 ± 0.04
	ΔPP-PLR ≥ 9%	79	85	79	85	5.24	0.25	0.86 ± 0.08
	ΔVF-PLR ≥ 8%	86	80	75	89	4.29	0.18	0.93 ± 0.04
Préau, 2012 [19]	ΔPP ≥ 10%	60	100	100	76		0.40	0.71. ± 0.12
	ΔPPdim ≥ 12%	90	100	100	93		0.10	0.95 ± 0.05
	ΔVF ≥ 10%	60	100	100	76		0.40	0.74 ± 0.11
	ΔVFdim ≥ 12%	90	100	100	93		0.10	0.95 ± 0.05
Hong, 2014 [20]	ΔPP_FB = 13.7%	90	87	87	90	6.72	0.12	0.91 (0.80–0.96)

Sens sensitivity, *Spec* specificity, *PPV* positive predictive value, *NPV* negative predictive value, *LR +* positive likelihood ratio, *LR −* negative likelihood ratio, *AUC* area under the receiver operating characteristics curve, *SD* standard deviation, *95% CI* 95% confidence intervals, *ΔPP* pulse pressure variation, *ΔSP* systolic pressure variation, *ΔPPf* ΔPP during forced inspiratory effort, *ΔSPf* ΔSP during forced inspiratory effort, *ΔPPV* ΔPP during the Valsalva maneuver, *ΔVSP* ΔSP during the Valsalva maneuver, *PPmin* lowest pulse pressure, *PLR* passive leg raising, *ΔSV-PLR* PLR-induced change in stroke volume, *ΔPP-PLR* PLR-induced change in radial pulse pressure, *ΔVF-PLR* PLR-induced change in the velocity peak of femoral artery flow, *ΔPPdim* deep inspiration maneuver-induced change in pulse pressure, *ΔVF* respiratory change in velocity peak of femoral artery flow, *ΔVFdim* deep inspiration maneuver-induced change in velocity peak of femoral artery flow, *ΔPP_FB* ΔPP during forced inspiratory breathing

Table 4 Performance of included studies that addressed echocardiography maneuvers, pulse contour analysis or noninvasive cardiac output monitor (NICOM®) to predict fluid responsiveness in spontaneously breathing patients

Author, year	Maneuver	Sens (%)	Spec (%)	PPV (%)	NPV (%)	LR+	LR−	AUC ± SD or (95% CI)
Lamia, 2007 [21]	SVi-PLR ≥ 12.5%	77	100	100	78		0.23	0.95 ± 0.04
Maizel, 2007 [22]	ΔCO > 12%	63	89	83	73	6.00	0.40	0.89 ± 0.06
	ΔSV > 12%	69	89	85	76	6.00	0.40	0.90 ± 0.06
Biais, 2009 [23]	ΔSV-PLR_TE > 13%	100	80	91	100	5.00		0.96 ± 0.03
	ΔSV-PLR_FloT > 16%	85	90	94	75	8.50	0.17	0.92 ± 0.05
Muller, 2012 [24]	cIVC = 40%	70	80	72	83	3.50	0.37	0.77 (0.60–0.88)
	E wave velocity of 0.7	67	90	84	83	6.67	0.37	0.83 (0.68–0.93)
Brun, 2013 [25]	ΔVTI-PLR > 12%	75	100	100	79		0.25	0.93 (0.83–1.00)
	VTI ≤ 21 cm	67	100	100	75		0.33	0.82 (0.64–1.00)
Lanspa, 2013 [26]	cIVC ≥ 15%	100	67	62	100	3.00		0.83 (0.58–1.00)
	ΔSV ≥ 17%	60	100	100	82		0.40	0.92 (0.73–1.00)
	AoVV ≥ 25%	75	67	50	85	2.25	0.37	0.67 (0.32–1.00)
Airapetian, 2015 [27]	cIVC > 42%	31	97	90	60	9.31	0.71	0.62 (0.66–0.88)
	IVCmax < 2.1 cm	93	33	57	83	1.40	0.21	0.62 (0.49–0.75)
	ΔCO-PLR > 10%	52	87	79	65	3.88	0.56	0.78 (0.66–0.88)
Duus, 2015 [29]	ΔSV-PLR	80	61	79	65	2.09	0.31	0.74 (0.65–0.83)
Corl, 2017 [28]	cIVC of 25%	87	81	81	87	4.56	0.16	0.84 (0.77–0.90)

Sens sensitivity, *Spec* specificity, *PPV* positive predictive value, *NPV* negative predictive value, *LR +* positive likelihood ratio, *LR −* negative likelihood ratio, *AUC* area under the receiver operating characteristics curve, *SD* standard deviation, *95% CI* 95% confidence intervals, *PLR* passive leg raising, *SVi-PLR* PLR-induced change in stroke volume index, *ΔCO* change in cardiac output, *ΔSV* stroke volume variation, *TE* transthoracic echocardiography, *FloT* FloTrac™, *cIVC* inferior vena cava collapsibility index, *VTI* aortic velocity–time integral, *ΔVTI-PLR* VTI variations during PLR, *AoVV* aortic velocity variation, *IVCmax* inferior vena cava maximum diameter, *ΔCO-PLR* change in cardiac output between baseline and after PLR

Discussion

The main finding of this systematic review is that, regardless of intrinsic limitations of each reported maneuver, fluid responsiveness can be assessed in spontaneously breathing patients with acceptable accuracy. Approximately two-thirds (19/29) of reported maneuvers were deemed adequate or excellent to predict fluid responsiveness in spontaneous breathing patients without ventilatory support and 60% (3/5) were deemed excellent in mechanically ventilated patients in a spontaneous mode. Moreover, approximately half of the patients included in this study were not fluid responsive. This finding reinforces the importance of assessing fluid responsiveness in critically ill patients prior to intravascular volume expansion, thus avoiding unnecessary exposure to additional fluids.

In patients with an invasive arterial line in place, dynamic parameters such as ΔPP in association with a maneuver that magnifies cyclic changes in intrathoracic pressures, i.e., deep inspiration or forced inspiratory breathing, represent important tools to assess fluid responsiveness continuously and with minimal inter-rater variability. [19, 20] Echocardiographic maneuvers such as ΔVF, ΔSV, cIVC represent important tools to assess fluid responsiveness in patients without availability of an invasive arterial line [19, 21, 23, 28]. Although it is operator-dependent, echocardiographic is a noninvasive technique that enables fluid responsiveness assessment with good accuracy in spontaneously breathing patients [19, 21, 23, 28]. The main disadvantages of echocardiographic measurements are non-continuous monitoring and high inter-rater variability [18, 24, 27].

Reversible and noninvasive maneuvers that magnify cyclic changes in intrathoracic pressures and on transpulmonary pressure, such as Valsalva or deep inspiration maneuver, in association with ΔPP or echocardiographic measurements, improve the accuracy of the maneuvers without adverse effects, allowing clinicians at the bedside to assess preload dependency [16, 19]. Nevertheless, it is important to emphasize that all reported methods to assess fluid responsiveness in spontaneously breathing patients have limitations [13, 14]. The need of patients cooperation, inability to sustain deep inspiration, presence of pain, intra-abdominal hypertension, major abdominal surgery, low diaphragm strength, higher respiratory rate, low reproducibility and lack of external validation are frequently reported limitations of available methods [16].

Furthermore, transforming a continuous diagnostic index, such as ΔPP and ΔSV, into binary variables (i.e., responders or non-responders) represents an important limitation of all methods to assess fluid responsiveness [37]. The decision of whether to support or avoid volume expansion in patients with intermediate values of continuous diagnostic index could be imprecise (gray zone) [37]. These patients may benefit from a reversible maneuver, such as PLR prior volume expansion to avoid unnecessary exposure to fluids [37].

Our study has limitations. First, it is important to emphasize that the results of this systematic review should be interpreted in the context of the included studies. Furthermore, studies with small sample size, carried out in different clinical scenarios and with a heterogeneous methodology, were included in this systematic review. Finally, systematic reviews are subject to publication bias, which may exaggerate the conclusion of the study if publication is related to the strengths of the results.

Conclusion

In conclusion, our systematic review suggests that regardless of the limitations of each maneuver, fluid responsiveness could be assessed in spontaneously breathing patients. Further research with adequate sample size and power are necessary to confirm the real accuracy of the different methods available to assess fluid responsiveness in this population of critically ill patients.

Abbreviations

95% CI: 95% confidence interval; ΔCO: change in cardiac output; ΔCO-PLR: change in cardiac output between baseline and after PLR; ΔPP: pulse pressure variation; ΔPPdim: deep inspiration maneuver-induced change in pulse pressure; ΔPP-PLR: PLR-induced change in radial pulse pressure; ΔPPf: ΔPP during forced inspiratory effort; ΔPP$_{FB}$: ΔPP during forced inspiratory breathing; ΔPPV: ΔPP during the Valsalva maneuver; ΔSP: systolic pressure variation; ΔSPf: ΔSP during forced inspiratory effort; ΔVSP: ΔSP during the Valsalva maneuver; ΔSV: stroke volume variation; ΔSV-PLR: passive leg raising-induced change in stroke volume; ΔVF: respiratory change in velocity peak of femoral artery flow; ΔVFdim: deep inspiration maneuver-induced change in velocity peak of femoral artery flow; ΔVF-PLR: PLR-induced change in the velocity peak of femoral artery flow; ΔVTI-PLR: VTI variations during PLR; AoVV: aortic velocity variation; AUC: area under the receiver operating characteristics curve; CI: cardiac index; cIVC: inferior vena cava collapsibility index; CO: cardiac output; CVP: central venous pressure; ED: emergency department; HES: hydroxyethyl starch; I.V.: intravenous; ICU: intensive care unit; ITBVI: intrathoracic blood volume index; IVCmax: inferior vena cava maximum diameter; IVCmin: vena cava minimum diameters; LR −: negative likelihood ratio; LR +: positive likelihood ratio; NICOM®: noninvasive cardiac output monitor; NPV: negative predictive value; PEEP: positive end-expiratory pressure; PLR: passive leg raising; PPmax: pulse pressure maximal; PPmin: lowest pulse pressure; PPV: positive predictive value; ROC curve: receiver operating characteristics curve; SD: standard deviation; Sens: sensitivity; Spec: specificity; SV: stoke volume; SVi: stroke volume index; SVi-PLR: PLR-induced change in stroke volume index; VTI: aortic velocity–time integral.

Authors' contributions

RCFC and MSCS conceived the study hypothesis and design. RCFC and FTM identified studies through electronic literature search. RCFC and TDC made the first manuscript draft. RCFC, TDC, ASN, BAB, RLC, FTM, KTT and MSCS critically revised the manuscript for important intellectual content. All authors approved the final manuscript and assumed responsibility for the integrity of the data and the accuracy of the data analysis. All authors read and approved the final manuscript.

Author details

[1] Intensive Care Unit, Hospital Israelita Albert Einstein, Av. Albert Einstein, 627/701, 5th Floor, São Paulo, SP 05651-901, Brazil. [2] Intensive Care Unit, Hospital Municipal Dr. Moysés Deutsch - M'Boi Mirim, São Paulo, SP, Brazil. [3] Department of Intensive Care, Academic Medical Center, University of Amsterdam, Amsterdam, The Netherlands.

Acknowledgements

We thank Helena Spalic for proofreading this manuscript. The work was performed in the intensive care unit of Hospital Israelita Albert Einstein.

Competing interests

The authors declare that they have no competing interests.

Funding

This research did not receive any specific grant from funding agencies in the public, commercial or not-for-profit sectors.

References

1. Monnet X, Teboul JL. Assessment of volume responsiveness during mechanical ventilation: recent advances. Crit Care. 2013;17(2):217.

2. Michard F, Teboul JL. Predicting fluid responsiveness in ICU patients: a critical analysis of the evidence. Chest. 2002;121(6):2000–8.

3. Cecconi M, Hofer C, Teboul JL, Pettila V, et al. Fluid challenges in intensive care: the FENICE study: a global inception cohort study. Intensive Care Med. 2015;41(9):1529–37.

4. Vincent JL, Sakr Y, Sprung CL, Ranieri VM, et al. Sepsis in European intensive care units: results of the SOAP study. Crit Care Med. 2006;34(2):344–53.

5. Payen D, de Pont AC, Sakr Y, Spies C, et al. A positive fluid balance is associated with a worse outcome in patients with acute renal failure. Crit Care. 2008;12(3):R74.

6. Sakr Y, Rubatto Birri PN, Kotfis K, Nanchal R, et al. Higher fluid balance increases the risk of death from sepsis: results from a large international audit. Crit Care Med. 2017;45(3):386–94.

7. Michard F, Boussat S, Chemla D, Anguel N, et al. Relation between respiratory changes in arterial pulse pressure and fluid responsiveness in septic patients with acute circulatory failure. Am J Respir Crit Care Med. 2000;162(1):134–8.

8. Yang X, Du B. Does pulse pressure variation predict fluid responsiveness in critically ill patients? A systematic review and meta-analysis. Crit Care. 2014;18(6):650.

9. Takata M, Wise RA, Robotham JL. Effects of abdominal pressure on venous return: abdominal vascular zone conditions. J Appl Physiol. 1990;69(6):1961–72.

10. Pinsky MR. Heart-lung interactions. Curr Opin Crit Care. 2007;13(5):528–31.

11. Muller L, Louart G, Bengler C, Fabbro-Peray P, et al. The intrathoracic blood volume index as an indicator of fluid responsiveness in critically ill patients with acute circulatory failure: a comparison with central venous pressure. Anesth Analg. 2008;107(2):607–13.

12. Eskesen TG, Wetterslev M, Perner A. Systematic review including re-analyses of 1148 individual data sets of central venous pressure as a predictor of fluid responsiveness. Intensive Care Med. 2016;42(3):324–32.

13. Cherpanath TG, Hirsch A, Geerts BF, Lagrand WK, et al. Predicting fluid responsiveness by passive leg raising: a systematic review and meta-analysis of 23 clinical trials. Crit Care Med. 2016;44(5):981–91.

14. Monnet X, Marik PE, Teboul JL. Prediction of fluid responsiveness: an update. Ann Intensive Care. 2016;6:111.

15. Soubrier S, Saulnier F, Hubert H, Delour P, et al. Can dynamic indicators help the prediction of fluid responsiveness in spontaneously breathing critically ill patients? Intensive Care Med. 2007;33(7):1117–24.

16. Monge García MI, Gil Cano A, Diaz Monrove JC. Arterial pressure changes during the Valsalva maneuver to predict fluid responsiveness in spontaneously breathing patients. Intensive Care Med. 2009;35(1):77–84.

17. Monnet X, Osman D, Ridel C, Lamia B, et al. Predicting volume responsiveness by using the end-expiratory occlusion in mechanically ventilated intensive care unit patients. Crit Care Med. 2009;37(3):951–6.

18. Preau S, Saulnier F, Dewavrin F, Durocher A, Chagnon JL. Passive leg raising is predictive of fluid responsiveness in spontaneously breathing patients with severe sepsis or acute pancreatitis. Crit Care Med. 2010;38(3):819–25.

19. Preau S, Dewavrin F, Soland V, Bortolotti P, et al. Hemodynamic changes during a deep inspiration maneuver predict fluid responsiveness in spontaneously breathing patients. Cardiol Res Pract. 2012;2012:191807.

20. Hong DM, Lee JM, Seo JH, Min JJ, et al. Pulse pressure variation to predict fluid responsiveness in spontaneously breathing patients: tidal vs. forced inspiratory breathing. Anaesthesia. 2014;69(7):717–22.

21. Lamia B, Ochagavia A, Monnet X, Chemla D, et al. Echocardiographic prediction of volume responsiveness in critically ill patients with spontaneously breathing activity. Intensive Care Med. 2007;33(7):1125–32.

22. Maizel J, Airapetian N, Lorne E, Tribouilloy C, et al. Diagnosis of central hypovolemia by using passive leg raising. Intensive Care Med. 2007;33(7):1133–8.

23. Biais M, Vidil L, Sarrabay P, Cottenceau V, et al. Changes in stroke volume induced by passive leg raising in spontaneously breathing patients: comparison between echocardiography and Vigileo/FloTrac device. Crit Care. 2009;13(6):R195.

24. Muller L, Bobbia X, Toumi M, Louart G, et al. Respiratory variations of inferior vena cava diameter to predict fluid responsiveness in spontaneously breathing patients with acute circulatory failure: need for a cautious use. Crit Care. 2012;16(5):R188.

25. Brun C, Zieleskiewicz L, Textoris J, Muller L, et al. Prediction of fluid responsiveness in severe preeclamptic patients with oliguria. Intensive Care Med. 2013;39(4):593–600.

26. Lanspa MJ, Grissom CK, Hirshberg EL, Jones JP, et al. Applying dynamic parameters to predict hemodynamic response to volume expansion in spontaneously breathing patients with septic shock. Shock. 2013;39(2):155–60.

27. Airapetian N, Maizel J, Alyamani O, Mahjoub Y, et al. Does inferior vena cava respiratory variability predict fluid responsiveness in spontaneously breathing patients? Crit Care. 2015;19:400.

28. Corl KA, George NR, Romanoff J, Levinson AT, et al. Inferior vena cava collapsibility detects fluid responsiveness among spontaneously breathing critically-ill patients. J Crit Care. 2017;41:130–7.

29. Duus N, Shogilev DJ, Skibsted S, Zijlstra HW, et al. The reliability and validity of passive leg raise and fluid bolus to assess fluid responsiveness in spontaneously breathing emergency department patients. J Crit Care. 2015;30(1):217.e1-5.

30. Stewart LA, Clarke M, Rovers M, Riley RD, et al. Preferred reporting items for systematic review and meta-analyses of individual participant data: the PRISMA-IPD statement. JAMA. 2015;313(16):1657–65.

31. Zarychanski R, Abou-Setta AM, Turgeon AF, Houston BL, et al. Association of hydroxyethyl starch administration with mortality and acute kidney injury in critically ill patients requiring volume resuscitation: a systematic review and meta-analysis. JAMA. 2013;309(7):678–88.

32. Zhang Z, Xu X, Ye S, Xu L. Ultrasonographic measurement of the respiratory variation in the inferior vena cava diameter is predictive of fluid responsiveness in critically ill patients: systematic review and meta-analysis. Ultrasound Med Biol. 2014;40(5):845–53.

33. Aya HD, Ster IC, Fletcher N, Grounds RM, et al. Pharmacodynamic analysis of a fluid challenge. Crit Care Med. 2016;44(5):880–91.

34. Whiting P, Rutjes AW, Reitsma JB, Bossuyt PM, et al. The development of QUADAS: a tool for the quality assessment of studies of diagnostic accuracy included in systematic reviews. BMC Med Res Methodol. 2003;3:25.

35. Zamora J, Abraira V, Muriel A, Khan K, et al. Meta-DiSc: a software for meta-analysis of test accuracy data. BMC Med Res Methodol. 2006;6:31.

36. Marik PE, Baram M, Vahid B. Does central venous pressure predict fluid responsiveness? A systematic review of the literature and the tale of seven mares. Chest. 2008;134(1):172–8.

37. Cannesson M. The "grey zone" or how to avoid the binary constraint of decision-making. Can J Anesth/J Can Anesth. 2015;62:1139–42.

9

Hyperchloraemia in sepsis

Christos Filis[1], Ioannis Vasileiadis[2*] and Antonia Koutsoukou[2]

Abstract

Chloride represents—quantitatively—the most prevalent, negatively charged, strong plasma electrolyte. Control of chloride concentration is a probable major mechanism for regulating the body's acid–base balance and for maintaining homeostasis of the entire internal environment. The difference between the concentrations of chloride and sodium constitutes the major contributor to the strong ion difference (SID); SID is the key pH regulator in the body, according to the physicochemical approach. Hyperchloraemia resulting from either underlying diseases or medical interventions is common in intensive care units. Recent studies have demonstrated the importance of hyperchloraemia in metabolic acidosis and in other pathophysiological disorders present in sepsis. The aim of this narrative review is to present the current knowledge about the effects of hyperchloraemia, in relation to the underlying pathophysiology, in septic patients.

Keywords: Hyperchloraemia, Chloride, Sepsis, Critically ill patients, Metabolic acidosis

Background

Sepsis and septic shock affect over 26 million people worldwide and remain the leading causes of death in the US hospitals, despite progress in early recognition and treatment [1]. Acidosis is a frequently identified acid–base disorder in patients with sepsis and is linked to different pathophysiological routes (type II respiratory failure, renal failure, lactic acidosis, ketoacidosis). Chloride (Cl^-) is the body's major anion, representing two-thirds of all negative charges in plasma and is also responsible for one-third of plasma tonicity [2]. Its role and significance in acid–base balance, osmosis, muscular activity and immunomodulation has been overshadowed by other serum electrolytes, even though chloride abnormalities have been detected in 25% of patients in the critical care setting [3]. Aggressive fluid resuscitation, with chloride-rich crystalloids, during the treatment of sepsis-induced hypoperfusion, may lead to iatrogenic hyperchloraemic acidosis [4]. The present review focuses on the effects of hyperchloraemia in septic patients (metabolic acidosis, haemodynamics, inflammatory response,

renal and gastrointestinal function, haemostatic disorders, mortality) and their underlying pathophysiology.

Main text

Hyperchloraemic metabolic acidosis

The major pathophysiological mechanisms leading to hyperchloraemic metabolic acidosis after fluid resuscitation with saline remain controversial. Van Slyke described the phenomenon of "dilution acidosis" almost 100 years ago [5], but the term was proposed after the Second World War [6]. He was the first to suggest that intravenous saline infusion leads to metabolic acidosis due to dilution of total body base. Further studies in non-intubated dogs showed that dilution acidosis was not related to the type of the solution used (0.9% saline, dextrose water 5%, mannitol 5%), since bicarbonate (HCO_3^-) dilution by the medium water produced acidosis of the same degree [7]. In the early 1980s Stewart [8] proposed an innovative model of acid–base balance regulation: changes in Cl^- concentration were suggested to be of particular importance, since it is the main negatively charged strong (fully dissociated) electrolyte in the extracellular space. According to Stewart's approach pH is determined by three independent variables: (i) strong ion difference (SID), which is the difference between the sum of all strong cations (Na^+, K^+, Ca^{2+}, Mg^{2+}) and the

*Correspondence: ioannisvmed@yahoo.gr
[2] Intensive Care Unit, 1st Department of Respiratory Medicine, "Sotiria" Hospital, National and Kapodistrian University of Athens, 152 Mesogion Av., 115 27 Athens, Greece

sum of all strong anions (Cl^-, other strong anions as lactate and ketones), (ii) partial pressure of carbon dioxide (PCO_2) and (iii) concentrations of non-volatile weak acids (A_{tot}), mainly albumin and phosphate. These variables change the degree of water dissociation into hydrogen and hydroxide ions according to three fundamental physicochemical principles that must be met simultaneously: (a) the law of mass preservation, (b) the law of electrical neutrality in aqueous solutions and thus in body fluids and (c) the law of mass action (i.e. the dissociation constant magnitude of weak electrolytes). The Cl^- concentration changes—due to either regulatory adaptations or underlying disorders of acid–base balance in the organism—may occur independently of sodium (Na^+) changes. Na^+ concentration is under hormonal control for the maintenance of plasma osmolality and water balance. Cl^- concentration can change by moving through cell membranes under the control of Donnan forces and by altered renal excretion depending on the acid–base status of the body [9]. Our knowledge about the function of Cl^- channels has grown considerably in recent years: for example renal excretion and reabsorption are mediated by Cl^- channels [10]; this knowledge has contributed to our understanding of the corresponding disorders by elucidating the pathophysiological mechanisms. In hyperchloraemia, increased Cl^- concentration decreases SID, which in turn leads to an increase in free H^+ ions [8]. The importance of Stewart's approach is clear in septic patients with low SID acidosis, who would have remained undiagnosed by changes in base excess, due to the alkalizing effect of hypoalbuminaemia [11].

However, there are indications that hyperchloraemia is not exclusively iatrogenic, but constitutes part of the pathophysiology of sepsis. Kellum and colleagues treated experimental shock (post-*E. coli* endotoxin infusion) in dogs with saline infusion. In this model it was demonstrated that the exogenous Cl^- administration could account for only one-third of the Cl^- serum increase, representing 38% of the total acid load; lactate contributed less than 10% of the acidic load at the end of the experimental period. The excess Cl^- was attributed to the activation of mechanisms that led to differential movements of Na^+ and Cl^- from intracellular to extracellular spaces or from extravascular to intravascular compartments; the endothelial injury and the extravasation of albumin might represent a scenario for this Cl^- movement [12].

Hyperchloraemia has been studied in children with meningococcal septic shock and was found to be the main cause of metabolic acidosis post-resuscitation [13]; this observation was confirmed 2 years later in critically ill, adult patients with severe sepsis and septic shock [14]. Szrama and Smuszkiewicz [15], analysing 990 arterial blood gas results from 43 septic intensive care unit (ICU) patients, found that low SID acidosis (increased Cl^-/Na^+ ratio) was the most frequent cause of acidosis, being present in 93.5% of blood samples. In a pilot study from our centre, the most important cause of metabolic acidosis in septic patients was hyperchloraemia and low SID [16]. In particular, the causes of metabolic acidosis were investigated in 94 patients with sepsis and septic shock on the day of ICU admission. Cl^- levels were significantly elevated, resulting in a low SID, in the metabolic acidosis group (BE < − 2 mEq/L), while lactic acid levels did not differ significantly among the subgroups of patients with low (< − 2 mEq/L), normal (between − 2 and + 2 mEq/L) or elevated (> 2 mEq/L) base excess values. Of note is the fact that in this ICU balanced crystalloid solutions (Ringer's lactate) are used for resuscitation, except for those cases requiring saline use (i.e. severe hyponatraemia).

Hyperchloraemia and inflammatory response during sepsis
Sepsis represents a state of hyperimmune response to an infection, with both pro-inflammatory (systemic inflammatory response syndrome—SIRS) and anti-inflammatory (compensatory anti-inflammatory response syndrome—CARS) pathways being activated [17]. The possible effects of hyperchloraemic acidosis on the host's immunity have been studied in experimental models.

Several studies [18–20] document that hydrochloric acid (HCl)-induced acidosis influences the TNF-α levels by enhancing TNF-α gene transcription [19]. However, a reduced TNF-α secretion is observed when pH reaches 7.0 or less [18] and the major pH-sensitive step(s) in TNF-α production appears to be located at a post-transcriptional level [21].

The upregulation of inducible nitric oxide synthase (iNOS) and the consequent overproduction of nitric oxide is associated with systemic hypotension and decreased vascular reactivity in septic patients [22]. Pedoto et al. [23, 24] reported the correlation of HCl-induced acidosis with increased iNOS activity, along with lung and intestinal injury in healthy rats. A previous study by Bellocq et al. [20] had suggested that lowering pH from 7.4 to 7.0 amplifies the nuclear factor-κB (NF-κB)-dependent iNOS pathway, by upregulating mRNA expression. However, extreme acidic conditions (pH 6.5) do not increase nitrite production [25], since the intracellular pH falls below 7.0, which has been suggested to be optimal for iNOS function [24].

The observed increase in both NF-κB binding activity in the nucleus and NF-κB-driven reporter gene expression under acidic conditions [20, 25] has been demonstrated to affect other inflammatory pathways. Kellum and co-workers studied the release of IL-6 and IL-10 in murine cell cultures stimulated with *E. coli* lipopolysaccharide after acidification with HCl. Extreme acidosis (pH 6.5) was associated with reduced release of both IL-6 and IL-10 as well as attenuated NF-κB DNA binding activity. However, the greater reduction in IL-10 levels led to a significant increase in IL-6 to IL-10 ratio from 5:1 at pH 7.4 to 55:1 at pH 6.5 [25]. In contrast to these in vitro results, data from experimental sepsis in rats suggest that both pro-inflammatory (TNF, IL-6) and anti-inflammatory (IL-10) mediators were increased by HCl infusion. The above results illustrate the major differences between ex vivo and in vivo models [26] due to a number of other parameters triggered by acidaemia (catecholamine synthesis, stimulation of vasopressin, adrenocorticotropic hormone and aldosterone).

In conclusion, hyperchloraemic acidification appears to have a main pro-inflammatory effect based on NO release, IL-6-to-IL-10 ratios and NF-κB binding activity demonstrated ex vivo. The reduced TNF-α secretion [18] and NF-κB binding activity [25] in severe acidosis suggest that not all pro-inflammatory pathways are preserved at the extremes of the acid–base homeostasis. In contrast, lactic acidosis appears to exhibit anti-inflammatory action by decreasing cytokine expression and NF-κB binding activity [25].

Hyperchloraemia and haemodynamics

Severe acidosis in sepsis is associated with haemodynamic instability through many different pathophysiologic mechanisms (reduced left ventricular contractility, diastolic dysfunction and right ventricular failure, predisposition to cardiac arrhythmias, arterial vasodilation, impaired responsiveness to catecholamines, reduced hepatic blood flow, impaired oxygen tissue delivery) [27]. Kellum et al. [28] demonstrated that hyperchloraemic acidosis reduced the mean arterial pressure (MAP) in normotensive septic rats; the decrease in MAP showed a higher correlation to plasma Cl^- elevation as compared to pH reduction. Moderate acidosis enhanced plasma nitrite levels, a result confirming previous studies by Pedoto et al. [24] who reported an increase in serum nitrite levels and a significant decrease in blood pressure in healthy rats after HCl-induced acidosis.

Hyperchloraemia and renal function

Among critically ill patients who develop acute kidney injury (AKI) almost 50% are septic. Furthermore, septic AKI is identified as an independent predictor of hospital death [29]. The administration of chloride-rich solutions and the probable adverse effects on kidney function have been studied in both animal and human trials.

An animal study performed by Wilcox indicated that intrarenal infusion of chloride-containing solutions led to renal vasoconstriction and fall in glomerular filtration rate (GFR). Chloride-induced vasoconstriction—which appeared to be specific for the renal vessels—was potentiated by previous salt depletion and related to tubular Cl^- reabsorption [30]. Pathophysiologically, this observation is attributed to high Cl^- sensitivity of K^+-induced smooth muscle cell contraction in the afferent arterioles [31] and also to the activation of tubuloglomerular negative feedback provoked by higher levels of Cl^- transport across the macula densa cells [32]. The chloride-induced thromboxane release—and its actions on the afferent and efferent arterioles that contribute to renal vascular resistance—offers an additional, hypothetical mechanism for the fall in GFR during hyperchloraemia [33]. An experimental study by Quilley suggested that exposure of isolated rat kidney to higher Cl^- concentration increased vasoconstrictor responses to angiotensin II (Ang II) [34]. However, a previous study in greyhounds had shown that hyperchloraemia also decreases generation of Ang II, questioning the role of intrarenal renin–angiotensin system in chloride-induced renal vasoconstriction in intact animals [35].

Studies in animals [36] and human volunteers [37] have shown a correlation between higher levels of inflammatory markers in sepsis with the development of AKI. The observed increase in IL-6 levels following saline resuscitation in septic animals and its association with increased AKI risk provide an additional explanation for renal dysfunction during sepsis resuscitation treatment [38].

Moving from animal to human studies, Williams and colleagues conducted a trial in healthy human volunteers and reported that infusion of large volumes of 0.9% saline (50 mL/kg) within 1 h resulted in lower pH and significantly prolonged the time until first urination compared to infusion of Ringer's lactate (RL) solution; the effect of acidosis persisted for 1 h beyond the end of infusion [39]. Other studies involving humans showed that the intravenous infusion of 2 L of 0.9% saline over 60 min resulted in a reduction in renal blood flow velocity and renal cortical tissue perfusion; such changes were not observed after infusion of balanced crystalloids [40]. The delayed time to first micturition in human volunteers, who had received 2 L intravenous infusions of 0.9% saline comparing to Hartman's solution (within 1 h, on separate occasions), was associated with the development of hyperchloraemia in all subjects; hyperchloraemia was recorded for 6 h from the beginning of the infusion. In contrast, serum chloride concentrations remained normal after Hartmann's infusion [41]. Although the infusion of a lower osmolality solution could relate to lower antidiuretic hormone secretion leading to earlier diuresis, the greater natriuresis observed could not support this theory [10]. A probable explanation might relate to chloride's vasoconstrictive action, boosted by the previously reported slower excess chloride excretion during administration of saline solutions [42].

Most studies examining the pathophysiological effects of hyperchloraemia on kidney function have not been performed in septic patients exclusively, but include a heterogeneous population of ICU patients. In a meta-analysis of studies relating intravenous resuscitation fluids administration to patient outcomes in the perioperative or intensive care setting, high-chloride fluids were associated with a significantly higher risk of acute kidney injury [43]. Two out of the 21 meta-analysed trials, that included general ICU patients, gave conflicting results. Yunos and colleagues studied a rather diverse population ($\sim 50\%$ post-operative, $\sim 7\%$ severe sepsis/septic shock patients) and demonstrated that chloride-restrictive intravenous fluids strategy was associated with a significant decrease in the incidence of (a) AKI, including the use of renal replacement therapy [44], (b) metabolic acidosis, (c) severe hyperchloraemia and (d) hypernatraemia [45]. On the contrary, the SPLIT trial (comparing saline vs balanced crystalloid) concluded that the type of crystalloid infused did not affect the incidence of AKI [46]. However, this study involved predominantly ICU post-operative population and sepsis was diagnosed in only 4% of the cases. In addition, the median volume of crystalloids infused was only 2000 cc, which might have affected the results as shown in the recently published SALT study. In this randomized trial on ICU patients the incidence of AKI did not differ between the two study arms (balanced crystalloids vs 0.9% saline). However, among patients who received larger volumes of fluids, those assigned to saline appeared to experience more major adverse kidney events [47]. The negative effect of the infused saline volume on kidney function has also been confirmed by two recent studies—a retrospective one by Sen et al. [48] and the SMART randomized trial [49]—involving critically ill patients. Furthermore, the SMART trial being a randomized study including 15,802 patients demonstrated a negative impact on renal function of saline infusion versus balanced crystalloids; this effect was even greater in the subgroup of 2336 septic patients.

Additional data from a retrospective cohort study suggest that maximal serum Cl^- concentration in the first 48 h after resuscitation of septic patients is associated with AKI. The increase in serum Cl^- exhibited a dose-dependent relationship with the severity of AKI, and remarkably, an increase in serum $Cl^- \geq 5$ mmol/L was associated with the development of AKI even among patients who remained normochloraemic [50]. These results are consistent with those of an earlier retrospective analysis of data from general ICU population. Zhang et al. demonstrated—for the first time—that higher maximal and mean Cl^- concentration values were associated

with the subsequent development of AKI, but the severity of AKI correlated only with the former [51]. Nevertheless, in a retrospective cohort study on septic patients published a year later [52] it was found that the prevalence of acute renal failure was independent of the crystalloid solution infused (balanced or isotonic saline). Therefore, large-scale randomized trials focusing on low versus high Cl^- strategy during fluid resuscitation in sepsis—as the ongoing FISSH trial [53]—must be undertaken for valid conclusions.

Effects of hyperchloraemia on the gastrointestinal tract

Experimental models have demonstrated the association of HCl-induced metabolic acidosis with reduced gastric motility in pigs [54] and intestinal injury in rats [23]. A trial among elderly surgical patients revealed a significant trend towards increased nausea and vomiting when saline infusion was compared to balanced fluids; two-third of the saline-treated patient group developed hyperchloraemic metabolic acidosis [55]. This information and the abdominal discomfort provoked in healthy subjects by saline infusion [39] suggest that hyperchloraemic acidosis could be associated with complications such as gastroparesis, emesis and altered intestinal permeability; further investigation on this subject is required.

Effects of hyperchloraemia on haemostasis and haemopoiesis

Coagulation activation during sepsis represents an important component of the overall response against invading pathogens [56]. This beneficial process can be reversed to a life-threatening event during severe inflammatory responses, since excessive thrombosis activation may lead to disseminated intravascular coagulation (DIC) and consumption of multiple clotting factors [57]. The correlation of hyperchloraemia during sepsis with coagulation has not been studied yet. A limited number of experimental and clinical studies [58, 59] suggest that large volumes of chloride-rich solutions lead to coagulation disorders and increased tendency for bleeding. However, coagulation abnormalities in substantial blood loss and haemorrhagic shock (and this was the case in the above-mentioned studies) are influenced by several factors—hormonal, immunological, extent of blood loss, hypoxia, acidosis, hypothermia—[60] that differ or may not be present in septic patients. On the other hand, the reduced coagulation proteases' activity observed in acidic pH [61] could affect the progression of sepsis in patients with hyperchloraemic acidosis by undermining coagulation activation; this hypothesis should be further investigated.

Anaemia is common in septic patients and is caused by shortening of red blood cell (RBC) circulatory lifespan (haemolysis, phlebotomy losses, invasive procedures, gastrointestinal bleeding, etc.) and/or diminished RBC production due to nutritional deficiencies, iron metabolism, inflammatory processes leading to impaired RBC proliferation, impaired erythropoietin production and signalling [62]. The results of a cohort study by Neyra et al. [63] in septic patients suggest that anaemia is more frequent in hyperchloraemic patients, requiring more blood transfusions compared to normochloraemic patients. A probable mechanism explaining this observation might relate to inhibition of erythropoietin production by pro-inflammatory cytokines [64] since the latter predominate in hyperchloraemic acidosis [25].

Hyperchloraemia and mortality in sepsis

The negative impact of hyperchloraemia on the mortality of septic [14] and critically ill [65] patients was first reported less than a decade ago. In contrast, data from a single-centre observational retrospective cohort study of critically ill septic patients suggested that Cl^- levels upon ICU admission were not related to hospital mortality. However, in subjects with deteriorating hyperchloraemia, higher levels of Cl^- (≥ 5 mEq/L) 72 h later were associated with increased hospital mortality [63]. Since the study population was limited to ICU patients, the acid–base balance could have been manipulated by fluid administration in the emergency room. Rochwerg et al. performed a meta-analysis of the effect different resuscitative fluids (crystalloids and colloids) had on the mortality rate in septic patients. A trend towards improved survival of patients resuscitated with balanced crystalloids compared to patients who received saline was noted at a 6-node meta-analysis level (crystalloids vs albumin vs hydroxyethyl starch vs gelatin, with crystalloids divided into balanced or unbalanced and hydroxyethyl starch divided into low or high molecular weight) [66]. Studies that compared chloride-rich versus balanced crystalloid solutions were designed and confirmed the previous findings. Shaw and colleagues conducted a retrospective cohort study that demonstrated an association between lower Cl^- load and lower mortality in hospitalized patients with SIRS; this observation was independent of the total fluid volume administered and remained significant after adjustment for illness severity [67]. Raghunathan et al. [52] confirmed the previous observation in septic patients who received greater proportions of balanced crystalloids. The retrospective study of Sen et al. [48] showed a negative association between higher Cl^- load and survival rate among ICU patients who had received large-volume fluids; this effect extended to at least 1 year post-ICU admission. The SMART randomized trial demonstrated a statistically significant higher 30-day in-hospital mortality in septic patients

treated with saline compared to those treated with balanced crystalloids [49].

Chloride-restrictive fluid administration

Saline 0.9% is the most commonly used crystalloid solution globally [50], even though doubts regarding its physiological effects had been raised as early as the end of the nineteenth century [68]; these observations led to the production of the first buffered solutions. The drastic changes in the pathophysiology of metabolic acidosis in sepsis within 8 h post-aggressive isotonic fluid resuscitation—from acidosis due to unmeasured anions to hyperchloraemic acidosis—[13] is an effect many clinicians are not aware of. This common condition among ICU patients [69] has probably influenced the clinical practice of intensivists, who favour the use of buffered crystalloid solutions over saline according to the FENICE study [70]. The latest Surviving Sepsis Campaign guidelines do not recommend balanced crystalloids over saline; however, close monitoring of chloride levels is advised for avoidance of hyperchloraemia [71]. Raised concerns about iatrogenic metabolic acidosis in critically ill patients are fully justified, because of the inadequate respiratory compensation and the anticipated exhaustion of buffering reserves [12]. It should be noted that from the studies mentioned, it cannot be safely ascertained whether the adverse events observed in the case of hyperchloraemia are due to elevated levels of Cl^- or acidosis per se.

The beneficial effect of balanced crystalloids is supported by the probable harmful effects of saline on MAP, renal haemodynamics and the gastrointestinal tract, particularly in the setting of sepsis-induced systemic hypoperfusion and lastly the higher mortality rates of patients receiving saline [49, 72]. Furthermore, among the ten studies (involving 15,000 critically ill patients) subjected to meta-analysis, none demonstrated superiority of saline in organ function or mortality rate over balanced crystalloids [43, 73]. The lower transfusion rate in patients receiving low-chloride balanced fluids supports the chloride-restrictive practice, although an incompatibility of calcium-containing buffered solutions and citrated blood cannot be excluded [43]. Buffered solutions have been associated with lower prevalence of SIRS and C-reactive protein levels—compared to saline in patients with acute pancreatitis [74]—and a lower risk of postoperative infections after open abdominal surgeries [75]; such observations are compatible with the pro-inflammatory effects of saline-induced hyperchloraemic acidosis demonstrated in experimental models. Up to date, saline remains the fluid of choice in septic patients with comorbidities such as severe hyponatraemia, cerebral oedema and brain injury [76].

Conclusions

Chloride, as the major anion of the extracellular fluid, constitutes an important element in the homeostasis of the human organism. Hyperchloraemia, whether a result of the sepsis process or a consequence of its treatment with supraphysiologic chloride fluids, appears to have a negative impact on the clinical outcome of septic patients. The detrimental effect of hyperchloraemic acidosis on the inflammatory response, on haemodynamics and also upon the homeostasis of organs or systems, demonstrated by studies in humans and some experimental models of sepsis, should keep clinicians alert. Close monitoring of chloride levels and acid–base homeostasis pertains to all levels of hospitalization, starting with the early resuscitation treatment in the emergency room. Balanced crystalloids appear to improve the sepsis outcome, when compared to saline. Large-scale randomized trials analysing more than one endpoint (mortality, haemodynamics, AKI, haemostatic disorders, other organ damage, length of ICU and hospital stay) are urgently needed in order to confirm the possible beneficial effect of chloride restriction strategies.

Abbreviations

Cl^-: chloride; SID: strong ion difference; PCO_2: partial pressure of carbon dioxide; A_{tot}: non-volatile weak acids; Na^+: sodium; ICU: intensive care unit; SIRS: systemic inflammatory response syndrome; CARS: compensatory anti-inflammatory response syndrome; HCl: hydrochloric acid; iNOS: inducible nitric oxide synthase; NF-κB: nuclear factor-κB; MAP: mean arterial pressure; AKI: acute kidney injury; GFR: glomerular filtration rate; Ang II: angiotensin II; RL: Ringer's lactate; DIC: disseminated intravascular coagulation; RBC: red blood cell.

Authors' contributions

CF drafted the majority of the manuscript. IV conceived the idea, contributed to manuscript drafting and revised critically the manuscript. AK was responsible for the final review of the manuscript. All authors read and approved the final manuscript.

Author details

[1] 3rd Department of Internal Medicine, "Sotiria" Hospital, National and Kapodistrian University of Athens, 152 Mesogion Av., 115 27 Athens, Greece.
[2] Intensive Care Unit, 1st Department of Respiratory Medicine, "Sotiria" Hospital, National and Kapodistrian University of Athens, 152 Mesogion Av., 115 27 Athens, Greece.

Acknowledgements

None.

Competing interests

The authors declare that they have no competing interests.

Funding

No funding was obtained for the creation of this review.

References

1. Liu V, Escobar GJ, Greene JD, Soule J, Whippy A, Angus DC, et al. Hospital deaths in patients with sepsis from 2 independent cohorts. JAMA. 2014;312(1):90–2.
2. Berend K, Van Hulsteijn LH, Gans ROB. Chloride: the queen of electrolytes? Eur J Intern Med. 2012;23(3):203–11.
3. Tani M, Morimatsu H, Takatsu F, Morita K. The incidence and prognostic value of hypochloremia in critically ill patients. Sci World J. 2012;2012:474185.
4. Kellum JA. Metabolic acidosis in patients with sepsis: epiphenomenon or part of the pathophysiology? Crit Care Resusc. 2004;6(3):197–203.
5. Van Slyke DD, Wu H, McLean FC. Studies of gas and electrolyte equilibria in the blood. V. Factors controlling the electrolyte and water distribution in the blood. J Biol Chem. 1923;56:765–849.
6. Shires GT, Holman J. Dilution acidosis. Ann Intern Med. 1948;28(3):557–9.
7. Asano S, Kato E, Yamauchi M, Ozawa Y, Iwasa M, Wada T, et al. The mechanism of the acidosis caused by infusion of saline solution. Lancet. 1966;287(7449):1245–6.
8. Stewart PA. Modern quantitative acid–base chemistry. Can J Physiol Pharmacol. 1983;61(12):1444–61.
9. Stewart PA. Whole-body acid–base balance. In: Kellum JA, Elbers P, editors. Stewart's textbook of acid–base. 2nd ed. Morrisville: Lullu Enterprises; 2009. p. 181–97.
10. Yunos NM, Bellomo R, Story D, Kellum J. Bench-to-bedside review: chloride in critical illness. Crit Care. 2010;14(4):226.
11. Mallat J, Michel D, Salaun P, Thevenin D, Tronchon L. Defining metabolic acidosis in patients with septic shock using Stewart approach. Am J Emerg Med. 2012;30(3):391–8.
12. Kellum JA, Bellomo R, Kramer DJ, Pinsky MR. Etiology of metabolic acidosis during saline resuscitation in endotoxemia. Shock. 1998;9(5):364–8.
13. O'Dell E, Tibby SM, Durward A, Murdoch IA. Hyperchloremia is the dominant cause of metabolic acidosis in the postresuscitation phase of pediatric meningococcal sepsis. Crit Care Med. 2007;35(10):2390–4.
14. Noritomi DT, Soriano FG, Kellum JA, Cappi SB, Biselli PJC, Libório AB, et al. Metabolic acidosis in patients with severe sepsis and septic shock: a longitudinal quantitative study. Crit Care Med. 2009;37(10):2733–9.
15. Szrama J, Smuszkiewicz P. An acid–base disorders analysis with the use of the Stewart approach in patients with sepsis treated in an intensive care unit. Anesthesiol Intensive Ther. 2016;48(3):180–4.
16. Vasileiadis I, Kompoti M, Tripodaki ES, Rovina N, Pontikis K, Ntouka E, et al. Metabolic acidosis in patients with sepsis. ESICM LIVES 2017. Intensive Care Med Exp. 2017;5(S2):542.
17. Ward NS, Casserly B, Ayala A. The compensatory anti-inflammatory response syndrome (CARS) in critically ill patients. Clin Chest Med. 2008;29(4):617–25.
18. Bidani A, Wang C-Z, Saggi SJ, Heming TA. Evidence for pH sensitivity of tumor necrosis factor-alpha release by alveolar macrophages. Lung. 1998;176(2):111–21.
19. Heming TA, Davé SK, Tuazon DM, Chopra AK, Peterson JW, Bidani A. Effects of extracellular pH on tumour necrosis factor-alpha production by resident alveolar macrophages. Clin Sci. 2001;101(3):267–74.
20. Bellocq A, Suberville S, Philippe C, Bertrand F, Perez J, Fouqueray B, et al. Low environmental pH is responsible for the induction of nitric-oxide synthase in macrophages. Evidence for involvement of nuclear factor-kappaB activation. J Biol Chem. 1998;273(9):5086–92.
21. Heming TA, Tuazon DM, Davé SK, Chopra AK, Peterson JW, Bidani A. Post-transcriptional effects of extracellular pH on tumour necrosis factor-a production in RAW 246.7 and J774 A.1 cells. Clin Sci. 2001;100(3):259–66.
22. Nava E, Palmer RMJ, Moncada S. Inhibition of nitric oxide synthesis in septic shock: how much is beneficial? Lancet. 1991;338(8782–8783):1555–7.

23. Pedoto A, Nandi J, Oler A, Camporesi EM, Hakim TS, Levine RA. Role of nitric oxide in acidosis-induced intestinal injury in anesthetized rats. J Lab Clin Med. 2001;138(4):270–6.

24. Pedoto A, Caruso JE, Nandi J, Oler A, Hoffman SP, Tassioupolos AK, et al. Acidosis stimulates nitric oxide production and lung damage in rats. Am J Respir Crit Care Med. 1999;159(2):397–402.

25. Kellum JA, Song M, Li J. Lactic and hydrochloric acids induce different patterns of inflammatory response in LPS-stimulated RAW 264.7 cells. AJP Regul Integr Comp Physiol. 2004;286(4):R686–92.

26. Kellum JA, Song M, Almasri E. Hyperchloremic acidosis increases circulating inflammatory molecules in experimental sepsis. Chest. 2006;130(4):962–7.

27. Velissaris D, Karamouzos V, Ktenopoulos N, Pierrakos C, Karanikolas M. The use of sodium bicarbonate in the treatment of acidosis in sepsis: a literature update on a long term debate. Crit Care Res Pract. 2015;2015:605830.

28. Kellum JA, Song M, Venkataraman R. Effects of hyperchloremic acidosis on arterial pressure and circulating inflammatory molecules in experimental sepsis. Chest. 2004;125(1):243–8.

29. Bagshaw SM, Uchino S, Bellomo R, Morimatsu H, Morgera S, Schetz M, et al. Septic acute kidney injury in critically ill patients: clinical characteristics and outcomes. Clin J Am Soc Nephrol. 2007;2(3):431–9.

30. Wilcox CS. Regulation of renal blood flow by plasma chloride. J Clin Invest. 1983;71(3):726–35.

31. Hansen PB, Jensen BL, Skott O. Chloride regulates afferent arteriolar contraction in response to depolarization. Hypertension. 1998;32(6):1066–70.

32. Schnermann J, Ploth DW, Hermle M. Activation of tubulo-glomerular feedback by chloride transport. Pflugers Arch. 1976;362(3):229–40.

33. Bullivant EM, Wilcox CS, Welch WJ, Mary E, Bullivant A, Wilcox CS, et al. Intrarenal vasoconstriction during hyperchloremia: role of thromboxane. Am J Physiol Renal Physiol. 1989;256(1 Pt 2):F152–7.

34. Quilley CP, Lin YR, McGiff JC. Chloride anion concentration as a determinant of renal vascular responsiveness to vasoconstrictor agents. Br J Pharmacol. 1993;108(1):106–10.

35. Wilcox CS, Peart WS. Release of renin and angiotensin II into plasma and lymph during hyperchloremia. Am J Physiol. 1987;253(4 Pt 2):F734–41.

36. Peng Z-Y, Wang H-Z, Srisawat N, Wen X, Rimmelé T, Bishop J, et al. Bactericidal antibiotics temporarily increase inflammation and worsen acute kidney injury in experimental sepsis. Crit Care Med. 2012;40(2):538–43.

37. Murugan R, Karajala-Subramanyam V, Lee M, Yende S, Kong L, Carter M, et al. Acute kidney injury in non-severe pneumonia is associated with an increased immune response and lower survival. Kidney Int. 2010;77(6):527–35.

38. Zhou F, Peng Z-Y, Bishop JV, Cove ME, Singbartl K, Kellum JA. Effects of fluid resuscitation with 0.9% saline versus a balanced electrolyte solution on acute kidney injury in a rat model of sepsis. Crit Care Med. 2014;42(4):e270–8.

39. Williams EL, Hildebrand KL, McCormick SA, Bedel MJ. The effect of intravenous lactated Ringer's solution versus 0.9% sodium chloride solution on serum osmolality in human volunteers. Anesth Analg. 1999;88(5):999–1003.

40. Chowdhury AH, Cox EF, Francis ST, Lobo DN. A, randomized, controlled, double-blind crossover study on the effects of 2-L infusions of 0.9% saline and plasma-lyte® 148 on renal blood flow velocity and renal cortical tissue perfusion in healthy volunteers. Ann Surg. 2012;256(1):18–24.

41. Reid F, Lobo DN, Williams RN, Rowlands BJ, Allison SP. (Ab)normal saline and physiological Hartmann's solution: a randomized double-blind crossover study. Clin Sci. 2003;104(1):17–24.

42. Veech RL. The toxic impact of parenteral solutions on the metabolism of cells: a hypothesis for physiological parenteral therapy. Am J Clin Nutr. 1986;44(4):519–51.

43. Krajewski ML, Raghunathan K, Paluszkiewicz SM, Schermer CR, Shaw AD. Meta-analysis of high- versus low-chloride content in perioperative and critical care fluid resuscitation. Br J Surg. 2015;102(1):24–36.

44. Yunos NM, Bellomo R, Hegarty C, Story D, Ho L, Bailey M. Association between a chloride-liberal vs chloride-restrictive intravenous fluid administration strategy and kidney injury in critically ill adults. JAMA. 2012;308(15):1566–72.

45. Yunos NM, Kim IB, Bellomo R, Bailey M, Ho L, Story D, et al. The biochemical effects of restricting chloride-rich fluids in intensive care. Crit Care Med. 2011;39(11):2419–24.

46. Young P, Bailey M, Beasley R, Henderson S, Mackle D, McArthur C, et al. Effect of a buffered crystalloid solution vs saline on acute kidney injury among patients in the intensive care unit: the SPLIT Randomized Clinical Trial. JAMA. 2015;314(16):1701–10.

47. Semler MW, Wanderer JP, Ehrenfeld JM, Stollings JL, Self WH, Siew ED, et al. Balanced crystalloids versus saline in the intensive care unit. The SALT Randomized Trial. Am J Respir Crit Care Med. 2017;195(10):1362–72.

48. Sen A, Keener CM, Sileanu FE, Foldes E, Clermont G, Murugan R, et al. Chloride content of fluids used for large-volume resuscitation is associated with reduced survival. Crit Care Med. 2017;45(2):e146–53.

49. Semler MW, Self WH, Wanderer JP, Ehrenfeld JM, Wang L, Byrne DW, et al. Balanced crystalloids versus saline in critically ill adults. N Engl J Med. 2018;378(9):829–39.

50. Suetrong B, Pisitsak C, Boyd JH, Russell JA, Walley KR. Hyperchloremia and moderate increase in serum chloride are associated with acute kidney injury in severe sepsis and septic shock patients. Crit Care. 2016;20(1):315.

51. Zhang Z, Xu X, Fan H, Li D, Deng H. Higher serum chloride concentrations are associated with acute kidney injury in unselected critically ill patients. BMC Nephrol. 2013;14(1):235.

52. Raghunathan K, Shaw A, Nathanson B, Stürmer T, Brookhart A, Stefan MS, et al. Association between the choice of IV crystalloid and in-hospital mortality among critically ill adults with sepsis. Crit Care Med. 2014;42(7):1585–91.

53. Rochwerg B, Millen T, Austin P, Zeller M, D'Aragon F, Jaeschke R, et al. Fluids in Sepsis and Septic Shock (FISSH): protocol for a pilot randomised controlled trial. BMJ Open. 2017;7(7):e017602.

54. Tournadre JP, Allaouchiche B, Malbert CH, Chassard D. Metabolic acidosis and respiratory acidosis impair gastro-pyloric motility in anesthetized pigs. Anesth Analg. 2000;90(1):74–9.

55. Wilkes NJ, Woolf R, Mutch M, Mallett SV, Peachey T, Stephens R, et al. The effects of balanced versus saline-based hetastarch and crystalloid solutions on acid–base and electrolyte status and gastric mucosal perfusion in elderly surgical patients. Anesth Analg. 2001;93(4):811–6.

56. Fiusa MML, Carvalho-Filho MA, Annichino-Bizzacchi JM, De Paula EV. Causes and consequences of coagulation activation in sepsis: an evolutionary medicine perspective. BMC Med. 2015;13(1):105.

57. Levi M, van der Poll T. Inflammation and coagulation. Crit Care Med. 2010;38(Suppl 2):S26–34.

58. Todd SR, Malinoski D, Muller PJ, Schreiber MA. Lactated Ringer's is superior to normal saline in the resuscitation of uncontrolled hemorrhagic shock. J Trauma Inj Infect Crit Care. 2007;62(3):636–9.

59. Waters JH, Gottlieb A, Schoenwald P, Popovich MJ, Sprung J, Nelson DR. Normal saline versus lactated Ringer's solution for intraoperative fluid management in patients undergoing abdominal aortic aneurysm repair: an outcome study. Anesth Analg. 2001;93(4):817–22.

60. Cap A, Hunt BJ. The pathogenesis of traumatic coagulopathy. Anaesthesia. 2015;70(Suppl 1):96–101.

61. Meng ZH, Wolberg AS, Monroe DM, Hoffman M. The effect of temperature and ph on the activity of factor VIIa: implications for the efficacy of high-dose factor VIIa in hypothermic and acidotic patients. J Trauma Inj Infect Crit Care. 2003;55(5):886–91.

62. Hayden SJ, Albert TJ, Watkins TR, Swenson ER. Anemia in critical illness: insights into etiology, consequences, and management. Am J Respir Crit Care Med. 2012;185(10):1049–57.

63. Neyra JA, Canepa-Escaro F, Li X, Manllo J, Adams-Huet B, Yee J, et al. Association of hyperchloremia with hospital mortality in critically ill septic patients. Crit Care Med. 2015;43(9):1938–44.

64. Jelkmann W. Proinflammatory cytokines lowering erythropoietin production. J Interf Cytokine Res. 1998;8(8):555–9.

65. Boniatti MM, Cardoso PRC, Castilho RK, Vieira SRR. Is hyperchloremia associated with mortality in critically ill patients? A prospective cohort study. J Crit Care. 2011;26(2):175–9.

66. Rochwerg B, Alhazzani W, Sindi A, Heels-Ansdell D, Thabane L, Fox-Robichaud A, et al. Fluid resuscitation in sepsis: a systematic review and network meta-analysis. Ann Intern Med. 2014;161(5):347–55.

67. Shaw AD, Raghunathan K, Peyerl FW, Munson SH, Paluszkiewicz SM, Schermer CR. Association between intravenous chloride load during resuscitation and in-hospital mortality among patients with SIRS. Intensive Care Med. 2014;40(12):1897–905.

68. Hahn RG II. Should anaesthetists stop infusing isotonic saline? Br J Anaesth. 2014;112(1):4–6.

69. Klemz K, Ho L, Bellomo R. Daily intravenous chloride load and the acid–base and biochemical status of intensive care unit patients. J Pharm Pract Res. 2008;38(4):296–9.

70. Cecconi M, Hofer C, Teboul J-L, Pettila V, Wilkman E, Molnar Z, et al. Fluid challenges in intensive care: the FENICE study. Intensive Care Med. 2015;41(9):1529–37.

71. Rhodes A, Evans LE, Alhazzani W, Levy MM, Antonelli M, Ferrer R, et al. Surviving sepsis campaign. Crit Care Med. 2017;45(3):486–552.

72. Rochwerg B, Alhazzani W, Gibson A, Ribic CM, Sindi A, Heels-Ansdell D, et al. Fluid type and the use of renal replacement therapy in sepsis: a systematic review and network meta-analysis.

73. Semler MW, Rice TW. Saline is not the first choice for crystalloid resuscitation fluids. Crit Care Med. 2016;44(8):1541–4.

74. Wu BU, Hwang JQ, Gardner TH, Repas K, Delee R, Yu S, et al. Lactated Ringer's solution reduces systemic inflammation compared with saline in patients with acute pancreatitis. Clin Gastroenterol Hepatol. 2011;9(8):710–7.

75. Shaw AD, Bagshaw SM, Goldstein SL, Scherer LA, Duan M, Schermer CR, et al. Major complications, mortality, and resource utilization after open abdominal surgery. Ann Surg. 2012;255(5):821–9.

76. Myburgh JA, Mythen MG. Resuscitation fluids. N Engl J Med. 2013;369(13):1243–51.

10

Internal jugular vein variability predicts fluid responsiveness in cardiac surgical patients with mechanical ventilation

Guo-guang Ma[†], Guang-wei Hao[†], Xiao-mei Yang, Du-ming Zhu, Lan Liu, Hua Liu, Guo-wei Tu[*] and Zhe Luo[*]

Abstract

Background: To evaluate the efficacy of using internal jugular vein variability (IJVV) as an index of fluid responsiveness in mechanically ventilated patients after cardiac surgery.

Methods: Seventy patients were assessed after cardiac surgery. Hemodynamic data coupled with ultrasound evaluation of IJVV and inferior vena cava variability (IVCV) were collected and calculated at baseline, after a passive leg raising (PLR) test and after a 500-ml fluid challenge. Patients were divided into volume responders (increase in stroke volume $\geq$ 15%) and non-responders (increase in stroke volume < 15%). We compared the differences in measured variables between responders and non-responders and tested the ability of the indices to predict fluid responsiveness.

Results: Thirty-five (50%) patients were fluid responders. Responders presented higher IJVV, IVCV and stroke volume variation (SVV) compared with non-responders at baseline ($P < 0.05$). The relationship between IJVV and SVV was moderately correlated ($r = 0.51$, $P < 0.01$). The areas under the receiver operating characteristic (ROC) curves for predicting fluid responsiveness were 0.88 (CI 0.78–0.94) for IJVV compared with 0.83 (CI 0.72–0.91), 0.97 (CI 0.89–0.99), 0.91 (CI 0.82–0.97) for IVCV, SVV, and the increase in stroke volume in response to a PLR test, respectively.

Conclusions: Ultrasound-derived IJVV is an accurate, easily acquired noninvasive parameter of fluid responsiveness in mechanically ventilated postoperative cardiac surgery patients, with a performance similar to that of IVCV.

Keywords: Internal jugular veins, Inferior vena cava, Stroke volume variation, Fluid responsiveness, Cardiac surgery

Background

Fluid management is one of the most important treatments for stabilizing hemodynamics in patients after cardiac surgery. Hypovolemia may lead to inadequate organ perfusion, whereas fluid overload may lead to postoperative complications such as congestive heart failure or pulmonary edema [1–3]. In addition, patients who underwent cardiac surgery have a certain degree of myocardial stunning [4], and hence, caution should be taken regarding fluid management in patients with a limited cardiac reserve.

It is imperative to predict the patient's fluid responsiveness before volume expansion [5]. Several parameters have been introduced in clinical practice to predict fluid responsiveness and to guide therapy [2]. Based on the influence of cycling intra-thoracic pressure on arterial pulse pressure or stroke volume, dynamic indicators such as arterial pulse pressure variation (PPV) or stroke volume variation (SVV) have been widely used as reliable predictors of fluid responsiveness [6–8]. However, these dynamic parameters have several limitations and can only be used under strict conditions.

Recently, noninvasive and point-of-care ultrasound seems to meet the criteria of an ideal bedside tool for fluid status assessment. Several studies have confirmed

*Correspondence: tu.guowei@zs-hospital.sh.cn; luo.zhe@zs-hospital.sh.cn
[†]Guo-guang Ma and Guang-wei Hao have contributed equally to this work
Department of Critical Care Medicine, Zhongshan Hospital, Fudan University, No. 180 Fenglin Road, Shanghai 200032, Xuhui District, People's Republic of China

that respiratory variations of the superior and inferior vena cava diameters (collapsibility index [CI] and distensibility index [DI]) accurately reflect volume responsiveness in mechanically ventilated patients [9, 10]. Unfortunately, measurements of the inferior vena cava (IVC) and superior vena cava (SVC) may fail to predict fluid responsiveness following cardiac surgery due to methodological problems such as poor subcostal caval image quality caused by mediastinal air, surgical drains, dressings, abdominal distension or morbid obesity [11–13]; a more accurate measurement would require transoesophageal echocardiography (TEE). It is well known that pressure and volume changes within the intra-thoracic systemic venous compartment can transmit to the extrathoracic veins, for example, the intra-abdominal IVC or extrathoracic internal jugular vein (IJV) [14–16]. The IJV is, technically, much more easily accessible for sonographic visualization than the IVC, and measurement of the IJV does not require TEE. Internal jugular vein variability (IJVV) has been studied in several studies [17–19], but its reliability has not been well confirmed in patients after cardiac surgery. The aim of this study was to evaluate the reliability of IJVV, as visualized by ultrasound, to predict fluid responsiveness in mechanically ventilated patients after cardiac surgery.

Methods

This study was approved by the Ethical Committee of Zhongshan Hospital affiliated to Fudan University (No. B2016077), and informed consent was obtained from all study participants. This trial has been registered at clinicaltrials.gov as NCT02852889.

Patient selection

Patients who underwent cardiac surgery between August and December 2016 in the Cardiac Surgery Intensive Care Unit (CSICU) of the Zhongshan Hospital of Fudan University were screened for inclusion by research personnel. All patients routinely underwent a TEE during the operation and a postoperative (after admission to ICU and prior to study enrollment) comprehensive transthoracic echocardiography (TTE). The TEE was used to monitor the hemodynamics and confirm the postoperative effect of surgery. TTE was used to identify different causes of hypotension in postoperative period such as obstructive shock, hypovolemia and reduced ventricular systolic function. The patients were included when they presented with circulatory instability and required a rapid fluid challenge based on the clinical judgment of the attending physician. The physician's decision was principally based on the presence of clinical signs of acute circulatory failure (low blood pressure or urine output, tachycardia, or mottling) and/or clinical signs of organ

hypoperfusion (renal dysfunction or hyperlactatemia). The exclusion criteria included age < 18 years; evidence of cardiac arrhythmia (e.g., atrial fibrillation); evidence of jugular vein thrombosis; bilaterally inserted venous catheters (jugular or subclavian vein); echocardiographic examination that showed the existence of severe tricuspid or mitral regurgitation or right heart dysfunction (right ventricular fractional area change < 40% examined by TEE; tricuspid annular plane systolic excursion < 16 mm examined by TTE); a history of radiotherapy or surgery of the neck region or back (making it impossible to put the patient in a supine position with the head elevated to 30°); a contraindication to the passive leg raising (PLR) test; and the inability to obtain interpretable ultrasound images due to a difficult acoustic window.

All enrolled patients were sedated via propofol and morphine infusion, and with absence of inspiratory efforts according to the ventilator waveform and monitoring parameters. No muscular blocking agents were used in this study. All patients were ventilated in the intermittent positive pressure ventilation (IPPV) mode in the supine position with the head elevated to 30°. The ventilatory parameters were adjusted to the following criteria: tidal volume (Vt): 8 ml/kg predicted body weight (PBW), Pplat < 30 cmH$_2$O, positive end-expiratory pressure (PEEP): 5 cmH$_2$O, respiratory rate: 12–16 breaths per minute, PaCO$_2$ ≤ 45 mmHg and oxygen saturation (SaO$_2$) > 96%. The following baseline data were recorded for each patient: age (years), weight (kg), height (cm), diagnosis, type of cardiac surgery, acute physiology and chronic health evaluation (APACHE) II score, European system for cardiac operative risk evaluation (Euro-SCORE), vasoactive drug infusion rates and preoperative echocardiographic parameters [left ventricular ejection fraction (LVEF), presence of left ventricular hypertrophy, right ventricular end-diastolic diameter, and tricuspid regurgitation grade].

Measurements

We analyzed a series of measured hemodynamic variables from an indwelling radial arterial catheter and central venous catheter in each patient. These data included heart rate (HR) (beats/minute), mean arterial pressure (MAP) (mmHg), central venous pressure (CVP) (mmHg), stroke volume (SV) (ml), PLR-induced increase in stroke volume (PLR-ΔSV) (ml), and stroke volume variation (SVV) using the FloTrac/Vigileo (Edwards Lifesciences, Irvine, CA, USA) continuous hemodynamic monitoring system. The pressure transducers were consistently adjusted to the level of the patient's right atrium.

Intensivists with a certification of ultrasound evaluation performed all of the ultrasound examinations. An associate critical care professor supervised the entire course of examinations. The intensivists performing the ultrasound examinations were blinded to the hemo-dynamic data. (These were collected by another inves-tigator.) Sonographic measurements of the IJV and IVC diameters were taken using a Philips CX50 ultra-sound device (Philips Healthcare, Hamburg, Germany) equipped with a linear transducer (L12-3 Broadband Lin-ear Array Transducer) and a transthoracic phased array transducer (S5-1 Phased Array Transducer), respectively.

Patients admitted at the ICU after cardiac surgery had a conventional right IJV catheter. To avoid any risk of infec-tion at the puncture site, sonographic measurements were taken on the left IJV. The IJV was visualized by placing the ultrasound transducer perpendicular to the skin in the transverse plane on the patient's neck at the level of the cricoid cartilage in order to avoid interference from the probe-to-vein angle. The vein was identified by compres-sion as well as by color Doppler imaging. To avoid any influence of external compression on the IJV diameter during the examination, sufficient ultrasound gel was used to prevent direct skin contact with the transducer [20], and thus, the least amount of pressure was applied (Fig. 1a).

An M-mode scan was recorded over a whole respira-tory cycle (Fig. 1b, c), and then, the image was frozen. The maximum antero-posterior diameter of the IJV was measured at the end of inspiration [diamax (cm)], and the minimum diameter was measured at the end of expira-tion [diamin (cm)]. The IJV variability (IJVV) was calcu-lated using the formula: IJVV (%) = (diamax − diamin)/ [(diamax + diamin)/2] × 100. Using similar methods, the IVC was visualized longitudinally in the subxyphoid long-axis view, and its M-mode cursor was used to measure the IVC variability (IVCV) approximately 3 cm from the right atrium.

Study design

Ultrasound examinations and the collection of hemody-namic data were performed at baseline (T0, in a supine position with the head elevated to 30° for baseline measurements), 1 min after a PLR test (T1, the bed was automatically moved to a position with the head ele-vated to 0° and the legs up to 45°) and after a 500-mL Gelofusine challenge (T2, the bed was returned to the initial position, and fluid was infused over 30 min). PLR was performed in order to compare the predictive value of different parameters in predicting fluid responsive-ness. Vasoactive drug infusion rates and ventilation set-tings were kept constant during the study procedures. Patients were classified as "volume responders" if there was an increase in SV ≥ 15% after the fluid challenge, and the remaining patients were classified as "volume non-responders" [21, 22].

Statistical analysis

The number of the enrolled patients was referred to similar studies evaluating the prediction ability of IJVV [17–19]. All continuous variables except the doses of nor-epinephrine and dobutamine were normally distributed (Kolmogorov–Smirnov test). The results are expressed as the mean ± SD (standard deviation) or median (25–75% inter-quartile range, IQR) as appropriate. After check-ing the homogeneity of variance for each parameter, the difference between values was compared using the inde-pendent sample t test, and the comparisons of hemo-dynamic variables between the different study times were assessed using paired Student t tests. Comparisons between responders and non-responders were assessed using two-sample Student's t tests. P values < 0.05 were considered statistically significant. Correlations were assessed by Pearson coefficient. Receiver operating char-acteristic (ROC) curves were constructed to establish the sensitivity and specificity of dynamic and static indica-tors in predicting fluid responsiveness. The areas under the ROC curves (AUCs) were compared using DeLong and colleagues' test. The optimal cutoff of each variable was estimated by maximizing the Youden index. A differ-ence between two AUCs was considered statistically sig-nificant, when the P value of DeLong and colleagues' test

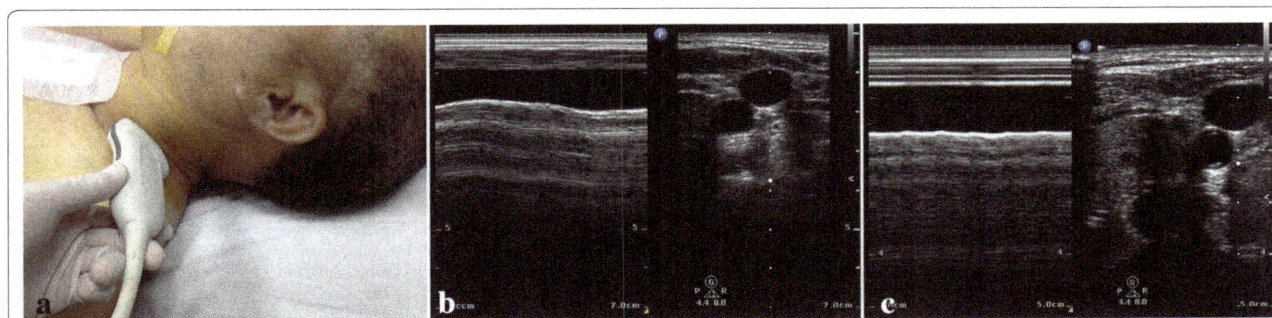

Fig. 1 Ultrasound probe position for IJV detection at the cricoid cartilage level (**a**). The patient is in the supine position at 30°. M-mode assessment of the antero-posterior diameter of the IJV in a responsive patient (**b**, a high variability of IJV diameter is seen) and in a non-responsive patient (**c**, lack of variation of the IJV diameter is seen) while on mechanical ventilation

was < 0.05. Statistical analyses were performed with the MedCalc 8.1.0.0 (Mariakerke, Belgium) and SPSS software (19.0).

Results

A total of seventy-five postoperative cardiac surgery patients were enrolled during a period of 5 months. Five patients were excluded because visualization of the IVC via ultrasound was technically difficult. Seventy patients (44 males and 26 females) were included in the final analysis. The reasons for hemodynamic instability were related to the hypovolemia (35 patients), cardiac dysfunction (27 patients) and vasoplegic shock (8 patients). The mean age of the patients was 61 ± 10 years, and the APACHE II scores were 9 ± 5. All patients were sedated and were in sinus rhythm. The patients' mean LVEF (Simpson's method) before surgery was 50%. Baseline patient characteristics and clinical data are shown in Table 1. Hemodynamic and ultrasound data in responders and non-responders at all study times [baseline

(T0), during PLR (T1), and after fluid challenge (T2)] are reported in Table 2. Fluid challenge significantly increased SV by more than 15% in 35 (50%) patients (responders, from 39.87 ± 13.67 to 58.72 ± 22.16 ml, $P < 0.05$). The remaining 35 (50%) patients did not exhibit a significant change in SV (non-responders, from 49.86 ± 17.71 to 54.81 ± 16.53 ml). The results of PLR and fluid challenge in this study are shown in Additional file 1.

Table 1 Baseline characteristics of the patients ($n = 70$)

Characteristic	
Age (years)	61 ± 10
Male sex, n (%)	44 (62.86)
Body mass index (kg/m^2)	22 ± 3
Left ventricular ejection fraction (%)	50
Cardiac surgery category, n (%)	
Valve	37 (52.86)
CABG	12 (17.14)
CABG + valve	7 (10.00)
Aortic surgery	9 (12.86)
Others	5 (7.14)
Postoperative day, n (%)	
d0	62 (88.57%)
d1	8 (11.43%)
APACHE II scores	9 ± 5
EuroSCORE	4 ± 2
Tidal volume (mL)	520 ± 28
PEEP (cm H$_2$O)	5
PaO$_2$/FiO$_2$ (mmHg)	123 ± 57
Lactate (mmol/L)	3.23 ± 3.39
Patients receiving norepinephrine, n (%)	45 (64.29)
Patients receiving dobutamine, n (%)	9 (12.86)
Dose of norepinephrine (µg kg^{-1} min^{-1})	0.24 (0.15–0.35)
Dose of dobutamine (µg kg^{-1} min^{-1})	0.33 (0.28–0.43)

Values are expressed as mean $\pm$ SD, median (25–75% inter-quartile range) or number and frequency in %

CABG coronary artery bypass grafting, APACHE II acute physiology and chronic health evaluation, EuroSCORE European system for cardiac operative risk evaluation, PEEP positive end-expiratory pressure, PaO$_2$ arterial partial pressure of oxygen, FiO$_2$ inspiratory fraction of oxygen

Table 2 Hemodynamic parameters measured in responders and non-responders

	T0	T1	T2
HR (beats min^{-1})			
Responders	91 ± 20	89 ± 18	87 ± 14
Non-responders	88 ± 17	88 ± 17	87 ± 16
SBP (mmHg)			
Responders	87 ± 19	95 ± 29	119 ± 26^c
Non-responders	111 ± 17^a	116 ± 19^a	112 ± 23
DBP (mmHg)			
Responders	46 ± 8	53 ± 7^b	58 ± 8^c
Non-responders	55 ± 11^a	58 ± 9^a	54 ± 8^a
MAP (mmHg)			
Responders	58 ± 10	67 ± 9^b	73 ± 11^c
Non-responders	71 ± 10^a	75 ± 10^a	70 ± 9
CVP (mmHg)			
Responders	11 ± 4	11 ± 3	12 ± 3
Non-responders	12 ± 4	$14 \pm 4^{a,b}$	13 ± 4
CO (L/min)			
Responders	3.60 ± 1.54	4.68 ± 1.79^b	5.11 ± 2.15^c
Non-responders	4.17 ± 0.93	4.50 ± 1.17	4.69 ± 1.44
SV (ml)			
Responders	39.87 ± 13.67	52.99 ± 16.22^b	58.72 ± 22.16^c
Non-responders	49.86 ± 17.71^a	53.52 ± 18.14	54.81 ± 16.53
SVV (%)			
Responders	14.94 ± 1.85	10.34 ± 5.26^b	8.71 ± 4.59^c
Non-responders	9.49 ± 2.67^a	7.74 ± 4.83^a	7.03 ± 2.67^c
IJVV (%)			
Responders	23.04 ± 16.76	9.88 ± 13.76^b	7.96 ± 8.72^c
Non-responders	9.90 ± 5.63^a	6.38 ± 2.37^b	5.73 ± 2.02^c
IVCV (%)			
Responders	15.97 ± 4.08	8.98 ± 4.52^b	8.08 ± 7.70^c
Non-responders	8.78 ± 5.42^a	8.14 ± 4.94	6.41 ± 2.76^c

Values are expressed as mean $\pm$ SD

HR heart rate, BP, SBP systolic blood pressure, DBP diastolic blood pressure, MAP mean arterial pressure, CVP central venous pressure, CO cardiac output, SV stroke volume, SVV stroke volume variation, IJVV internal jugular venous variability, IVCV inferior vena cava variability

T0 baseline, T1 after passive leg raising test, T2 after fluid expansion

[a] $P < 0.05$ non-responders versus responders

[b] $P < 0.05$ T1 versus T0

[c] $P < 0.05$ T2 versus T0

Basal HR was not different between the responders and non-responders either at T1 or T2 (T1 89 ± 18 vs. 88 ± 17 beats min^{-1}, T2 87 ± 14 vs. 87 ± 16 beats min^{-1}), although HR tended to decrease after the PLR test or fluid challenge in responders. Responders displayed an increase in SBP, DBP and MAP from T0 to T2 (87 ± 19 vs. 119 ± 26 mmHg, $P < 0.05$; 46 ± 8 vs. 58 ± 8 mmHg, $P < 0.05$; and 58 ± 10 vs. 73 ± 11 mmHg, $P < 0.05$, respectively), and the same changes are also observed from T0 to T1 in DBP and MAP but not in SBP. No significant change in arterial pressure or HR was observed in non-responders. Non-responders generally displayed a higher CVP than responders after PLR (T1 14 ± 4 vs. 11 ± 3 mmHg, $P < 0.05$, Table 2). Although CVP tended to increase after the PLR test or fluid challenge in non-responders, we found a significant increase in CVP only after PLR (12 ± 4 vs. 14 ± 4 mmHg, $P < 0.05$); a difference was not observed after volume expansion (12 ± 4 vs. 13 ± 4 mmHg). In responders, a significant change in CVP was not observed after the PLR test nor the fluid challenge (11 ± 4 vs. 11 ± 3 mmHg; 11 ± 4 vs. 12 ± 3 mmHg).

In volume responders, IJVV, IVCV and SVV were significantly higher compared with non-responders at baseline. All of these values significantly decreased after the PLR test or fluid administration in responders. However, we found that both responders and non-responders exhibited a significant reduction in IJVV from baseline to the PLR test time or post-volume expansion, and similar findings were also presented for IVCV after fluid challenge (Table 2). We determined that the relationship between IJVV and SVV was moderately correlated (Fig. 2a, $r = 0.51$, $P < 0.01$). IVCV and SVV were significantly correlated (Fig. 2b, $r = 0.75$, $P < 0.01$).

The AUCs established for SVV and PLR-ΔSV were comparable (0.97 vs. 0.91, $P = 0.61$). The AUC of SVV was significantly greater than that of IVCV (0.97 vs. 0.83, $P < 0.01$) and IJVV (0.97 vs. 0.88, $P = 0.03$) (Fig. 3a). The AUCs for static indicators (CVP, IVC diameter and IJV diameter) were significantly lower than that of dynamic indicators (Fig. 3b). An SVV value > 12% was able to identify volume responders with a sensitivity of 91.43%, a specificity of 94.29% and an AUC of 0.97 (CI 0.89–0.99). The PLR-ΔSV > 12.84% for the prediction of fluid responsiveness was associated with a sensitivity of 100%, a specificity of 82.86% and an AUC of 0.91 (CI 0.82–0.97). IJVV > 12.99% predicted fluid responsiveness with a sensitivity of 91.43%, a specificity of 82.86% and an AUC of 0.88 (CI 0.78–0.94). IVCV showed an AUC of 0.83 (CI 0.72–0.91) with a cutoff value of 13.39% (sensitivity 85.71% and specificity 85.71%) (Table 3). A significant difference between IJVV and IVCV was not observed (0.88 vs. 0.83, $P = 0.43$).

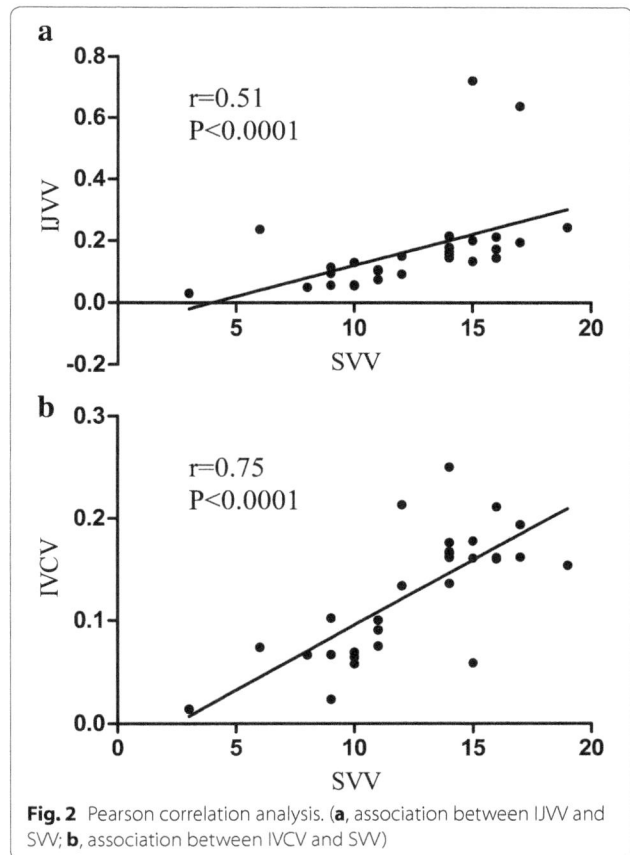

Fig. 2 Pearson correlation analysis. (**a**, association between IJVV and SVV; **b**, association between IVCV and SVV)

The intra-observer variability and inter-observer variability of IJVV measurement were further investigated in 30 patients. The results showed good concordance between estimation of IJVV by the two investigators, with a mean bias of − 0.01 and limits of agreement between − 0.1 and 0.08. The reliability of the measurements was also analyzed with intraclass correlation coefficients (ICCs) assessing intra-observer and inter-observer correlation (Additional file 2).

Discussion

The objective of this study was to evaluate whether ultrasound assessment of IJV respiratory diameter changes can serve as a simple indicator of fluid responsiveness in mechanically ventilated patients after cardiac surgery. Our data showed that IJVV was comparable to IVCV in predicting fluid responsiveness. There was a positive correlation between SVV and ventilator-induced IJVV. It was also found that the predictive value of PLR-ΔSV and SVV was superior to that of IVCV and IJVV.

Correcting hypovolemia is of paramount importance during the postoperative critical care of cardiac surgical patients. However, its correction should be carefully

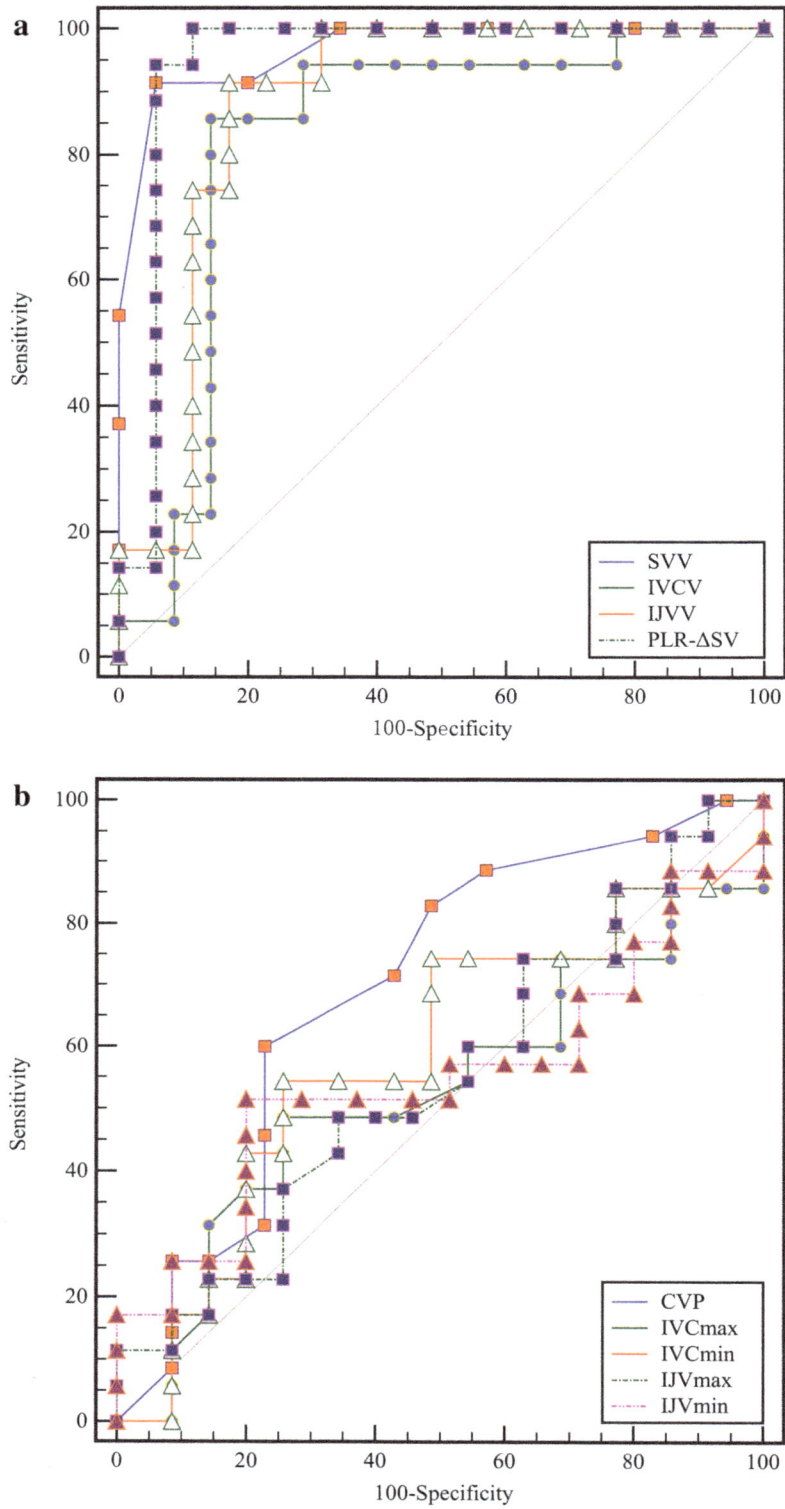

Fig. 3 Comparison of the areas under the ROC curves for the indicators used for predicting fluid responsiveness (**a**, dynamic indicators; and **b**, static indicators)

Table 3 Diagnostic ability of the different indices of fluid responsiveness

	AUC (95% CI)	Optimal cutoff (%)	Sensitivity (%)	Specificity (%)	Youden index	Positive predictive value	Negative predictive value	Positive likelihood ratio	Negative likelihood ratio
Dynamic indicators									
SVV	0.97 (0.89–0.99)	12.00	91.43	94.29	0.86	0.94	0.92	16.00	0.09
PLR-ΔSV	0.91 (0.82–0.97)	12.84	100.00	82.86	0.83	0.85	1.00	5.83	0.00
IJVV	0.88 (0.78–0.94)	12.99	91.43	82.86	0.74	0.84	0.91	5.33	0.10
IVCV	0.83 (0.72–0.91)	13.39	85.71	85.71	0.71	0.86	0.86	6.00	0.17
Static indicators									
CVP	0.70 (0.57–0.80)	11.00	60.00	77.14	0.37	0.72	0.66	2.63	0.52
IVCmax	0.53 (0.40–0.65)	1.57	48.57	74.29	0.23	0.65	0.59	1.89	0.69
IVCmin	0.58 (0.46–0.70)	1.40	54.29	74.29	0.29	0.68	0.62	2.11	0.62
IJVmax	0.55 (0.43–0.67)	0.86	48.57	65.71	0.14	0.59	0.56	1.42	0.78
IJVmin	0.55 (0.43–0.67)	0.64	51.43	80.00	0.31	0.72	0.62	2.57	0.61

AUC area under the receiver operating characteristic curve, *CI* confidence interval, *SVV* respiratory variation of stroke volume, *PLR-ΔSV* the increase in stroke volume in response to a passive leg raising test, *IJVV* internal jugular venous variability, *IVCV* inferior vena cava variability, *CVP* central venous pressure, *IVCmax* the maximum inferior vena cava diameter, *IVCmin* the minimum inferior vena cava diameter, *IJVmax* the maximum internal jugular venous diameter, *IJVmin* the minimum internal jugular venous diameter

guided to avoid unnecessary volume expansion [23]. Therefore, many investigators have explored reliable techniques with the goal of predicting fluid responsiveness in critically ill patients. Static parameters, such as CVP, are poor predictors of fluid responsiveness as previously reported and as shown in our study [23–25]. Based on the hemodynamic consequences of the heart–lung interactions, the use of dynamic indices of preload that result from respiratory variations is well-accepted bedside parameters of fluid responsiveness [7]. It was worth mentioning that tidal volume should be large enough to promote adequate preload variations. Fluid responsiveness cannot be reliably predicted if the tidal volume is < 8 ml/kg PBW [26]. Therefore, a Vt 8 mL/kg PBW was set in the present study. As higher PEEP may have adverse effects such as overinflation and hemodynamic deterioration, a PEEP of 5 cm H_2O was set initially after cardiac surgery according to our routine practice.

Mechanical ventilation-induced cyclic variations in vena cava diameter have been shown to be accurate predictors of fluid responsiveness. In our study, we have shown that the IVCV was a good predictor of fluid responsiveness for mechanically ventilated patients following cardiac surgery. IVCV threshold values of 13.39% have been reported in the literature to be able to discriminate between responders and non-responders with a sensitivity of 85.71% and a specificity of 85.71%. Based on the associations of intra-thoracic venous pressure and volume with extrathoracic venous pressure, we hypothesized that fluid responsiveness may also be reflected by changes in IJV pressure as assessed by IJVV. Measuring IJV diameter change is easily achieved with ultrasound with minimal training, as this approach is frequently

used for ultrasound-guided central vein catheterization. We demonstrated the reliability of IJVV with a value of 12.99% in detecting fluid responsiveness, having a sensitivity of 91.43% and a specificity of 82.86% in mechanically ventilated cardiac surgical patients.

Several studies have investigated the ability of respiratory variations in IJV diameter to evaluate hypovolemia or a hemodynamic response to a fluid challenge. Guarracino et al. have reported that IJV distensibility [(diamax − diamin)/diamin × 100] accurately predicts volume responsiveness in mechanically ventilated septic patients [19]. A cutoff value of 18% IJV distensibility resulted in 80% sensitivity and 85% specificity for predicting a fluid response, which was defined as an increase in cardiac index ≥ 15%. However, this study did not include patients with cardiac disease who have different hemodynamic characteristics. Moreover, the authors did not compare the predictive values of IVCV and IJVV. Thudium et al. showed that ultrasound evaluation of IJV extensibility can change in response to preload-altering orthostatic maneuvers and pulse pressure variation alterations [17]. However, this study was conducted at the cardiac surgery intensive care unit, and all of the patients were included after elective cardiac surgery; the reporters did not perform the standard fluid challenge, and the subgroup analysis showed that different surgery categories had different results. Broilo et al. verified the hypothesis that respiratory variations of the IVC and IJV were correlated [18]. These two indicators showed a significant agreement in evaluating fluid responsiveness. However, they did not identify changes in cardiac output following a fluid challenge, and they did not evaluate changes in the vein diameters before and after a fluid challenge.

There were other studies demonstrating its utility, using measurements of the IJV to detect early hemorrhage in healthy volunteers that were donating blood [27, 28]. To our knowledge, this was the first study to evaluate the value of IJVV in predicting fluid responsiveness based on a standard fluid challenge in mechanically ventilated cardiac surgical patients.

Our study has several limitations. First, all subjects were on mechanical ventilation and absence of spontaneous breathing under sedation. Whether the conclusions can be extrapolated to patients with spontaneous breathing remains uncertain. Second, an uncalibrated system for hemodynamic monitoring was used in this study. Although the validation of FloTrac/vigileo system in measuring cardiac output has been assessed by numerous studies, the reliability of uncalibrated devices is still under debate [29–31]. Compared with pulmonary artery catheter (PAC) or transpulmonary thermodilution devices, FloTrac/vigileo system can be directly connected to the arterial catheter and has the advantage of auto-calibration. It theoretically meets the needs for rapidly assessing hemodynamic changes. Moreover, the dynamic indicator of SVV that could continuously displayed by the FloTrac/Vigileo system has also been shown to be able to predict fluid responsiveness in cardiac surgical patients [32–34]. Third, we did not enroll patients with right heart failure, as severe right heart failure or high CVP could influence IJV pressure and diameter and may decrease the relative variability even in the presence of preload responsiveness. Fourth, technical errors were possible, because even a slight pressure could have caused a great change in the cross-sectional image and diameter of the IJV during the acquisition of the measurements. We have made further efforts on the reproducibility and agreement of IJVV in 30 patients. The results showed good concordance between estimation of IJVV by the two investigators. Fifth, the initial semirecumbent position of the patient was 30° head of the bed (HOB) elevated instead of 45° (standard baseline position of PLR), because this was the recommended position for supine ventilated patient in the ICU. It was believed that this was more consistent with clinical scenario. Furthermore, taking sonographic measurements of the IVC diameters seems more easily in the position with HOB 30° than HOB 45°. The predict value of IJVV in other positions (such as the horizontal position) remains to be assessed.

Conclusions

Ultrasound evaluation of IJVV is a simple, easy and readily accessible bedside measurement that predicts volume responsiveness in mechanically ventilated cardiac surgical patients. The respiratory variations of the IJV and IVC showed comparable value in the prediction of fluid responsiveness.

Abbreviations
HR: Heart rate; MAP: Mean arterial pressure; CVP: Central venous pressure; SV: Stroke volume; SVV: Stroke volume variation; IJV: Internal jugular venous; IJVV: Internal jugular venous variability; IVC: Inferior vena cava; IVCV: Inferior vena cava variability; PLR: Passive leg raising; PLR-ΔSV: The increase in stroke volume in response to a passive leg raising test; CSICU: Cardiac surgery intensive care unit; PEEP: Positive end-expiratory pressure; PBW: Predicted body weight; IPPV: Intermittent positive pressure ventilation; LVEF: Left ventricular ejection fraction; ROC: Receiver operating characteristic.

Authors' contributions
G-gM, G-wH, G-wT performed the literature search, extracted date and drafted the manuscript. X-mY, LL and HL reviewed studies for inclusion and extracted data. G-wT, D-mZ and ZL performed the analysis and helped draft the manuscript. G-wT and ZL conceived the idea, participated in manuscript writing and revision. All authors read and approved the final manuscript.

Acknowledgements
None.

Competing interests
The authors declare that they have no competing interests.

Funding
This article was supported by grants from the National Natural Science Foundation of China (81500067), Natural Science Foundation of Shanghai (16ZR1405600), Health and Family Planning Commission of Shanghai (20154Y011) and the research funds of Zhong Shan Hospital (2017ZSYXQN23 and 2016ZSQN23).

References
1. Lee J, de Louw E, Niemi M, Nelson R, Mark RG, Celi LA, et al. Association between fluid balance and survival in critically ill patients. J Intern Med. 2015;277:468–77.
2. Carsetti A, Cecconi M, Rhodes A. Fluid bolus therapy: monitoring and predicting fluid responsiveness. Curr Opin Crit Care. 2015;21:388–94.
3. Kalus JS, Caron MF, White CM, Mather JF, Gallagher R, Boden WE, et al. Impact of fluid balance on incidence of atrial fibrillation after cardiothoracic surgery. Am J Cardiol. 2004;94:1423–5.
4. Mentzer RM Jr. Myocardial protection in heart surgery. J Cardiovasc Pharmacol Ther. 2011;16:290–7.
5. Donati A, Carsetti A, Damiani E, Adrario E, Romano R, Pelaia P. Fluid responsiveness in critically ill patients. Indian J Crit Care Med. 2015;19:375–6.
6. Suzuki S, Woinarski NC, Lipcsey M, Candal CL, Schneider AG, Glassford NJ, et al. Pulse pressure variation-guided fluid therapy after cardiac surgery: a pilot before-and-after trial. J Crit Care. 2014;29:992–6.
7. Marik PE, Cavallazzi R, Vasu T, Hirani A. Dynamic changes in arterial waveform derived variables and fluid responsiveness in mechanically ventilated patients: a systematic review of the literature. Crit Care Med. 2009;37:2642–7.
8. Michard F, Boussat S, Chemla D, Anguel N, Mercat A, Lecarpentier Y, et al. Relation between respiratory changes in arterial pulse pressure and fluid responsiveness in septic patients with acute circulatory failure. Am J Respir Crit Care Med. 2000;162:134–8.
9. Vieillard-Baron A, Chergui K, Rabiller A, Peyrouset O, Page B, Beauchet A, et al. Superior vena caval collapsibility as a gauge of volume status in ventilated septic patients. Intensive Care Med. 2004;30:1734–9.

10. Barbier C, Loubieres Y, Schmit C, Hayon J, Ricome JL, Jardin F, et al. Respiratory changes in inferior vena cava diameter are helpful in predicting fluid responsiveness in ventilated septic patients. Intensive Care Med. 2004;30:1740–6.

11. Tavazzi G, Price S, Fletcher N. Bedside ultrasonographic measurement of the inferior vena cava. J Cardiothorac Vasc Anesth. 2015;29:e54–5.

12. Sobczyk D, Nycz K, Andruszkiewicz P. Bedside ultrasonographic measurement of the inferior vena cava fails to predict fluid responsiveness in the first 6 hours after cardiac surgery: a prospective case series observational study. J Cardiothorac Vasc Anesth. 2015;29:663–9.

13. Nagdev AD, Merchant RC, Tirado-Gonzalez A, Sisson CA, Murphy MC. Emergency department bedside ultrasonographic measurement of the caval index for noninvasive determination of low central venous pressure. Ann Emerg Med. 2010;55:290–5.

14. Chua Chiaco JM, Parikh NI, Fergusson DJ. The jugular venous pressure revisited. Cleve Clin J Med. 2013;80:638–44.

15. Conn RD, O'Keefe JH. Simplified evaluation of the jugular venous pressure: significance of inspiratory collapse of jugular veins. Mo Med. 2012;109:150–2.

16. Constant J. Using internal jugular pulsations as a manometer for right atrial pressure measurements. Cardiology. 2000;93:26–30.

17. Thudium M, Klaschik S, Ellerkmann RK, Putensen C, Hilbert T. Is internal jugular vein extensibility associated with indices of fluid responsiveness in ventilated patients? Acta Anaesthesiol Scand. 2016;60:723–33.

18. Broilo F, Meregalli A, Friedman G. Right internal jugular vein distensibility appears to be a surrogate marker for inferior vena cava vein distensibility for evaluating fluid responsiveness. Rev Bras Ter Intensiva. 2015;27:205–11.

19. Guarracino F, Ferro B, Forfori F, Bertini P, Magliacano L, Pinsky MR. Jugular vein distensibility predicts fluid responsiveness in septic patients. Crit Care. 2014;18:647.

20. Prekker ME, Scott NL, Hart D, Sprenkle MD, Leatherman JW. Point-of-care ultrasound to estimate central venous pressure: a comparison of three techniques. Crit Care Med. 2013;41:833–41.

21. Cecconi M, Parsons AK, Rhodes A. What is a fluid challenge? Curr Opin Crit Care. 2011;17:290–5.

22. Vincent JL, Weil MH. Fluid challenge revisited. Crit Care Med. 2006;34:1333–7.

23. Preisman S, Kogan S, Berkenstadt H, Perel A. Predicting fluid responsiveness in patients undergoing cardiac surgery: functional haemodynamic parameters including the Respiratory Systolic Variation Test and static preload indicators. Br J Anaesth. 2005;95:746–55.

24. Marik PE, Baram M, Vahid B. Does central venous pressure predict fluid responsiveness? A systematic review of the literature and the tale of seven mares. Chest. 2008;134:172–8.

25. Osman D, Ridel C, Ray P, Monnet X, Anguel N, Richard C, et al. Cardiac filling pressures are not appropriate to predict hemodynamic response to volume challenge. Crit Care Med. 2007;35:64–8.

26. De Backer D, Heenen S, Piagnerelli M, Koch M, Vincent JL. Pulse pressure variations to predict fluid responsiveness: influence of tidal volume. Intensive Care Med. 2005;31:517–23.

27. Unluer EE, Kara PH. Ultrasonography of jugular vein as a marker of hypovolemia in healthy volunteers. Am J Emerg Med. 2013;31:173–7.

28. Akilli NB, Cander B, Dundar ZD, Koylu R. A new parameter for the diagnosis of hemorrhagic shock: jugular index. J Crit Care. 2012;27(530):e13–8.

29. Marque S, Gros A, Chimot L, Gacouin A, Lavoue S, Camus C, et al. Cardiac output monitoring in septic shock: evaluation of the third-generation Flotrac-Vigileo. J Clin Monit Comput. 2013;27:273–9.

30. Monnet X, Anguel N, Jozwiak M, Richard C, Teboul JL. Third-generation FloTrac/Vigileo does not reliably track changes in cardiac output induced by norepinephrine in critically ill patients. Br J Anaesth. 2012;108:615–22.

31. De Backer D, Marx G, Tan A, Junker C, Van Nuffelen M, Huter L, et al. Arterial pressure-based cardiac output monitoring: a multicenter validation of the third-generation software in septic patients. Intensive Care Med. 2011;37:233–40.

32. Krige A, Bland M, Fanshawe T. Fluid responsiveness prediction using Vigileo FloTrac measured cardiac output changes during passive leg raise test. J Intensive Care. 2016;4:63.

33. Kim SY, Song Y, Shim JK, Kwak YL. Effect of pulse pressure on the predictability of stroke volume variation for fluid responsiveness in patients with coronary disease. J Crit Care. 2013;28(318):e1–7.

34. Cannesson M, Musard H, Desebbe O, Boucau C, Simon R, Henaine R, et al. The ability of stroke volume variations obtained with Vigileo/FloTrac system to monitor fluid responsiveness in mechanically ventilated patients. Anesth Analg. 2009;108:513–7.

11

Ultrasound assessment of rectus femoris and anterior tibialis muscles in young trauma patients

Maria Giuseppina Annetta[1], Mauro Pittiruti[2], Davide Silvestri[1], Domenico Luca Grieco[1]* (iD), Alessio Maccaglia[1], Michele Fabio La Torre[3], Nicola Magarelli[3], Giovanna Mercurio[1], Anselmo Caricato[1] and Massimo Antonelli[1]

Abstract

Purpose: Quantitative and qualitative changes of skeletal muscle are typical and early findings in trauma patients, being possibly associated with functional impairment. Early assessment of muscle changes—as evaluated by muscle ultrasonography—could yield important information about patient's outcome.

Methods: In this prospective observational study, we used ultrasonography to evaluate the morphological changes of rectus femoris (RF) and anterior tibialis (AT) muscles in a group of young, previously healthy trauma patients on enteral feeding.

Results: We studied 38 severely injured patients (median Injury Severity Score = 34; median age = 40 y.o.) over the course of the ICU stay up to 3 weeks after trauma. We found a progressive loss of muscle mass from day 0 to day 20, that was more relevant for the RF (45%) than for the AT (22%); this was accompanied by an increase in echogenicity (up to 2.5 by the Heckmatt Scale, where normal echogenicity = 1), which is an indicator of myofibers depletion.

Conclusions: Ultrasound evaluation of skeletal muscles is inexpensive, noninvasive, simple and easily repeatable. By this method, we were able to quantify the morphological changes of skeletal muscle in trauma patients. Further studies may rely on this technicque to evaluate the impact of different therapeutic strategies on muscle wasting.

Keywords: Muscle mass, Muscle ultrasonography, Enteral feeding, Trauma

Background

Muscle wasting is a frequent finding in critically ill patients and is associated with worse short- and long-term outcomes. Loss of mass and function of skeletal muscles starts early—in the first 24 h after admission to intensive care unit (ICU)—and may persist for years ('post-ICU syndrome'). Loss of muscle mass is a major cause of ICU-acquired muscle weakness and is associated with delayed weaning, prolonged ICU and hospital stay and is an independent predictor of 1-year mortality [1–3]. Long-term muscle impairment may be responsible of physical, mental and cognitive dysfunction, which affects the quality of life of ICU survivors and increases the costs of the healthy care services [4–6]. Early physical rehabilitation has been associated with conflicting results in terms of functional outcome [7, 8], so that the best strategy would theoretically be to avoid or minimize muscle loss during ICU stay, for example delivering an appropriate nutritional support. Unfortunately, limited data clarify the possible impact of adequate calories and protein delivery on skeletal muscle preservation and long-term outcome of muscular function [9–11]; also, the conclusions of the few available clinical studies are controversial. Some studies have even suggested that increasing protein intake in the early phase of critical illness may accelerate muscle loss during the first week [4, 12].

The sequential assessment of quantitative and qualitative changes of muscle mass may help identify critically ill patients with high risk of muscle dysfunction, as well

*Correspondence: dlgrieco@ymail.com
[1] Department of Anesthesia and Intensive Care, Fondazione Policlinico Universitario 'A.Gemelli', Largo A.Gemelli, 8, 00168 Rome, Italy

as verify the effects of different nutritional regimens. In this regard, B-mode ultrasonographic evaluation of skeletal muscles (in particular, rectus femoris and anterior tibialis) is an emerging and reliable tool to assess muscle changes over time. It is a bedside technique, easy to use and inexpensive [13]. Its cost-effectiveness is higher than CT scan evaluation, which has been used for the same purpose [2].

In this prospective clinical study, we evaluated the feasibility of detecting the quantitative and qualitative changes of rectus femoris and anterior tibialis muscles over the course of the ICU stay up to 20 days from admission in a cohort of young trauma patients.

Methods

This was a prospective observational study performed in a cohort of severe multiple trauma patients admitted to the 20-bed ICU of our institution (Fondazione Policlinico 'A.Gemelli'—University Hospital) in a period of 10 consecutive months. All subjects were on enteral feeding.

Patients

We enrolled exclusively young trauma patients with an injury severity score(ISS) exceeding 25, who were admitted to our ICU within few hours after the injury. We recruited only well-nourished, previously healthy subjects, aged 18–59 y.o, with no past history of nutritional problems, chronic use of drugs nor orthopedic issues (such as skeletal fractures or immobilization) in the previous 2 years. Trauma patients not fulfilling this criteria were not considered for the enrollment. Exclusion criteria were: relevant comorbidities (renal, liver or heart disease or COPD), previous immune abnormalities (including treatment with corticosteroids), neuromuscular disease, past or recent history of cancer.

For each patient, demographics and clinical data were recorded: age, height, weight, body mass index (BMI), ISS, APACHE II score, Sequential Organ Failure Assessment score (SOFA), Glasgow Coma Scale (GCS)—both total and motor (GCS-M)—Glasgow Outcome Scale (GOS), number of days on mechanical ventilation, ICU length of stay, incidence of secondary infections, daily provision of calories and protein, blood levels of albumin, total protein and creatinine, blood urea nitrogen (BUN) and other laboratory data. Among mechanically ventilated patients, weaning was classified as simple, difficult or prolonged, as previously described [14]. Infections were classified according to definitions by the Center for Disease Control and Prevention [15].

Nutritional support

Enteral feeding was started as soon as the patient was hemodynamically stable and fully resuscitated,

usually within 24 h. Our nutritional target was to achieve a minimal protein intake of 0.8 g/kg/day within day 5 after admission. Patients who did not reach this target for any reason (gastrointestinal intolerance or contraindication to enteral feeding or repeated forced suspensions of enteral feeding because of multiple surgical procedures) were excluded from the final analysis. We used either a standard feeding formula (1.5 total kcal/ml, protein 60 g/L) or a high-protein formula (1.35 total kcal/ml, protein 75 g/L): These different regimens were not assigned by randomization, but they were the result of a change of nutritional policies in our ICU during the period of the study; though, the two groups of patients—nourished by a standard formula (SF) or nourished by a high-protein formula (HPF)—were similar in terms of age, Injury Severity Score (ISS), Acute Physiology and Chronic Health Evaluation (APACHE II score), height and weight. Tube feeding was started at a very low rate (10–20 ml/h) and increased at each 24-h interval as tolerated, in order to meet a minimal protein intake of 0.8 g/kg/day. The patient's intolerance to feeding was defined on the basis of clinical signs (abdominal distention, vomiting, increase in serum lactate, high gastric residual volume).

Ultrasonography of skeletal muscles

An ultrasound (US) evaluation of the rectus femoris (RF) and anterior tibialis (AT) muscles was performed in all patients at day 0 (within 24 h from trauma), 5, 10, 15 and 20. We used an US device with a 5- to 7.5-MHz linear probe (Esaote MyLab). According to a previously described methodology [13, 16], skeletal muscles were evaluated by US scan, collecting both quantitative and qualitative data. The transducer was placed perpendicular to the long axis of the muscle (i.e., perpendicular to the major axis of the limb), at 3/5 of the distance between the anterior superior iliac spine and the superior border of patella (i.e., about 15 cm from the patella) for the RF and 5 cm below the peroneal head for the AT muscle. The measurement points were marked with indelible ink to ensure day-to-day consistency and facilitate subsequent measurements. Visualization was consistently obtained, while the patients were supine with both legs in passive extension. Two measurements were taken for each muscle in each leg. In the presence of lower limb fractures, measurements were taken on the contralateral leg only. Excess contact gel was applied so to minimize underlying soft tissue distortion. One operator only (specifically trained in muscle ultrasonography) performed all measurements. US settings (depth, gain and focus) were standardized for both RF and AT examinations. After freezing the US image, quantitative parameters were recorded for both muscles: anterior–posterior diameter (AP diam); lateral–lateral diameter (LL diam); and cross-sectional area (CSA) (computed from the perimetral contour of the muscle section). The value of CSA is considered to be proportional to the total mass of the skeletal muscle [13, 16]. We also recorded one qualitative parameter—echogenicity—that was expressed according to the Heckmatt Scale [17]. Echogenicity of normal muscle is expected to be 1 on this scale. Increased echogenicity is usually regarded as an index of myofibers depletion [18].

Primary endpoints of our study were the qualitative and quantitative changes of skeletal muscles during 3 weeks of ICU stay, taking into consideration the role of protein intake. The study protocol was approved by the Ethics Committee of our institution (Prot. 10917/15).

Statistical analysis

Qualitative data are expressed as number of events (%) and continuous data as median [interquartile range]. Difference in the distribution of qualitative variables in SF versus HPF group was investigated with the Chi-square test or Fisher's exact test, as appropriate. Difference in the distribution of quantitative and ordinal variables in SF versus HPF group was assessed with the Mann–Whitney test. In the overall population, the significance of changes in the quantitative variables over time was determined with the one-way ANOVA test for repeated measures; paired comparisons between 2 consecutive timepoints were then analyzed with the Wilcoxon sum of ranks test. The effect of SF versus HPF on the change in the quantitative variables over time was determined with the two-way ANOVA. Paired comparisons between the distribution of quantitative variable in SF versus HPF group at each time point were also assessed with the Mann–Whitney test.

The entire analysis was conducted applying a bilateral null hypothesis; accordingly, results with two-tailed $p \le 0.05$ were considered significant.

Statistical analysis was conducted with SPSS 20.0.

Results

A total of 120 trauma patients admitted to our ICU were screened for possible inclusion in our prospective study, and only 52 met the requirements. Nine patients did not reach the minimal protein intake by enteral feeding. Of the remaining patients, five died during the first 3 weeks. The final analysis was conducted on 38 patients, whose characteristics are listed in Table 1. All patients were young (median age 40 year old); most were male (76%), and all of them had a good nutritional status on admission (median BMI = 25). All patients were severely injured (ISS = 34, APACHE II score = 16), and most of them had associated brain injury (84%). There were no significant differences between patients on SF versus HPF.

Muscular changes are shown in Table 2.

Results concerning muscular changes over the course of the study are reported in table 2. The RF muscle mass changed significantly during the ICU stay in all patients. Its AP diameter decreased progressively (ANOVA for repeated measures: $p = 0.03$), in particular from day 5 to day 20 ($p < 0.05$), though such decrease was not significant between day 0 and day 5 ($p = 0.24$). The LL diameter did not show a significant progressive decrease (ANOVA for repeated measures: $p = 0.25$), but the difference between day 0 and day 20 was significant ($p = 0.04$). The CSA of RF muscle progressively decreased during the ICU stay (ANOVA for repeated measures: $p = 0.03$), with a statistically significant difference among all time points between day 5 and day 20 (all $p < 0.05$), but not between day 0 and day 5 ($p = 0.13$). In particular, there was an overall 45% reduction in CSA during the first 20 days of ICU stay (15% loss from day 5 to 10, 12% from day 10 to 15, 21% from day 15 to 20).

As regards the AT muscle, its AP diameter decreased progressively during the ICU stay (ANOVA for repeated measures: $p = 0.03$) in all patients, with a statistically significant reduction among all time points between day 0 and day 20 ($p < 0.05$). Its LL diameter did not decrease significantly during the ICU stay (ANOVA for repeated measures: $p = 0.63$) but only between day 5 and 10 ($p = 0.03$). The 22% decrease in CSA of AT muscle during the overall ICU stay was not significant (ANOVA for repeated measures: $p = 0.30$).

There was a progressive increase in both RF and AT echogenicity—as evaluated with the Heckmatt Scale—from day 0 on ($p < 0.05$), with the main increase from day 0 to day 5.

None of these quantitative and qualitative muscular changes showed any significant difference between the groups SF versus HPF.

Nutritional intake is shown in Table 3. We had 20 patients in the SF and 18 in the HPF group. Mean protein intake after day 5 was of 0.87 g/kg/day in the SF group and 1.6 g/kg/day in the HPF group. Mean total calories were 19 kcal/kg in the SF group and 30 kcal/kg in the HPF group. No major differences were detected in the main laboratory values (Table 4), though HPF patients had nonsignificantly higher blood protein levels ($p < 0.07$) and significantly higher albumin levels ($p < 0.03$) at day 20.

Discussion

In our study, we adopted ultrasonography for the evaluation of quantitative and qualitative changes of skeletal muscles in a homogeneous group of young trauma patients who were previous healthy, well nourished and physically active. A previous similar study published

Table 1 Demographics

	ALL	SF *n* 20	HPF *n* 18
Female sex, *n* (%)	9 (24)	5 (25)	4 (22)
Age (years)	40 [31–54]	47 [37–58]	37 [29–46]
Height (cm)	175 [167–180]	175 [168–180]	170 [167–180]
Weight (k)	75 [70–81]	80 [70–90]	75 [67–85]
BMI	25 [23–28]	26 [23–29]	23 [24–26]
GCS at inclusion	7 [3–9]	7 [3–9]	6 [3–10]
GCS-M at inclusion	4 [1–5]	4 [1–5]	4 [1–5]
Injury Severity Score (ISS)	34 [27–42]	34 [28–40]	34 [27–45]
Apache II score	16 [13–20]	16 [13–19]	18 [12–22]
SOFA	7 [5–9]	8 [5–10]	6 [5–9]
Brain injury *n* (%)	32 (84)	17 (85)	15 (83)
Thoracic trauma *n* (%)	30 (79)	16 (80)	14 (78)
Abdominal trauma *n* (%)	17 (45)	9 (45)	8 (44)
Pelvic trauma *n* (%)	15 (40)	8 (40)	7 (40)
Spinal trauma *n* (%)	21 (55)	10 (50)	11 (61)
GOS 28 days	3 [3, 4]	3 [3, 4]	3 [3, 4]
GCS-M at discharge	6 [4–6]	6 [5, 6]	6 [4–6]
Tracheostomy *n* (%)	24 (63)	12 (60)	12 (67)
Weaning			
Simple, *n* (%)	21 (55)	10 (50)	11 (61)
Difficult, *n* (%)	11 (29)	6 (30)	5 (28)
Prolonged, *n* (%)	6 (16)	4 (20)	2 (11)
Days of mechanical ventilation	13 [11–19]	14 [9–22]	13 [11–17]
Patients with at least one documented infection, *n* (%)	34 (90)	19 (95)	15 (83)
Patients with at least one documented infection MDR infection, *n* (%)	23 (61)	13 (65)	10 (56)
Patients with septic shock during the ICU stay, *n* (%)	7 (18)	5 (25)	2 (11)
ICU length of stay	22 (17–33)	22 (16–37)	22 (17–31)
ICU outcome, died, *n* (%)	3 (8)	2 (10)	1 (6)

Data expressed as median [interquartile range], if not otherwise specified

See abbreviations in the text

few years ago [4] was focused on a heterogeneous group of critically ill patients with only 25% of them being trauma victims. All previous clinical studies with muscle ultrasonography have been conducted in mixed ICU populations that included medical and surgical, as well as acute and chronic, critically ill patients [4, 13, 19]. On the contrary, in our study there were no confounding factors such as old age, comorbidities, cancer and long-term use of medications.

Quantitative changes of skeletal muscles

In ICU patients, the daily amount of muscle loss—as estimated by US—is reported to range between 6 [20] and 12.5% between day 1 and 7 [4]. Muscle wasting correlates with the ICU length of stay [16] and can be predictive of long-term functional disability [21]. Several factors contribute to muscle wasting over the course of the critical illness, both in the acute and chronic phase:

inflammation, neuroendocrine stress response, immobilization, impaired microcirculation and denervation (in the acute phase); infections, nutritional deficiency, hyperglycemia, drugs [22] (in the late phase). Other predisposing factors are: age, baseline muscle function, nutritional status, comorbidities (COPD, renal and heart disease, cancer) [22, 23]. Finally, some data suggest that also parenteral nutrition may worsen muscle function [24].

A retrospective study demonstrated a correlation between hospital mortality and skeletal muscle mass, as estimated by abdominal CT scan [2]: this is particularly evident in trauma patients [25], but apparently not in ICU patients with acute lung injury [26].

Ultrasound has been used to rate the loss of skeletal muscles in patients with orthopedic trauma, COPD, cancer and neuromuscular disorders [13, 27, 28]; indeed, it appears as an emerging field of interest in ICU. Ultrasonography is more accurate than anthropometric

Table 2 Muscle ultrasound

	Day 0	Day 5	Day 10	Day 15	Day 20
RF: AP diam (mm)					
All pts	17 [15–20]	17 [15–20]	16 [13–19]	14 [12–17]	13 [9–15]
SF	17 [15–20]	18 [16–20]	19 [14–20]	15 [12–17]	14 [9–17]
HPF	17 [15–19]	16 [15–20]	16 [12–18]	13 [12–17]	9 [9–12]
RF: LL diam (mm)					
All pts	43 [40–46]	41 [38–44]	40 [37–45]	40 [36–44]	38 [34–41]
SF	41 [40–44]	41 [37–42]	39 [35–42]	40 [34–44]	35 [34–40]
HPF	43 [40–47]	44 [37–46]	44 [37–47]	40 [37–47]	41 [37–43]
RF: CSA (cm^2)					
All pts	6.1 [5.1–7.3]	5.9 [4.8–6.3]	5.1 [4.3–6.2]	4.6 [3.8–5.3]	3.5 [3.2–4.7]
SF	6.1 [5.1–7.3]	5.9 [4.9–6.3]	5.6 [4.2–6.2]	4.7 [3.9–5.4]	3.5 [3.2–4.8]
HPF	6.3 [4.7–7.3]	5.9 [4.3–6.5]	5 [4.2–6.6]	4.4 [3.5–5.1]	3.5 [2.8–4.4]
RF: echogenicity, Heckmatt Scale					
All pts	1 [1, 2]	2 [1, 2]	2 [1–2.5]	2 [1–3]	2.5 [1.5–3]
SF	1 [1, 2]	2 [1, 2]	2 [1.3–2.8]	2.3 [1.6–3.5]	2.5 [2, 3]
HPF	1.3 [1, 2]	1.5 [1, 2]	1 [1, 2]	1.5 [1–2.5]	2.5 [1–3]
AT: AP diam (mm)					
All pts	22 [20–25]	21 [19–23]	20 [17–22]	19 [17–22]	18 [16–20]
SF	22 [20–24]	21 [19–24]	20 [18–23]	20 [17–23]	19 [15–21]
HPF	24 [20–26]	22 [19–23]	21 [17–22]	18 [17–20]	18 [18]
AT: LL diam (mm)					
All pts	25 [22–26]	24 [21–26]	23 [21–25]	22 [20–25]	22 [20–27]
SF	25 [23–27]	24 [21–27]	23 [21–26]	23 [19–26]	25 [21–28]
HPF	23 [22–26]	24 [21–26]	22 [21–25]	21 [20–24]	22 [20–22]
AT: CSA (cm^2)					
All pts	5.6 [4.5–6.4]	4.8 [3.7–5.6]	4 [3.7–5.2]	4 [3.3–4.8]	4.2 [3.4–4.7]
SF	5.7 [4.7–6.8]	4 [3.6–6]	3.9 [3.7–5.2]	4 [3.3–5.7]	4 [3.2–5.2]
HPF	5.5 [4.5–6.2]	4.9 [4.2–5.9]	4.2 [3.6–5.3]	3.9 [3.3–4.5]	4.3 [3.4–4.6]
AT: echogenicity, Heckmatt Scale					
All pts	2 [1, 2]	2 [1–3]	2 [1–3]	1.5 [1–3]	2.5 [1–4]
SF	1.8 [1–2.1]	2.3 [1.3–3]	2 [1.3–3]	2 [1–3.4]	3.5 [1–4]
HPF	2 [1, 2]	2 [1–3]	1.3 [1–3]	1.3 [1–2.5]	1.5 [1–3]

Data expressed as median [interquartile range]

See abbreviations in the text

See statistical significance in the text

measurements and has been shown to closely correlate with the data obtained by MRI and CT scan [19, 29], with the advantage of being less expensive, less time-consuming and safer, since it does not imply radiation exposure. Though some studies have shown a good intra-rater and inter-rater reliability for US measurement of muscle CSA or thickness in adult critically ill patients [4, 30], the matter is still somehow controversial [31, 32].

All of our trauma patients (100%) experienced severe muscle mass loss, as estimated by CSA. Almost half (45%) of RF muscle mass was lost by day 20 with the greatest reduction (21%) occurring after day 15. In a previous work [4], a 17.7% reduction in RF cross-sectional area was shown in a group of mixed ICU patients from day 1 to day 10, with the major loss occurring during the first 7 days. We found a less important reduction in AT cross-sectional area (22%) by day 20.

The exact underlying mechanisms of dissimilar magnitudes of losses in different muscle groups are still unknown. In both rodent and human models, the rate and magnitude of muscle loss seem to depend on both muscle type and degree of inactivity [33, 34]. In experimental and clinical models of lower limb immobilization, muscle loss is greater in the extensor muscles (soleus and gastrocnemius). This is consistent with the greater muscle loss we report in RF (extensor muscle) as compared

Table 3 Nutritional intake

	Day 0–5	Day 5–10	Day 10–15	Day 15–20	SF versus HPF p value
Enteral nutrition (ml/day)					
SF	850 [625–900]	1000 [1000–1400]*	1050 [950–1500]*	1350 [1000–1500]*	0.007
HPF	1000 [700–1200]	1500 [1175–1500]*	1500 [1500–1700]*	1500 [1500–2000]*	
Proteins (g/day)					
SF	47 [32–63]*	67 [50–91]*	70 [48–90]*	70 [50–90]*	0.001
HPF	74 [40–93]*	112 [99–136]*	136 [112–136]*	120 [106–136]*	
Total calories (kcal/day)					
SF	1059 [763–1200]*	1500 [1160–1915]*	1500 [1050–2062]*	1500 [1250–2200]*	0.005
HPF	1326 [934–1564]*	1958 [1762–2250]*	2250 [1920–2341]*	2250 [1920–2560]*	

Data expressed as median [interquartile range]

The overall p value refers to the comparison between the whole time series of changes SF versus HPF

* p < 0.05 for the comparison of SF versus HPF at each time point

See abbreviations in the text

Table 4 Laboratory data

	Day 0	Day 5	Day 10	Day 15	Day 20	SF versus HPF p value
BUN (mg/dl)						
SF	12 [10–15]	17 [13–26]	20 [17–30]	25 [17–35]	24 [18–47]	0.51
HPF	13 [11–17]	18 [12–22]	23 [19–29]	20 [16–24]	30 [23–37]	
Creatinine (mg/dl)						
SF	0.8 [0.7–1]	0.6 [0.5–0.8]	0.6 [0.5–0.8]	0.6 [0.5–0.7]	0.6 [0.5–1.6]	0.46
HPF	1 [0.6–1.2]	0.7 [0.5–0.8]	0.6 [0.5–0.7]	0.6 [0.4–0.7]	0.7 [0.5–0.8]	
Phosphate (mg/dl)						
SF	2.7 [2–3.5]	2.9 [2.3–3.4]	3 [2.5–3.3]	3.5 [2.7–3.8]	3.5 [2.8–4.1]	0.41
HPF	3.1 [2.5–4]	2.9 [2.1–3.6]	3.5 [2.5–4]	3.4 [2.6–4.1]	3.6 [3.3–4]	
Proteins (g/L)						
SF	4.7 [3.9–6.1]	5.2 [4.7–5.6]	5.8 [5.2–6.3]	6.1 [5.3–6.5]	5.8 [5.2–6.4]	0.07
HPF	5.3 [5–5.7]	5.4 [5, 6]	5.8 [5.2–6.6]	6.4 [5.7–7.3]	7.3 [5.6–8.3]	
Albumin (g/L)						
SF	2.9 [2.4–3.4]*	2.6 [2.2–2.9]	2.6 [2.1–2.9]	2.8 [2.3–3]	2.5 [2.1–2.9]*	0.03
HPF	3.3 [3–3.6]*	2.7 [2.5–3.1]	2.7 [2.3–3.1]	3 [2.8–3.3]	3.1 [2.6–3.7]*	

Data expressed ad median [interquartile range]

The overall p value refers to the comparison between the whole time series of changes SF versus HPF

* p < 0.05 for the comparison of SF versus HPF at each time point

See abbreviations in the text

to AT (flexor muscle). Also, RF is a power muscle made up predominantly of type II fast-twitch fibers, while AT muscle composition is mainly made of type I slow-twitch fibers [35]. The preferential loss of a certain kind of muscle fibers might be a crucial determinant of long-term outcome, especially in the development of ICU-acquired weakness and in success of physical rehabilitation. Muscle weakness is usually symmetric and predominates in the proximal part of the limbs (shoulders and ankles) [36]. Laboratory model of ischemic injury has shown that muscle with predominance of fast-twitch fibers had significantly greater necrosis than those richer in

slow-twitch fibers [37]. Immobilization studies have shown a preferential loss of type II fibers and conversion of fiber typing from type I to type II in postural muscles [38].

Qualitative changes of skeletal muscles

Several studies have demonstrated that pathological muscle changes (such as fatty infiltration, atrophy and intramuscular fibrosis) can be detected by ultrasound. Alteration of muscle echogenicity may be ascribed to muscle edema (in the early phase) but also to fibrosis and fatty degeneration (in the late phase). These latter findings may be an indicator of quantitative loss of muscular myofibers and disruption of muscle architecture and may correlate with impaired muscle function [18]. Since edema cannot alter the bone signal in contrast to fibrous tissue, changes in muscle echogenicity are related to the fibrous tissue content and with specific structural damage in muscle architecture as seen with muscle biopsies [4] or with muscle magnetic resonance imaging [18]. Structural muscle changes detected by the increased echogenicity have been correlated with measures of muscle strength and function [39].

In our study, echogenicity was quantified by the Heckmatt Scale (Table 5), previously used in the critically ill setting by Grimm [18]. A higher grade of echogenicity with reduced bone signal correlates with the severity of myopathy [17]. Of course, the use of a semiquantitative method such as the Heckmatt Scale may be biased by observer dependency and technical misinterpretation in contrast to objective, user-independent algorithms for image analysis such as computer-assisted quantitative grayscale analysis [40]. Though, the Heckmatt Scale has the relevant advantage of being a rapid and inexpensive bedside technique that can be easily used in the intensive care setting.

Changes in muscle architecture have been documented in previous studies on ICU patients and are associated with increased length of stay in ICU [4, 16, 18, 27, 29]. Changes in muscle echogenicity [4, 18] suggest an alteration of myofibers content, secondary to edema from capillary leak or inflammation. These data are confirmed by muscle biopsies on day 1 and 7 after ICU admission, showing muscle necrosis and macrophage infiltrate [4].

In our study, we found a progressive increase in both RF and AT echogenicity from day 5 on. An alteration of echogenicity was already evident in AT muscle soon after admission and tended to increase in the following weeks. The early alteration of echogenicity in AT but not in RF may have many explanations; probably, post-traumatic edema was more pronounced in the muscles of the lateral/posterior part of the limb (AT) than in the anterior area (RF).

Table 5 Heckmatt Scale: visual grading scale to classify muscle echo intensity (Ref 17)

Grade	Ultrasound appearance
Grade 1	Normal
Grade 2	Increased muscle echo intensity with distinct bone echo
Grade 3	Marked increased muscle echo intensity with a reduced bone echo
Grade 4	Very strong muscle echo and complete loss of bone echo

Muscle wasting and nutrition

An optimal provision of energy and protein has been regarded as an important factor improving the patient's chance of survival and satisfactory clinical outcome [41]. Provision of an optimal amount of protein has been shown to improve the rate of protein synthesis in tissues with rapid turnover, though it did not reduce the catabolic response to injury [42, 43]. In one recent multicenter study [44], provision of at least 80% of the prescribed protein (i.e., 1 g/kg/day) reduced mortality in a ICU population. In patients on parenteral nutrition, protein delivery may be more important than caloric support in terms of short-term outcome [11].

In our study, we found no difference in muscle mass loss or in muscle echogenicity between patients fed with standard (SF) versus high-protein formulas (HPF): though, no conclusion can be drawn in this regard, since the study was not designed or powered to verify such hypothesis. Nonetheless, this finding may be consistent with previous studies showing that depletion of lean body mass, particularly skeletal muscle, is not influenced by nutritional support [45–47] and with studies showing an inverse correlation between the amount of protein delivery and the cross-sectional area of RF [4].

Immobilization and inflammation—rather than inadequate nutritional support—might be major determinants of loss of muscle. Inactivity is a potent stimulus to muscle protein breakdown and activation of the ubiquitin–proteasome pathway of proteolysis [48]. Immobility of limbs is quite common in ICU patients and is related to bed rest and sedation. Acute and chronic activation of inflammatory pathway is another potent stimulus for proteolysis [49]. Though, in our study we did not measure any index of inflammatory activity and we could not verify such contention.

Conclusions

In conclusion, we found that ultrasonography was an easy, effective and practical tool for the daily estimate of changes in skeletal muscles and we confirmed the feasibility of such methodology in trauma patients. Our data show that early loss of muscle mass is particularly relevant also in young trauma patients and that extensor muscles such as rectus femoris are much more affected than flexor muscles (anterior tibialis). Such quantitative muscle loss is associated with an increased echogenicity, possibly associated with progressively impaired muscle function.

Abbreviations

AP diam: anterior–posterior diameter; APACHE: acute physiologic and chronic health evaluation; AT: anterior tibialis; BMI: body mass index; BUN: blood urea nitrogen; COPD: chronic obstructive pulmonary diseases; CSA: cross-sectional area; CT: computerized tomography; GCS: Glasgow Coma Scale; GCS-M: Glasgow Coma Scale (motor); GOS: Glasgow Outcome Scale; HPF: high-protein feeding formula; ICU: intensive care unit; ISS: Injury Severity Score; LL diam: latero-lateral diameter; MDR: multiple drug resistant; RF: rectus femoris; SF: standard feeding formula; SOFA: sequential organ failure assessment; US: ultrasound.

Authors' contributions

MGA, MP and MA designed the study and drafted the manuscript. DLG, DS, MFLT and NM participated in the acquisition of data. AM, AC and GM participated in the data analysis. All authors edited the manuscript and approved the final manuscript. All authors read and approved the final manuscript.

Author details

[1] Department of Anesthesia and Intensive Care, Fondazione Policlinico Universitario 'A.Gemelli', Largo A.Gemelli, 8, 00168 Rome, Italy. [2] Department of Surgery, Fondazione Policlinico Universitario 'A.Gemelli', Rome, Italy. [3] Department of Radiology, Fondazione Policlinico Universitario 'A.Gemelli', Rome, Italy.

Acknowledgements

None.

Competing interests

The authors declare that they have no competing interests and that they have full control of all primary data.

References

1. De Jonghe B, Bastuji-Garin S, Durand MC, Malissin I, Rodriguez P, Cerf C, et al. Respiratory weakness is associated with limb weakness and delayed weaning in critical illness. Crit Care Med. 2007;35:2007–15.
2. Weijs PMJ, Looijaard WGPM, Dekker IM, Stapel SN, Girbes AR, et al. Low skeletal muscle area is a risk factor for mortality in mechanically ventilated critically ill patients. Crit Care. 2014;18:R12.
3. Hermans G, Van Mechelen H, Clerckx B, Vanhullebush T, Mesotten D, et al. Acute outcome and 1-year mortality of ICU-acquired weakness: a cohort study and propensity matched analysis. Am J Respir Crit Care Med. 2014;190:410–20.
4. Pathucheary ZA, Rawal J, McPhail M, Connolly B, Ratnayake G, et al. Acute skeletal muscle wasting in critical illness. JAMA. 2013;310(15):1591–600.
5. Fan E, Dowdy DW, Colantuoni E, Mendez-Tellez PA, Sevransky JE, Shanholtz C, et al. Physical complications in acute lung injury survivors: a 2-year longitudinal prospective study. Crit Care Med. 2013;42:849–59.
6. Herridge MS, Tansey CM, Mattè A, Tomlinson G, Diaz-Granados N, Cooper A, et al. Functional disability 5 years after acute respiratory distress syndrome. N Engl J Med. 2011;364:1293–304.
7. Schweickert WD, Pohlman MC, Pohlman AS, Nigos C, Pawlik AJ, Esbrook CL, et al. Early physical and occupational therapy in mechanically ventilated, critically ill patients: a randomized controlled trial. Lancet. 2009;373:1874–82.
8. Denehy L, Skinner EH, Edbrooke L, Haines K, Warrilow S, Hawthorne G, et al. Exercise rehabilitation for patients with critical illness: a randomized controlled trial with 12 months follow-up. Crit Care. 2013;17:R156.
9. Alberda C, Gramlich L, Jones N, Jeejeebhoy K, Day AG, Dhaliwal R, Heyland DK. The relationship between nutritional intake and clinical outcome in critically ill patients: results of an international observational study. Intensive Care Med. 2009;35:1728–37.
10. Weijs PJ, Stapel SN, de Groot SD, Driessen RH, de Jong E, Girbes AR, et al. Optimal protein and energy nutrition decreases mortality in mechanically ventilated, critically ill patients: a prospective observational cohort study. JPEN J Parenter Enteral Nutr. 2012;36:60–8.
11. Ferrie S, Allman-Farinelli M, Daley M, Smith K. Protein requirements in the critically ill: a randomized controlled trial using parenteral nutrition. JPEN J Parenter Enteral Nutr 2016;40(6):795–805.
12. Casaer MP, Wilmer A, Hermans G, Wouters PJ, Mesotten D, Van den Berghe G. Role of disease and macronutrient dose in the randomized controlled EPaNIC trial: a post hoc analysis. Am J Respir Crit Care Med. 2013;187:247–55.
13. Seymour JM, Ward K, Sidhu PS, Puthucheary Z, Steier J, et al. Ultrasound measurement of rectus femoris cross-sectional area and the relationship with quadriceps strength in COPD. Thorax. 2009;64:418–23.
14. Boles JM, Bion J, Connors A, Herridge M, Marsh B, Melot C, et al. Weaning from mechanical ventilation. Eur Respir J. 2007;29:1033–56.
15. Horan TC, Andrus M, Dudeck MA. CDC/NHSN surveillance definition of health care-associated infection and criteria for specific types of infections in the acute care setting. Am J Infect Control. 2008;36:309–32.
16. Gruther W, Benesch T, Zorn C, Paternostro-Sluga T, Quittan M, Fialka-Moser V, et al. Muscle wasting in intensive care patients: ultrasound observation of the m. quadriceps femoris muscle layer. J Rehabil Med. 2008;40:185–9.
17. Heckmatt JZ, Pier N, Dubowitz V. Real-time ultrasound imaging of the muscle. Muscle Nerve. 1988;11:56–65.
18. Grimm A, Teschner U, Porzelius C, Ludewig K, Zielske J, et al. Muscle ultrasound for early assessment of critical illness neuromyopathy in severe sepsis. Crit Care. 2013;17:R227.
19. Paris MT, Mourtzakis M, Day A, Leung R, Watharkar S, Kozar R, et al. Validation of bedside ultrasound of muscle layer thickness of the quadriceps in the critically ill patient (VALIDUM study): a prospective multicenter study. JPEN J Parenter Enteral Nutr. 2017;41(2):171–80.
20. Campbell IT, Watt T, Withers D, England R, Sukumar S, Keegan MA, et al. Muscle thickness, measured with ultrasound, may be an indicator of lean tissue wasting in multiple organ failure in presence of edema. Am J Clin Nutr. 1995;62:533–9.
21. dos Santos C, Hussain SNA, Marthur S, Picard M, Herridge M, Correa J, et al. Mechanism of chronic muscle wasting and dysfunction after an intensive care unit stay: a pilot study. Am J Respir Crit Care Med. 2016;194(7):821–30.
22. Fan E, Cheek F, Chlan L, Gosselink R, Hart N, Herridge MS, et al. An official American Thoracic Society Clinical Practice guideline: the diagnosis of intensive care unit-acquired weakness in adults. Am J Respir Crit Care Med. 2014;190:1437–46.
23. Farhan H, Moreno-Duarte I, Latronico N, Zafonte R, Eikermann M. Acquired muscle weakness in the surgical intensive care unit: Nosology, epidemiology, and prevention. Anesthesiol. 2016;124:207–34.
24. Hermans G, Casaer MP, Clerckx B, Guiza F, Vanhullebusch T, Derde S, et al. Effect of tolerating macronutrient deficit on the development of intensive- care unit acquired weakness: a subanalysis of the EPaNIC trial. Lancet Respir Med. 2013;1:621–9.
25. Moisey LL, Mourtzakis M, Cotton BA, Premji T, Heyland DK, Wade CE, et al. Skeletal muscle predict ventilator-free days, ICU-free days and mortality in elderly ICU patients. Crit Care. 2013;17:R206.
26. Sheean PM, Peterson SJ, Gomez Perez S, Troy KL, Patel A, Sclamberg JS, et al. The prevalence of sarcopenia in patients with respiratory failure classified as normally nourished using computed tomography and subjective global assessment. JPEN J Parenter Enteral Nutr. 2014;38:873–9.
27. Campbell SE, Adler R, Sofka CM. Ultrasound of muscle abnormalities. Ultrasound Q. 2005;21:87–94.
28. Pillen S, Zwartz MJ. Muscle ultrasound in neuromuscular disorders. Muscle Nerve. 2008;37:679–93.
29. Reeves ND, Maganaris CN, Narici MV. Ultrasonographic assessment of human skeletal muscle size. Eur J Appl Physiol. 2004;91:116–8.
30. Tillquist M, Kutsogiannis DJ, Wischmeyer PE, Kummerlen K, Leung R, et al. Bedside ultrasound is a practical and reliable measurement tool for assessing quadriceps muscle layer thickness. JPEN J Parenter Enteral Nutr. 2014;38(7):886–90.
31. Segers J, Hermans G, Charususin N, Fivez T, Vanhorebeek I, et al. Assessment of quadriceps muscle mass with ultrasound in critically ill patients: intra- and inter-observer agreement and sensitivity. Intensive Care Med. 2015;41(3):562–3.
32. Fivez T, Hendrickx A, Van Herpe T, Vlasselaers D, Desmet L, et al. An analysis of reliability and accuracy of muscle thickness ultrasonography in critically ill children and adults. JPEN J Parenter Enteral Nutr. 2016;40:944–9.
33. Zhong H, Roy RR, Siengthai B, Edgerton VR. Effects of inactivity on fiber size and myonuclear number in rat soleus muscle. J Appl Physiol. 2005;99:1494–9.

34. Psatha M, Wu Z, Gammie FM, Ratkevicius A, Wackerhage H, Lee JH, Redpath TW, Gilbert FJ, Ashcroft GP, Meakin JR, Aspden RM. A longitudinal MRI study of muscle atrophy during lower leg immobilization following ankle fracture. J Magn Reson Imaging. 2012;35:686–95.

35. Henriksson-Larsen KB, Lexell J, Sjostrom M. Distribution of different fibre types in human skeletal muscles. Method for the preparation and analysis of cross-sections of whole tibialis anterior. Histochem J. 1983;15:167–78.

36. De Jonghe B, Sharshar T, Lefaucheur JP, Authier FJ, Durand-Zaleski I, et al. Paresis acquired in the intensive care unit: a prospective multicenter study. JAMA. 2002;288:2859–67.

37. Petrasek PF, Homer-Vanniasinkam S, Walker PM. Determinants of ischemic injury to skeletal muscle. J Vasc Surg. 1994;19:623–31.

38. Krawiec BJ, Frost RA, Vary TC, Jefferson LS, Lang CH. Hindlimb casting decreases muscle mass in part by proteasome-dependent proteolysis but independent of protein synthesis. Am J Physiol Endocrinol Metab. 2005;289:E969–80.

39. Parry SM, El-Ansary D, Cartwright MS, Sarwal A, Berney S, et al. Ultrasonography in the intensive care setting can be used to detect changes in the quality and quantity of muscle and is related to muscle strength and function. J Crit Care. 2015;30:1151.e9–14.

40. Pillen S. Skeletal muscle ultrasound. Eur J Transl Myol. 2010;1(4):145–55.

41. Allingstrup MJ, Esmailzadeh N, Wilkens Knudsen A, Espersen K, Hartvig Jensen T, Wiis J, et al. Provision of protein and energy in relation to measured requirements in intensive care patients. Clin Nutr. 2012;31:462e8.

42. Mansoor O, Breuille D, Bechereau F, Buffiere C, Pouyet C, Beaufrere B, et al. Effect of an enteral diet supplemented with a specific blend of amino acid on plasma and muscle protein synthesis in ICU patients. Clin Nutr. 2007;26:30e40.

43. Hoffer LJ, Bistrian BR. Appropriate protein provision in critical illness: a systematic and narrative review. Am J Clin Nutr. 2012;96:591e600.

44. Nicolo M, Heyland DK, Chittams J, Sammarco T, Compher C. Clinical outcomes related to protein delivery in a critically ill population: a multicentre, multinational observational study. JPEN J Parenter Enteral Nutr. 2016;40:45–51.

45. Streat SJ, Beddoe AH, Hill GL. Aggressive nutritional support does not prevent protein losses despite fat gain in septic intensive care patients. J Trauma. 1987;27:262–6.

46. Hart DW, Wolf SE, Herndon DN, et al. Energy expenditure and caloric balance after burn. Increased feeding leads to fat rather than lean mass accretion. Ann Surg. 2002;235:152–61.

47. Casaer MP, Langouche L, Coudyzer W, Vanbeckevoort D, De Dobbelaer B, Guiza FG, et al. Impact of early parenteral nutrition on muscle and adipose tissue compartments during critical illness. Crit Care Med. 2013;41:2298–309.

48. Dock W. The evil sequelae of complete bed rest. JAMA. 1944;125:1083–5.

49. Reid MB, Moylan JS. Beyond atrophy: redox mechanisms of muscle dysfunction in chronic inflammatory disease. J Physiol. 2011;589:2171–9.

12

Acid–base status and its clinical implications in critically ill patients with cirrhosis, acute-on-chronic liver failure and without liver disease

Andreas Drolz[1,2]*[†] [iD], Thomas Horvatits[1,2†], Kevin Roedl[1,2], Karoline Rutter[1,2], Richard Brunner[1], Christian Zauner[1], Peter Schellongowski[3], Gottfried Heinz[4], Georg-Christian Funk[5], Michael Trauner[1], Bruno Schneeweiss[1] and Valentin Fuhrmann[1,2]

Abstract

Background: Acid–base disturbances are frequently observed in critically ill patients at the intensive care unit. To our knowledge, the acid–base profile of patients with acute-on-chronic liver failure (ACLF) has not been evaluated and compared to critically ill patients without acute or chronic liver disease.

Results: One hundred and seventy-eight critically ill patients with liver cirrhosis were compared to 178 matched controls in this post hoc analysis of prospectively collected data. Patients with and without liver cirrhosis showed hyperchloremic acidosis and coexisting hypoalbuminemic alkalosis. Cirrhotic patients, especially those with ACLF, showed a marked net metabolic acidosis owing to increased lactate and unmeasured anions. This metabolic acidosis was partly antagonized by associated respiratory alkalosis, yet with progression to ACLF resulted in acidemia, which was present in 62% of patients with ACLF grade III compared to 19% in cirrhosis patients without ACLF. Acidemia and metabolic acidosis were associated with 28-day mortality in cirrhosis. Patients with pH values < 7.1 showed a 100% mortality rate. Acidosis attributable to lactate and unmeasured anions was independently associated with mortality in liver cirrhosis.

Conclusions: Cirrhosis and especially ACLF are associated with metabolic acidosis and acidemia owing to lactate and unmeasured anions. Acidosis and acidemia, respectively, are associated with increased 28-day mortality in liver cirrhosis. Lactate and unmeasured anions are main contributors to metabolic imbalance in cirrhosis and ACLF.

Keywords: Acid–base, Cirrhosis, Acute-on-chronic liver failure, Mortality

Background

Derangements in acid–base balance are frequently observed in critically ill patients at the intensive care unit (ICU) and present in various patterns [1–4]. Severe acid–base disorders, especially metabolic acidosis, have been associated with increased mortality [5, 6]. As a consequence, acid–base status in critically ill patients with various disease entities has been extensively studied.

Yet, only a few studies assessed the impact of underlying chronic liver disease on acid–base equilibrium in critical illness [7, 8]. While a balance of offsetting acidifying and alkalinizing metabolic acid–base disorders with a resulting equilibrated acid–base status has been described in stable cirrhosis [9], severe derangements with resulting net acidosis owing to hyperchloremic, dilutional and lactic acidosis were observed when cirrhosis was accompanied by critical illness [7, 8]. Acute liver failure (ALF) is characterized by a different acid–base pattern with dramatically increased lactate levels [10]. The acidifying effect of this increase in lactate was neutralized by hypoalbuminemia in non-paracetamol-induced ALF [11].

*Correspondence: a.drolz@uke.de
[†]Andreas Drolz and Thomas Horvatits contributed equally to the work
[2] Department of Intensive Care Medicine, University Medical Center, Hamburg-Eppendorf, Martinistraße 52, 20246 Hamburg, Germany

Despite advantages in intensive care medicine, which have led to an improved outcome over the last decade [12], mortality in cirrhotic patients admitted to ICU is still high [13–15]. Measurement and knowledge of specific acid–base patterns and their implications in critically ill patients with liver cirrhosis may help to improve patient management, especially in the ICU setting [16]. However, to our knowledge, the acid–base profile of critically ill cirrhotic patients with acute-on-chronic liver disease (ACLF) has not been compared to critically ill patients without acute or chronic liver disease. Most information on the acid–base status of critically ill patients with cirrhosis was obtained by comparing these patients with healthy controls [8]. Yet, part of metabolic disturbances in critically ill patients with liver cirrhosis may be attributable to critical illness per se, rather than to the presence of chronic liver disease.

The aim of this study was to assess acid–base patterns of critically ill patients with liver cirrhosis and ACLF, respectively, in comparison with critically ill patients without acute or chronic liver disease.

Methods
Patients
All patients admitted to 3 medical ICUs at the Medical University of Vienna between July 2012 and August 2014 were screened for inclusion in the study. For the present study, only patients who had arterial blood samples drawn within 4 h after ICU admission were eligible for inclusion. Patients with acute liver injury in the absence of chronic liver disease were excluded. One hundred and seventy-eight patients with liver cirrhosis were identified as eligible for inclusion. The control group of 178 critically ill patients without acute or chronic liver disease was selected by propensity score matching (PSM).

On admission, Simplified Acute Physiology Score II (SAPS II) [17], SOFA [18], infections and organ dysfunctions were documented.

All patients were screened for the presence of acute kidney injury (AKI) defined by urine output and serum creatinine according to the Kidney Disease: Improving Global Outcomes (KDIGO) Clinical Practice Guidelines for Acute Kidney Injury [19].

The presence of liver cirrhosis was defined by a combination of characteristic clinical (ascites, caput medusae, spider angiomata, etc.), laboratory and radiological findings (typical morphological changes of the liver, sings of portal hypertension, etc., in ultrasonography or computed

tomography scanning), or via histology, if available. ACLF was identified and graded according to recommendations of the chronic liver failure (CLIF) consortium of the European Association for the Study of the Liver (EASL) [20]. CLIF-SOFA score [20] and CLIF-C ACLF score [21] were calculated. Septic shock was defined according to the recommendations of the Surviving Sepsis Campaign [22].

Twenty-eight-day mortality and 1-year mortality were assessed on site or by contacting the patient or the attending physician, respectively.

This study is based on a post hoc analysis of prospectively collected data [23]. The Ethics Committee of the Medical University of Vienna waived the need for informed consent due to the observational character of this study.

Sampling and blood analysis
On admission, arterial blood samples were collected from arterial or femoral artery and parameters for the assessment of acid–base status were instantly measured.

pH, partial pressure of carbon dioxide ($PaCO_2$), ionized calcium (Ca^{2+}) and lactate were measured with a blood gas analyzer (ABL 725; Radiometer, Copenhagen, Denmark). Samples of separated plasma were analyzed for concentrations of sodium (Na^+), potassium (K^+), chloride (Cl^-), magnesium (Mg^{2+}), inorganic phosphate (Pi), albumin (Alb), plasma creatinine, blood urea nitrogen (BUN), aspartate aminotransferase (AST) and alanine aminotransferase (ALT) by a fully automated analyzer (Hitachi 917; Roche Diagnostics GmbH, Mannheim, Germany). Na^+ and Cl^- were measured using ion-selective electrodes. Lactate was measured with an amperometric electrode.

Acid–base analysis
Arterial concentration of bicarbonate ($HCO3^-$) was calculated from measured pH and $PaCO_2$ values according to the Henderson–Hasselbalch equation [24, 25]. Base excess (BE) was calculated according to the formulae by Siggaard-Andersen [24–26].

Quantitative physical–chemical analysis was performed using Stewart's biophysical methods [27], modified by Figge and colleagues [28].

Apparent strong ion difference (SIDa) was calculated:

$$SIDa = Na^+ + K^+ + 2 \times Mg^{2+} + 2 \times Ca^{2+} - Cl^- - lactate$$
(SIDa in mEq/l; all concentrations in mmol/l)

Effective strong ion difference (SIDe) was calculated in order to account for the role of weak acids [29]:

$$SIDe = 1000 \times 2.46 \times 10^{-11} \times \frac{PaCO_2}{10^{-pH}} + Alb \times (0.123 \times pH - 0.631) + Pi \times (0.309 \times pH - 0.469)$$
(SIDe in mEq/l; $PaCO_2$ in mmHg, Alb in g/l and Pi in mmol/l)

The effect of unmeasured charges was quantified by the strong ion gap (SIG) [30]:

$$SIG = SIDa - SIDe$$

(all parameters in mEq/l)

Based on the concept that BE can be altered by plasma dilution/concentration reflected by sodium concentration (BE_{Na}), changes of chloride (BE_{Cl}), albumin (BE_{Alb}), lactate (BE_{Lac}) and unmeasured anions (BE_{UMA}), the respective components contributing to BE were calculated according to Gilfix et al. [31]. The detailed formulae for the BE subcomponents are shown in "Appendix."

Thus, total BE is calculated by the sum of the BE subcomponents:

$$BE = BE_{Na} + BE_{Cl} + BE_{Alb} + BE_{Lac} + BE_{UMA}$$

Reference values were obtained from a historical cohort of healthy volunteers, as published elsewhere [8]. Acidemia and alkalemia were defined by $pH < 7.36$ and > 7.44, respectively. $HCO3^- < 22$ and > 26 mmol/l, respectively, defined metabolic acidosis and alkalosis [2]. Respiratory acidosis and alkalosis were identified by $PaCO_2 > 45$ and < 35 mmHg, respectively. $BE_{Na} < -5$ and > 5 mmol/l defined dilutional acidosis and alkalosis, respectively. Hyperchloremic acidosis and hypochloremic alkalosis were defined by $BE_{Cl} < -5$ and > 5 mmol/l, respectively. $BE_{Alb} > 5$ mmol/l identified hypoalbuminemic alkalosis. Lactic acidosis was defined by $BE_{Lac} < -1.1$ mmol/l (calculated BE_{Lac} for lactate at the upper limit of normal) and metabolic acidosis owing to unmeasured anions by $BE_{UMA} < -5$ mmol/l.

Statistical analysis

Data are presented as median and interquartile range (25–75% IQR), if not otherwise specified. PSM was used to minimize the confounding effect of severity of disease on acid–base status when comparing cirrhosis to non-cirrhosis patients. One-to-one PSM (1:1) was done by cirrhosis versus non-cirrhosis based on the following variables: SOFA score, need for mechanical ventilation and the presence of AKI. IBM SPSS 22 (with SPSS Python essentials and FUZZY extension command) was used for PSM. McNemar test was used for the comparison of binary and Wilcoxon's signed-rank test for the comparison of metric variables between cirrhosis and matched controls. Nonparametric one-way ANOVA (Kruskal–Wallis test) with Dunn's post hoc analysis was performed to assess differences in acid–base parameters between matched controls, cirrhosis patients without ACLF and ACLF patients. Within each group, comparisons were made using Chi-squared test or Mann–Whitney U test, as appropriate. Spearman's rank correlation was used to assess correlations between metric variables. A receiver

operating curve (ROC) analysis was performed, and the area under the ROC curve (AUROC) was calculated to evaluate the prognostic value of different metric variables. Impact of acid–base disorders on mortality was assessed using Cox regression. A p value < 0.05 is considered statistically significant. Statistical analysis was conducted using IBM SPSS Statistics version 22.

Results

Patients' characteristics

One hundred and seventy-eight patients had liver cirrhosis, and 157 of these patients (88%) were admitted with ACLF. The remaining cirrhosis patients ($n = 21$, 12%) were admitted to ICU due to isolated non-kidney organ failure ($n = 9$), isolated cerebral failure ($n = 4$), bleedings ($n = 4$), infections ($n = 3$) and after surgery ($n = 1$); all of which did not fulfill criteria for ACLF. The control group consisted of 178 critically ill patients without acute or chronic liver disease. SAPS II score and SOFA score did not differ between patients with and without cirrhosis (Table 1).

Causes of liver cirrhosis were alcoholic liver disease ($n = 96$, 54%), viral hepatitis ($n = 31$, 17%), combined alcoholic viral ($n = 7$, 4%), cryptogenic ($n = 23$, 13%), primary biliary cholangitis ($n = 5$, 3%) and others ($n = 16$, 9%). Triggers for occurrence ACLF were infections/sepsis ($n = 110$, 70%), bleeding ($n = 23$, 15%) and others.

Clinical and laboratory features of critically ill patients with and without cirrhosis are shown in Table 1.

Acid–base disorders in critically ill patients with and without cirrhosis

Disturbances of acid–base balance were evident in the vast majority of our critically ill patients, irrespective of cirrhosis (Tables 2, 3). Critically ill patients (irrespective of cirrhosis) showed coexisting hyperchloremic acidosis and hypoalbuminemic alkalosis, mostly antagonizing each other in their contribution to total BE. In ACLF, we observed a marked metabolic acidosis owing to increased lactate levels, unmeasured anions and (to a lesser extent) dilutional acidosis. Both BE_{UMA} and SIG differed significantly between critically ill patients with ACLF and without liver disease, respectively, although the small difference in SIG may be clinically negligible (Table 2). In cirrhosis patients without ACLF, BE_{UMA} was significantly higher compared to patients with ACLF. The resulting metabolic acidosis in ACLF was partly compensated by coexisting respiratory alkalosis in its contribution to pH; however, increasing net metabolic acidosis is resulted in acidemia in patients with ACLF grade III (62%, Table 3). Metabolic differences between critically ill patients with and without cirrhosis tended to increase with the severity

Table 1 Baseline characteristics

Parameter	Propensity score-matched controls (n = 178)	Liver cirrhosis (n = 178)	p value
Age, years (IQR)	65 (55–75)	55 (48–62)	< 0.01
Male gender, n (%)	79 (44%)	82 (46%)	0.837
SOFA score (IQR)	12 (8–16)	13 (10–16)	0.084
SAPS II score (IQR)	59 (44–72)	62 (44–79)	0.101
CLIF-SOFA score (IQR)	–	14 (11–16)	
ACLF grade			
No ACLF, n (%)		21 (12%)	
Grade I, n (%)	–	27 (15%)	
Grade II, n (%)	–	45 (25%)	
Grade III, n (%)	–	85 (48%)	
CLIF-C ACLF score (IQR)	–	56.5 (48.8–63.3)	
MELD score (IQR)	–	26 (20–35)	
Child–Pugh score (IQR)	–	11 (10–13)	
Acute kidney injury, n (%)	133 (75%)	138 (78%)	0.575
Vasopressor support, n (%)	154 (87%)	158 (89%)	0.596
Mechanical ventilation, n (%)	116 (65%)	101 (57%)	0.120
Laboratory parameters			
AST, U/l (IQR)	51 (30–116)	94 (54–204)	< 0.01
ALT, U/l (IQR)	32 (19–71)	43 (24–85)	0.096
Bilirubin, mg/dl (IQR)	1.0 (0.6–1.9)	5.4 (2.9–14.4)	< 0.01
INR (IQR)	1.2 (1.1–1.4)	1.8 (1.5–2.5)	< 0.01
Creatinine, mg/dl (IQR)	1.8 (1.2–2.7)	1.8 (1.1–3.1)	0.851
Outcome			
28-Day mortality, n (%)	54 (30%)	105 (59%)	< 0.01

IQR interquartile range, *SOFA* Sequential Organ Failure Assessment, *SAPS* Simplified Acute Physiology Score, *CLIF-SOFA* Chronic Liver Failure—Sequential Organ Failure Assessment, *ACLF* acute-on-chronic liver failure, *CLIF-C ACLF* CLIF consortium ACLF score, *MELD* Model of End-Stage Liver Disease, *AST* aspartate aminotransferase, *ALT* alanine aminotransferase, *INR* international normalized ratio

of disease, as indicated by SOFA score (Additional file 1: Figure S1).

Both SIG and BE_{UMA} were associated with renal impairment (Additional file 2: Figure S2). Overall ($n = 356$), SIG was significantly higher and BE_{UMA} significantly lower in patients presenting with AKI as compared to those without [8.4 (IQR 6.0–11.1) mmol/l vs. 5.4 (IQR 2.7–7.5) mmol/l and −2.0 (IQR −6.0 to 1.4) mmol/l vs. 2.8 (IQR −0.3 to 5.6) mmol/l; $p < 0.01$ for both].

Lactate levels were significantly elevated in critically ill patients with liver cirrhosis compared to those without [3.0 (IQR 1.7–6.1) mmol/l vs. 1.4 (IQR 1.0–2.7) mmol/l; $p < 0.01$]. Additionally, lactate levels were higher in patients receiving vasopressors compared to those without [2.3 (IQR 1.3–4.6) mmol/l vs. 1.2 (IQR 0.9–1.8) mmol/l; $p < 0.01$]. Lactate levels increased with SOFA score in cirrhotic and non-cirrhotic patients (Additional file 1: Figure S1). Accordingly, highest lactate levels were observed in patients with ACLF (Table 2). Lactate levels correlated with bilirubin ($r = 0.41$) and international normalized ratio (INR, $r = 0.46$), respectively, but also weakly with serum creatinine ($r = 0.17$); $p < 0.01$ for all.

Metabolic acid–base characteristics of critically ill patients with and without liver disease are illustrated in Fig. 1 and Additional file 1: Figure S1.

Acid–base equilibrium and outcome in patients with liver cirrhosis

In particular, metabolic acidosis and acidemia, respectively, were linked to 28-day mortality in cirrhosis (Fig. 2, Additional file 3: Table S1). Accordingly, arterial pH values < 7.1 on admission were associated with 100% and HCO_3^- values < 10 mmol/l with 89% 28-day mortality, respectively (Fig. 2).

Similarly, BE showed a strong association with 28-day mortality (Additional file 3: Table S1). Analysis of the BE subgroups revealed that the impact on mortality in cirrhosis was primarily caused by lactate and unmeasured anions (Table 4). This effect remained significant after correction for demographics, ACLF grade and the presence of infection/sepsis (Table 4). AUROCs for admission lactate/BE_{Lac} and BE_{UMA} in prediction of 28-day mortality in critical ill patients with liver cirrhosis were 0.744 (95% CI 0.671–0.816) and 0.692 (95% CI 0.613–0.770),

Table 2 Acid–base parameters of critically ill patients with and without liver disease

Parameter	Propensity score-matched controls ($n = 178$)	Cirrhosis ($n = 178$)		Overall p value (Kruskal–Wallis)	Significant differences pairwise (Dunn's post hoc)
		No ACLF ($n = 21$)	ACLF ($n = 157$)		
pH	7.36 (7.27 to 7.43)	7.44 (7.37 to 7.47)	7.35 (7.23 to 7.45)	< 0.01	No ACLF versus ACLF $p < 0.01$, matched controls versus no ACLF $p < 0.01$
PaCO$_2$, mmHg	40.0 (33.1 to 49.0)	38.1 (30.0 to 44.2)	35.0 (28.5 to 44.6)	< 0.01	Matched controls versus ACLF $p < 0.01$
HCO$_3^-$	22.0 (19.0 to 25.3)	22.7 (20.3 to 24.0)	18.9 (14.7 to 24.0)	< 0.01	No ACLF versus ACLF $p < 0.01$, matched controls versus ACLF $p < 0.01$
BE	− 3.5 (− 7.4 to 0.8)	− 1.2 (− 3.9 to 1.7)	− 7.0 (− 12.6 to − 0.5)	< 0.01	No ACLF versus ACLF $p < 0.01$, matched controls versus ACLF $p < 0.01$
BE$_{Na}$	− 0.3 (− 1.5 to 0.9)	− 0.9 (− 1.8 to 0.3)	− 1.2 (− 3.0 to 0.3)	< 0.01	Matched controls versus ACLF $p < 0.01$
BE$_{Cl}$	− 5.7 (− 8.3 to − 2.7)	− 5.2 (− 8.5 to − 1.4)	− 4.5 (− 7.3 to 0.7)	0.062	
BE$_{Alb}$	4.2 (2.9 to 5.3)	5.2 (3.9 to 6.3)	4.9 (3.8 to 6.2)	< 0.01	Matched controls versus ACLF $p < 0.01$
BE$_{lactate}$	− 0.6 (− 1.9 to − 0.2)	− 0.9 (− 1.9 to − 0.4)	− 2.7 (− 6.0 to − 0.9)	< 0.01	No ACLF versus ACLF $p < 0.01$, matched controls versus ACLF $p < 0.01$
BE$_{UMA}$	− 0.3 (− 3.7 to 2.7)	1.5 (− 0.7 to 4.3)	− 1.8 (− 6.1 to 1.9)	< 0.01	No ACLF versus ACLF $p < 0.01$, matched controls versus ACLF $p < 0.01$
SIDe, mEq/l	33 (30 to 37)	32 (30 to 37)	29 (25 to 34)	< 0.01	No ACLF versus ACLF $p < 0.05$, matched controls versus ACLF $p < 0.01$
SIDa, mEq/l	41 (37 to 43)	40 (36 to 44)	39 (35 to 42)	< 0.01	Matched controls versus ACLF $p < 0.01$
SIG, mEq/l	7 (4 to 10)	7 (5 to 8)	8 (6 to 11)	< 0.01	No ACLF versus ACLF $p < 0.05$, matched controls versus ACLF $p < 0.01$
Na	138 (134 to 142)	136 (133 to 140)	135 (129 to 140)	< 0.01	Matched controls versus ACLF $p < 0.01$
Cl	106 (102 to 109)	105 (99 to 108)	102 (96 to 108)	< 0.01	Matched controls versus ACLF $p < 0.01$
Cl$_{Na corrected}$	107 (104 to 109)	106 (102 to 110)	106 (100 to 108)	0.075	
Ca total	2.1 (2.0 to 2.2)	2.0 (1.9 to 2.1)	2.0 (1.9 to 2.2)	0.191	
Ca ionized	1.1 (1.1 to 1.2)	1.2 (1.1 to 1.2)	1.1 (1.0 to 1.2)	< 0.01	No ACLF versus ACLF $p < 0.05$, matched controls versus ACLF $p < 0.01$
Mg	0.9 (0.7 to 1.0)	0.7 (0.7 to 0.9)	0.9 (0.7 to 1.0)	< 0.05	No ACLF versus ACLF $p < 0.05$
Albumin, g/l	28.5 (24.3 to 33.8)	25.8 (21.8 to 30.5)	25.6 (21.1 to 30.3)	< 0.01	Matched controls versus ACLF $p < 0.01$
Lactate	1.4 (1.0 to 2.7)	1.7 (1.2 to 2.7)	3.5 (1.7 to 6.8)	< 0.01	No ACLF versus ACLF $p < 0.01$, matched controls versus ACLF $p < 0.01$

ACLF acute-on-chronic liver failure, *PaCO$_2$* partial pressure of arterial carbon dioxide, *HCO$_3^-$* bicarbonate, *BE* base excess, *SBE* standard base excess, *BE$_{Na}$* BE caused by free water effect, *BE$_{Cl}$* BE caused by changes in chloride, *BE$_{Alb}$* BE caused by albumin effect, *BE$_{lactate}$* BE attributable to lactate elevation, *BE$_{UMA}$* BE attributable to unmeasured anions, *SIDe* effective strong ion difference, *SIDa* apparent strong ion difference, *SIG* strong ion gap, *Na* sodium, *Cl* chloride, *Ca* calcium, all values are given in mmol/l with interquartile range (IQR), unless otherwise indicated

respectively ($p < 0.001$ for both). Thus, the predictive potential of admission arterial lactate levels regarding 28-day mortality in critically ill cirrhosis patients at the ICU was comparable to SOFA score [AUROC 0.780 (95% CI 0.713–0.847)].

In our matched controls, we observed no significant effect of acidemia, alkalemia, lactic acidosis and net metabolic acidosis, respectively, on 28-day mortality. Yet, pH values differed significantly between non-cirrhosis 28-day survivors and non-survivors [7.37 (IQR

Table 3 Acid–base disorders stratified according to the presence of cirrhosis and ACLF

Metabolic disturbances on admission	Propensity score-matched controls (n = 178)	Cirrhosis (n = 178) Overall cirrhosis (n = 178)	ACLF category No ACLF (n = 21)	ACLF grade 1 and 2 (n = 72)	ACLF grade III (n = 85)	p value for over-all cirrhosis ver-sus matched controls	p value for the effect of ACLF category*
Acidemia	87 (49%)	86 (48%)	4 (19%)	29 (40%)	53 (62%)	1.00	<0.01
Alkalemia	35 (20%)	52 (29%)	11 (52%)	21 (29%)	20 (24%)	<0.05	<0.05
Respiratory acidosis	64 (36%)	41 (23%)	3 (14%)	13 (18%)	25 (29%)	<0.05	0.052
Respiratory alkalosis	55 (31%)	88 (49%)	10 (48%)	40 (56%)	38 (45%)	<0.01	0.338
Metabolic acidosis	89 (50%)	112 (63%)	7 (33%)	45 (63%)	60 (71%)	<0.05	<0.01
Metabolic alkalosis	38 (21%)	33 (19%)	4 (19%)	16 (22%)	13 (15%)	0.596	0.365
Dilutional acidosis	1 (0.6%)	11 (6%)	0	4 (6%)	7 (8%)	<0.01	0.205
Concentrational alkalosis	2 (1.1%)	6 (3%)	0	6 (8%)	0	0.289	0.136
Hyperchloremic acidosis	98 (55%)	78 (44%)	11 (52%)	32 (44%)	35 (41%)	<0.05	0.399
Hypochloremic alkalosis	7 (4%)	15 (8%)	0	8 (11%)	7 (8%)	0.134	0.702
Hypoalbuminemic alkalosis	58 (33%)	86 (48%)	11 (52%)	36 (50%)	39 (46%)	<0.01	0.516
Acidosis owing to unmeasured anions	32 (18%)	48 (27%)	1 (5%)	16 (22%)	31 (37%)	0.061	<0.01
Lactic acidosis	65 (37%)	118 (66%)	7 (33%)	44 (61%)	67 (79%)	<0.01	<0.01

All values are given in number (n) and percent (%)

ACLF acute-on-chronic liver failure

*p value calculated by univariate ordinal logistic regression

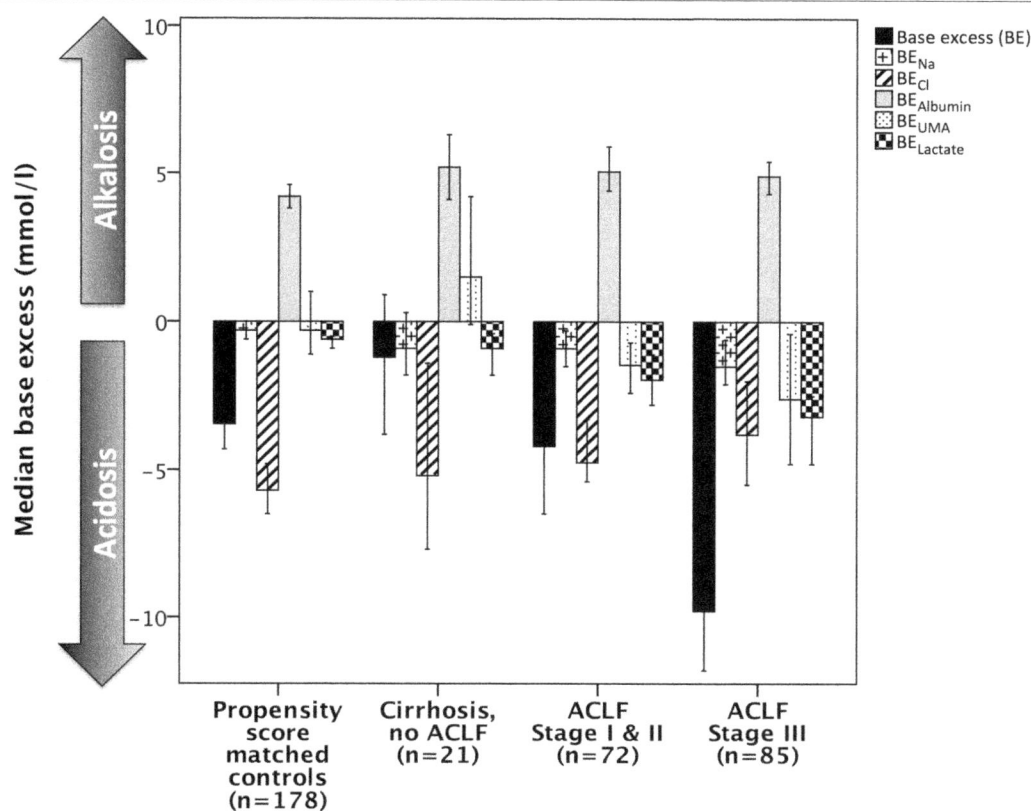

Fig. 1 Disequilibrium in acid–base status in critically ill patients with liver cirrhosis, acute-on-chronic liver failure (ACLF) and without chronic liver disease. Results displayed as median and 95% CI; associations of base excess and its subcomponents with ACLF stage in cirrhosis patients assessed by univariate ordinal regression: BE $p < 0.001$, BE_{Na} $p = 0.074$, BE_{Cl} $p = 0.728$, BE_{Alb} $p = 0.295$, BE_{Lac} $p < 0.001$, BE_{UMA} $p < 0.05$. Differences between cirrhosis and control patients are illustrated in Table 2

7.29–7.44) vs. 7.34 (IQR 7.22–7.34), $p < 0.05$, Additional file 3: Table S1]. Acidosis attributable to unmeasured anions was associated with 28-day mortality in our propensity score-matched controls; however, BE_{UMA} did not differ significantly between non-cirrhotic 28-day survivors and non-survivors (Additional file 3: Table S1). Moreover, admission arterial lactate levels differed significantly between non-cirrhosis 28-day survivors and non-survivors [1.4 (IQR 0.9–2.4) mmol/l vs. 1.7 (IQR 1–4.1) mmol/l; $p < 0.05$]. Yet, the association between metabolic derangement and outcome was more distinct in cirrhosis patients (Additional file 3: Table S1).

Discussion

Disturbances in acid–base equilibrium are common in critical illness [16]. In this study, we demonstrate that critically ill patients with cirrhosis and ACLF, respectively, differentiate considerably from patients without hepatic impairment in terms of acid–base balance.

In accordance with earlier reports, we observed in our cohort a marked hyperchloremic acidosis with coexisting

hypoalbuminemic alkalosis [8, 9, 11]. This phenomenon, however, was not limited to patients with cirrhosis and should therefore not be considered an exclusive acid–base pattern of liver disease. Instead, this seems to be a characteristic pattern of critical illness per se [3]. Yet, hypoalbuminemia and resulting alkalosis were most pronounced in patients with ACLF. However, the main distinguishing metabolic acid–base characteristic between critically ill patients with and without cirrhosis was a marked metabolic acidosis attributable to an increased lactate (and unmeasured anions). In cirrhosis, coexisting respiratory alkalosis partly compensated for metabolic acidosis, thereby resulting in almost normal pH values. However, respiratory alkalosis failed to compensate for net metabolic acidosis in patients with ACLF.

Increased lactate levels in critically ill patients can result from both increased production (e.g., tissue malperfusion, impaired cellular oxygen metabolism during sepsis, hypermetabolic states) and reduced lactate clearance (e.g., loss of functioning hepatocytes in acute hepatic injury or chronic liver disease) [32–34]. The liver

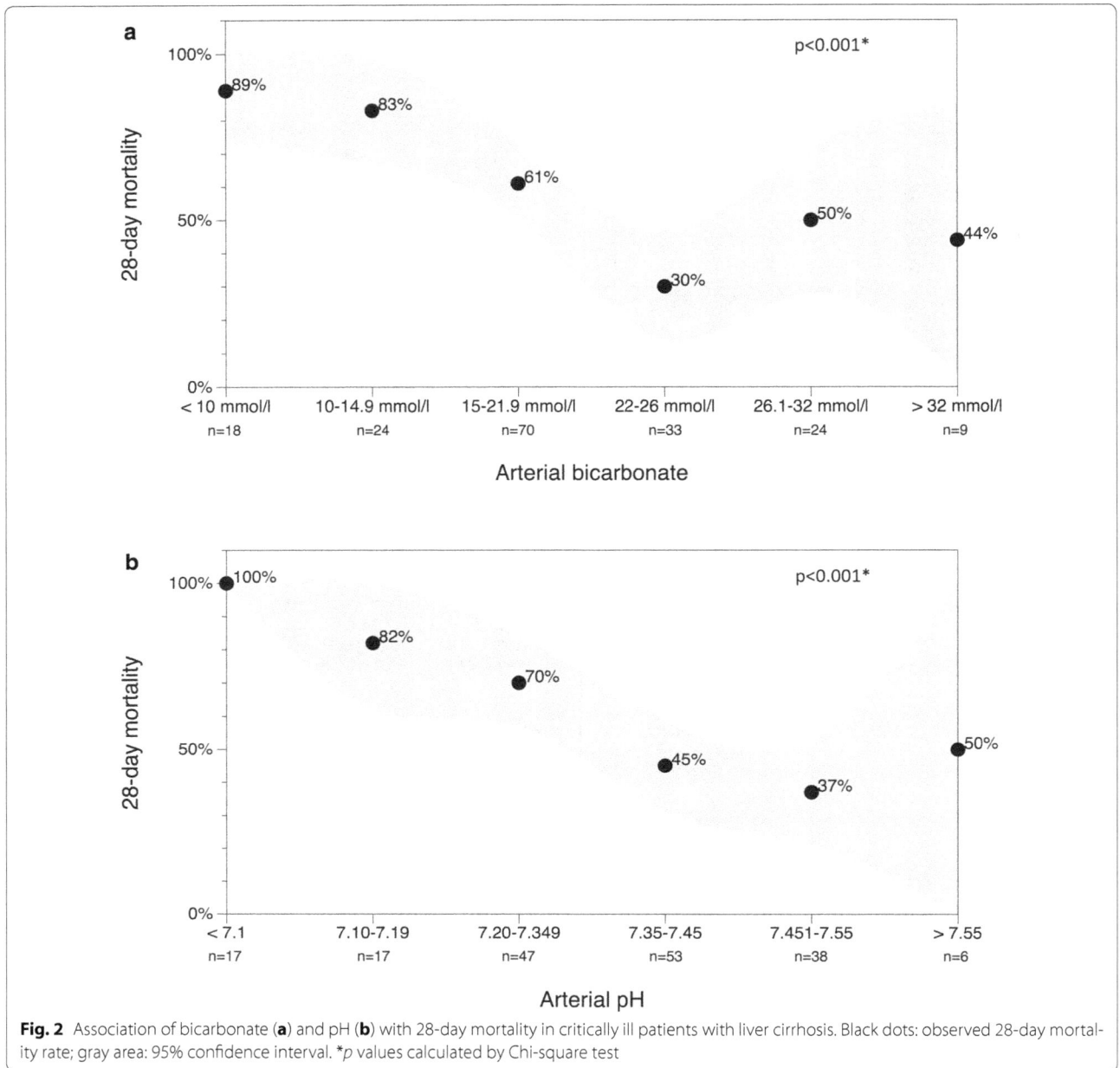

a

100% — 89%
                83%
                            61%
50% —   50%   44%
                                    30%
0% —

< 10 mmol/l   10-14.9 mmol/l   15-21.9 mmol/l   22-26 mmol/l   26.1-32 mmol/l   > 32 mmol/l
n=18   n=24   n=70   n=33   n=24   n=9

28-day mortality

p<0.001*

Arterial bicarbonate

b

100% — 100%
                82%
                            70%
50% —   45%   50%
                                                    37%
0% —

< 7.1   7.10-7.19   7.20-7.349   7.35-7.45   7.451-7.55   > 7.55
n=17   n=17   n=47   n=53   n=38   n=6

28-day mortality

p<0.001*

Arterial pH

Fig. 2 Association of bicarbonate (**a**) and pH (**b**) with 28-day mortality in critically ill patients with liver cirrhosis. Black dots: observed 28-day mortality rate; gray area: 95% confidence interval. *p values calculated by Chi-square test

not only is a crucial player in the disposal of lactate, but may also become a net producer of lactate, especially during hepatic parenchymal hypoxia. Although lactic acidosis has been described in the literature in critical ill patients with cirrhosis [7, 8], this is the first study investigating the association of metabolic disturbances with ACLF compared to a matched cohort of critically ill patients without liver disease. Indeed, the extent of lactic acidosis was directly associated with ACLF grade. Accordingly, lactic acidosis was present in almost 80% of all patients with ACLF grade III. Moreover, lactate levels

were correlated with INR and bilirubin, thereby suggesting that lactate levels are directly related to liver function. Vasopressor support and severity of disease (as reflected by SOFA score) were also significantly associated with increased lactate levels. In sum, our data suggest that a combination of hepatic impairment and tissue hypoxia may contribute to lactic acidosis in critically ill patients with liver cirrhosis.

Great effort has been put in revealing the nature of unmeasured anions in critical illness [2, 35–38]. Still, source and clinical implications of unmeasured anions

Table 4 Cox regression model for risk factors for mortality in critically ill patients with liver cirrhosis

Parameter	Hazard ratio (95% CI)	
	Univariate	Multivariate
Age	1.02 (1.00–1.04)*	1.02 (1.00–1.04)*
Sex (male gender)	0.75 (0.51–1.11)	0.77 (0.51–1.15)
Liver disease		
ACLF grade 1 versus no ACLF	1.80 (0.63–5.19)	1.36 (0.47–4.01)
ACLF grade 2 versus no ACLF	2.02 (0.76–5.37)	1.44 (0.53–3.94)
ACLF grade 3 versus no ACLF	5.52 (2.22–13.74)**	3.68 (1.42–9.52)**
Sepsis/infection	1.69 (1.09–2.61)*	1.21 (0.76–1.92)
Base excess		
BE_{Na}	0.96 (0.90–1.03)	0.96 (0.89–1.04)
BE_{Cl}	1.00 (0.98–1.03)	0.97 (0.93–1.00)
BE_{Alb}	0.91 (0.81–1.02)	0.89 (0.79–1.00)
BE_{UMA}	0.95 (0.93–0.97)**	0.96 (0.92–0.99)*
$BE_{lactate}$	0.88 (0.85–0.92)**	0.92 (0.88–0.97)**

ACLF acute-on-chronic liver failure, BE_{Na} BE caused by free water effect, BE_{Cl} BE caused by changes in chloride, BE_{Alb} BE caused by albumin effect, $BE_{lactate}$ BE attributable to lactate elevation, BE_{UMA} BE attributable to unmeasured anions

*p value < 0.05; **p value < 0.01

are incompletely understood [39, 40]. Recently, it was shown in a large cohort of critically ill patients that increased concentrations of unmeasured anions were independently associated with increased mortality [41]. Citrate, acetate, fumarate, α-ketoglutarate and urate have been identified as potential candidates contributing to acidosis associated with high SIG in hemorrhagic shock [36]. Apart from states of shock, renal failure has been linked to increased levels of unmeasured anions in several studies [8, 42, 43]. As compared to non-ACLF cirrhosis patients, the presence of ACLF was associated with an increase in unmeasured anions, as reflected by BE_{UMA} and SIG. Both variables were strongly associated with acute kidney injury. Patients with liver cirrhosis are especially susceptible to renal failure [44–47], and renal impairment constitutes a central criterion for ACLF [20]. In sum, our findings indicate that impairment of renal function, rather than "hepatic failure," may be responsible for the increase in levels of unmeasured anions observed in patients with ACLF.

In the present study, metabolic acidosis and acidemia, respectively, were associated with increased 28-day mortality in liver cirrhosis. Accordingly, 28-day mortality rate was 91% in cirrhosis patients with arterial pH values < 7.2 and 86% in those with arterial HCO_3^- values < 15 mmol/l. Lactic acidosis and acidosis attributable to unmeasured anions were identified as main contributors to acid–base imbalance in critically ill patients with liver cirrhosis. Earlier studies have challenged the prognostic

value of unmeasured anions or lactate in critically ill patients [40]. Yet, the relationship between lactate levels, unmeasured anions and mortality and poor outcome has been described multiply in the literature [7, 8, 32, 33, 48], and lactate levels have recently been suggested as a parameter, indicating severity of disease in patients with chronic liver disease [49]. In our critically ill cirrhosis patients, we observed a dramatic independent impact of both lactate and BE_{UMA} on 28-day mortality. Thus, acid–base status in critically ill patients with cirrhosis and ACLF, respectively, is an early and independent predictor of outcome (Fig. 2). By contrast, acid–base status was of poor prognostic value in our propensity score-matched controls. This may be attributable to the fact that our control patients were matched to critically ill cirrhosis patients, thereby resulting in the exclusion of less severely ill non-cirrhosis patients with better acid–base profiles and lower mortality rates.

This study has strengths and limitations. First, this is a post hoc analysis; however, our study comprises structured acid–base analyses from a large cohort of critically ill patients stratified according to the presence of liver cirrhosis. Second, this study was performed in patients admitted to the ICU. Thus, our findings may not entirely reflect acid–base status of cirrhotic patients treated at normal wards. However, our study also incorporates cirrhosis patients without ACLF and patients of all ACLF categories. Third, there are pros and cons of propensity score matching. In this study, we have decided to use propensity score-matched controls in order to minimize the confounding effect of severity of disease on acid–base balance. Although we were able to achieve good comparability, inherent differences between cirrhotic and non-cirrhotic patients affecting acid base balance cannot be entirely abolished by matching procedures. Moreover, the loss of heterogeneity (by selection of the most severely ill patients) hampers survival analyses in the control group. Fourth, residual confounding is, as always, a matter of concern and cannot be entirely excluded. Future studies should confirm these results and focus on therapeutic implications for patients with liver disease at the ICU.

Conclusions

In conclusion, we could demonstrate that hyperchloremic acidosis and hypoalbuminemic alkalosis coexist in critically ill patients, including those with liver cirrhosis. In cirrhosis, but particularly in ACLF, net metabolic acidosis was caused by lactate and unmeasured anions. Lactate was linked to liver function and vasopressor use, whereas unmeasured anions were strongly related to acute kidney injury. Metabolic differences between cirrhosis and non-cirrhosis critically ill patients increase with the severity of disease, resulting in pronounced acidemia in cirrhosis patients with ACLF. Acidemia and metabolic acidosis, respectively, were associated with poor outcome in cirrhosis patients. Lactate and BE_{UMA} were identified as independent predictors of 28-day mortality in critically ill patients with liver cirrhosis and ACLF.

Abbreviations

ICU: intensive care unit; ALF: acute liver failure; ACLF: acute-on-chronic liver failure; PSM: propensity score matching; SAPS II: Simplified Acute Physiology Score II; SOFA: Sequential Organ Failure Assessment; AKI: acute kidney injury; KDIGO: Kidney Disease: Improving Global Outcomes; CLIF: chronic liver failure; EASL: European Association for the Study of the Liver; CLIF-SOFA: Chronic Liver Failure Sequential Organ Failure Assessment; CLIF-C ACLF: chronic liver failure consortium acute-on-chronic liver failure score; $PaCO_2$: partial pressure of arterial carbon dioxide; Ca^{2+}: total calcium; K^+: potassium; Cl^-: chloride; Mg^{2+}: magnesium; Pi: inorganic phosphate; Alb: albumin; BUN: blood urea nitrogen; AST: aspartate aminotransferase; ALT: alanine aminotransferase; $HCO3^-$: bicarbonate; BE: base excess; SID_a: apparent strong ion difference; SID_e: effective strong ion difference; SIG: strong ion gap; UMA: unmeasured anions; BE_{Na}: base excess attributable to sodium; BE_{Cl}: base excess attributable to chloride; BE_{Alb}: base excess attributable to albumin; BE_{Lac}: base excess attributable to lactate; BE_{UMA}: base excess attributable to unmeasured anions; IQR: interquartile range; ROC: receiver operating characteristic; AUROC: area under the receiver operating characteristic curve.

Authors' contributions

AD, TH, BS and VF participated in conception and design of the study. KRo, KRu, RB, CZ, PS and GH contributed to acquisition and interpretation of data. AD, TH and VF performed the statistical analysis. AD and TH drafted the manuscript. GCF, MT, BS and VF critically read and revised the manuscript for important intellectual content. All authors read and approved the final manuscript.

Author details

[1] Division of Gastroenterology and Hepatology, Department of Internal Medicine III, Medical University of Vienna, Vienna, Austria. [2] Department of Intensive Care Medicine, University Medical Center, Hamburg-Eppendorf, Martinistraße 52, 20246 Hamburg, Germany. [3] Division of Oncology and Infectious Diseases, Department of Internal Medicine I, Medical University of Vienna, Vienna, Austria. [4] Division of Cardiology, Department of Internal Medicine II, Medical University of Vienna, Vienna, Austria. [5] Department of Respiratory and Critical Care Medicine, and Ludwig Boltzmann Institute for COPD, Otto-Wagner Hospital, Vienna, Austria.

Acknowledgements
Not applicable.

Competing interests
The authors declare that there are no competing interests.

Funding
No funding.

Appendix

BE subcomponents reflecting the contributions of sodium (BE_{Na}), chloride (BE_{Cl}), albumin (BE_{Na}), lactate (BE_{Lac}) and unmeasured anions (BE_{UMA}), according to Gilfix et al. [31]:

(A) Na^+ was used to assess BE caused by free water effect (dilution)

$$BE_{Na} = 0.3 \times \left(Na^+ - Na^+_{normal}\right)$$
$$\left(Na^+_{normal} = 139 \text{ mmol/l}\right)$$

(B) After correction Cl^- for changes in free water ($Cl^-_{Na \text{ corrected}}$)

$$Cl^-_{Na \text{ corrected}} = Cl^- \times \frac{Na^+_{normal}}{Na^+}$$

BE attributable to chloride (BE_{Cl}) was calculated:

$$BE_{Cl} = Cl^-_{normal} - Cl^-_{Na \text{ corrected}}$$
$$\left(Cl^-_{normal} = 101 \text{ mmol/l}\right)$$

(C) BE attributable to albumin was calculated as follows [28]:

$$BE_{Alb} = (0.148 \times pH - 0.818)$$
$$\times \left(Alb_{normal} - Alb_{observed}\right)$$
$$\left(Alb_{normal} = 44.4 \text{ g/l}\right)$$

(D) BE due to lactate was calculated:

$$BE_{Lac} = lactate_{normal} - lactate_{observed}$$
$$(lactate_{normal} = 0.8 \text{ mmol/l})$$

(E) Changes in BE not related to the aforementioned factors correspond to UMA, which are quantified as follows:

$$BE_{UMA} = BE - (BE_{Na} + BE_{Cl} + BE_{Alb} + BE_{Lac})$$

References

1. Kassirer JP. Serious acid–base disorders. N Engl J Med. 1974;291:773–6.
2. Kellum JA. Determinants of blood pH in health and disease. Crit Care. 2000;4:6–14.
3. Noritomi DT, Soriano FG, Kellum JA, Cappi SB, Biselli PJC, Libório AB, Park M. Metabolic acidosis in patients with severe sepsis and septic shock: a longitudinal quantitative study. Crit Care Med. 2009;37:2733–9.

4. Mæhle K, Haug B, Flaatten H, Nielsen E. Metabolic alkalosis is the most common acid–base disorder in ICU patients. Crit Care. 2014;18:420.

5. Neyra JA, Canepa-Escaro F, Li X, Manllo J, Adams-Huet B, Yee J, Yessayan L. Acute Kidney Injury in Critical Illness Study Group: association of hyperchloremia with hospital mortality in critically ill septic patients. Crit Care Med. 2015;43:1938–44.

6. Smith I, Kumar P, Molloy S, Rhodes A, Newman PJ, Grounds RM, Bennett ED. Base excess and lactate as prognostic indicators for patients admitted to intensive care. Intensive Care Med. 2001;27:74–83.

7. Moreau R, Hadengue A, Soupison T, Kirstetter P, Mamzer MF, Vanjak D, Vauquelin P, Assous M, Sicot C. Septic shock in patients with cirrhosis: hemodynamic and metabolic characteristics and intensive care unit outcome. Crit Care Med. 1992;20:746–50.

8. Funk G-C, Doberer D, Kneidinger N, Lindner G, Holzinger U, Schneeweiss B. Acid–base disturbances in critically ill patients with cirrhosis. Liver Int. 2007;27:901–9.

9. Funk G-C, Doberer D, Osterreicher C, Peck-Radosavljevic M, Schmid M, Schneeweiss B. Equilibrium of acidifying and alkalinizing metabolic acid–base disorders in cirrhosis. Liver Int. 2005;25:505–12.

10. Bihari D, Gimson AE, Lindridge J, Williams R. Lactic acidosis in fulminant hepatic failure. Some aspects of pathogenesis and prognosis. J Hepatol. 1985;1:405–16.

11. Funk G-C, Doberer D, Fuhrmann V, Holzinger U, Kitzberger R, Kneidinger N, Lindner G, Schneeweiss B. The acidifying effect of lactate is neutralized by the alkalinizing effect of hypoalbuminemia in non-paracetamol-induced acute liver failure. J Hepatol. 2006;45:387–92.

12. McPhail MJW, Shawcross DL, Abeles RD, Chang A, Patel V, Lee G-H, Abdulla M, Sizer E, Willars C, Auzinger G, Bernal W, Wendon JA. Increased survival for patients with cirrhosis and organ failure in liver intensive care and validation of the chronic liver failure-sequential organ failure scoring system. Clin Gastroenterol Hepatol. 2015;13(7):1353–60.

13. Weil D, Levesque E, McPhail M, Cavallazzi R, Theocharidou E, Cholongitas E, Galbois A, Pan HC, Karvellas CJ, Sauneuf B, Robert R, Fichet J, Piton G, Thevenot T, Capellier G, Di Martino V. METAREACIR Group: prognosis of cirrhotic patients admitted to intensive care unit: a meta-analysis. Ann Intensive Care. 2017;7:33.

14. Warren A, Soulsby CR, Puxty A, Campbell J, Shaw M, Quasim T, Kinsella J, McPeake J. Long-term outcome of patients with liver cirrhosis admitted to a general intensive care unit. Ann Intensive Care. 2017;7:37.

15. Piton G, Chaignat C, Giabicani M, Cervoni J-P, Tamion F, Weiss E, Paugam-Burtz C, Capellier G, Di Martino V. Prognosis of cirrhotic patients admitted to the general ICU. Ann Intensive Care. 2016;6:94.

16. Scheiner B, Lindner G, Reiberger T, Schneeweiss B, Trauner M, Zauner C, Funk G-C. Acid–base disorders in liver disease. J Hepatol. 2017;67:1062–73.

17. Le Gall JR, Lemeshow S, Saulnier F. A new Simplified Acute Physiology Score (SAPS II) based on a European/North American multicenter study. JAMA. 1993;270:2957–63.

18. Vincent JL, Moreno R, Takala J, Willatts S, De Mendonça A, Bruining H, Reinhart CK, Suter PM, Thijs LG. The SOFA (Sepsis-related Organ Failure Assessment) score to describe organ dysfunction/failure. On behalf of the Working Group on sepsis-related problems of the European Society of Intensive Care Medicine. Intensive Care Med. 1996;22:707–10.

19. Kidney Disease Improving Global Outcomes KDIGO Acute Kidney. Injury Work Group: KDIGO clinical practice guideline for acute kidney injury. Kidney Int Suppl. 2012;2012(2):1–138.

20. Moreau R, Jalan R, Gines P, Pavesi M, Angeli P, Cordoba J, Durand F, Gustot T, Saliba F, Domenicali M, Gerbes A, Wendon J, Alessandria C, Laleman W, Zeuzem S, Trebicka J, Bernardi M, Arroyo V. CANONIC Study Investigators of the EASL–CLIF Consortium: acute-on-chronic liver failure is a distinct syndrome that develops in patients with acute decompensation of cirrhosis. Gastroenterology. 2013;144:1426–37.

21. Jalan R, Saliba F, Pavesi M, Amorós À, Moreau R, Gines P, Levesque E, Durand F, Angeli P, Caraceni P, Hopf C, Alessandria C, Rodriguez E, Solis-Muñoz P, Laleman W, Trebicka J, Zeuzem S, Gustot T, Mookerjee R, Elkrief L, Soriano G, Cordoba J, Morando F, Gerbes A, Agarwal B, Samuel D, Bernardi M, Arroyo V. CANONIC Study Investigators of the EASL–CLIF Consortium: development and validation of a prognostic score to predict mortality in patients with acute-on-chronic liver failure. J Hepatol. 2014;61:1038–47.

22. Dellinger RP, Levy MM, Carlet JM, Bion J, Parker MM, Jaeschke R, Reinhart K, Angus DC, Brun-Buisson C, Beale R, Calandra T, Dhainaut J-F, Gerlach H, Harvey M, Marini JJ, Marshall J, Ranieri M, Ramsay G, Sevransky J, Thompson BT, Townsend S, Vender JS, Zimmerman JL, Vincent J-L. Surviving Sepsis Campaign: international guidelines for management of severe sepsis and septic shock: 2008. Intensive Care Med. 2008;34:17–60.

23. Drolz A, Horvatits T, Roedl K, Rutter K, Staufer K, Kneidinger N, Holzinger U, Zauner C, Schellongowski P, Heinz G, Perkmann T, Kluge S, Trauner M, Fuhrmann V. Coagulation parameters and major bleeding in critically ill patients with cirrhosis. Hepatology. 2016;64:556–68.

24. Siggaard-Andersen O, Fogh-Andersen N. Base excess or buffer base (strong ion difference) as measure of a non-respiratory acid–base disturbance. Acta Anaesthesiol Scand Suppl. 1995;107:123–8.

25. Siggaard-Andersen O, Gøthgen IH, Wimberley PD, Fogh-Andersen N. The oxygen status of the arterial blood revised: relevant oxygen parameters for monitoring the arterial oxygen availability. Scand J Clin Lab Invest Suppl. 1990;203:17–28.

26. Siggaard-Andersen O. The van Slyke equation. Scand J Clin Lab Invest Suppl. 1977;146:15–20.

27. Stewart PA. Modern quantitative acid–base chemistry. Can J Physiol Pharmacol. 1983;61:1444–61.

28. Figge J, Rossing TH, Fencl V. The role of serum proteins in acid–base equilibria. J Lab Clin Med. 1991;117:453–67.

29. Fencl V, Jabor A, Kazda A, Figge J. Diagnosis of metabolic acid–base disturbances in critically ill patients. Am J Respir Crit Care Med. 2000;162:2246–51.

30. Kellum JA. Closing the gap on unmeasured anions. Crit Care. 2003;7:219–20.

31. Gilfix BM, Bique M, Magder S. A physical chemical approach to the analysis of acid–base balance in the clinical setting. J Crit Care. 1993;8:187–97.

32. Mizock BA. Controversies in lactic acidosis. Implications in critically ill patients. JAMA. 1987;258:497–501.

33. Oster JR, Perez GO. Acid–base disturbances in liver disease. J Hepatol. 1986;2:299–306.

34. Mallat J, Lemyze M, Meddour M, Pepy F, Gasan G, Barrailler S, Durville E, Temime J, Vangrunderbeeck N, Tronchon L, Vallet B, Thevenin D. Ratios of central venous-to-arterial carbon dioxide content or tension to arteriovenous oxygen content are better markers of global anaerobic metabolism than lactate in septic shock patients. Ann Intensive Care. 2016;6:10.

35. Forni LG, McKinnon W, Lord GA, Treacher DF, Peron J-MR, Hilton PJ. Circulating anions usually associated with the Krebs cycle in patients with metabolic acidosis. Crit Care. 2005;9:R591–5.

36. Bruegger D, Kemming GI, Jacob M, Meisner FG, Wojtczyk CJ, Packert KB, Keipert PE, Faithfull NS, Habler OP, Becker BF, Rehm M. Causes of metabolic acidosis in canine hemorrhagic shock: role of unmeasured ions. Crit Care. 2007;11:R130.

37. Kneidinger N, Lindner G, Fuhrmann V, Doberer D, Dunkler D, Schneeweiss B, Funk GC. Acute phase proteins do not account for unmeasured anions in critical illness. Eur J Clin Invest. 2007;37:820–5.

38. Mizock BA, Belyaev S, Mecher C. Unexplained metabolic acidosis in critically ill patients: the role of pyroglutamic acid. Intensive Care Med. 2004;30:502–5.

39. Balasubramanyan N, Havens PL, Hoffman GM. Unmeasured anions identified by the Fencl–Stewart method predict mortality better than base excess, anion gap, and lactate in patients in the pediatric intensive care unit. Crit Care Med. 1999;27:1577–81.

40. Rocktaeschel J, Morimatsu H, Uchino S, Bellomo R. Unmeasured anions in critically ill patients: can they predict mortality? Crit Care Med. 2003;31:2131–6.

41. Masevicius FD, Rubatto Birri PN, Risso Vazquez A, Zechner FE, Motta MF, Valenzuela Espinoza ED, Welsh S, Guerra Arias EF, Furche MA, Berdaguer

FD, Dubin A. Relationship of at admission lactate, unmeasured anions, and chloride to the outcome of critically ill patients. Crit Care Med. 2017;45:e1233–9.

42. Naka T, Bellomo R. Bench-to-bedside review: treating acid–base abnormalities in the intensive care unit—the role of renal replacement therapy. Crit Care. 2004;8:108–14.

43. Naka T, Bellomo R, Morimatsu H, Rocktaschel J, Wan L, Gow P, Angus P. Acid–base balance during continuous veno-venous hemofiltration: the impact of severe hepatic failure. Int J Artif Organs. 2006;29:668–74.

44. Nadim MK, Durand F, Kellum JA, Levitsky J, O'Leary JG, Karvellas CJ, Bajaj JS, Davenport A, Jalan R, Angeli P, Caldwell SH, Fernández J, Francoz C, Garcia-Tsao G, Gines P, Ison MG, Kramer DJ, Mehta RL, Moreau R, Mulligan D, Olson JC, Pomfret EA, Senzolo M, Steadman RH, Subramanian RM, Vincent J-L, Genyk YS. Management of the critically ill patient with cirrhosis: a multidisciplinary perspective. J Hepatol. 2016;64:717–35.

45. Angeli P, Gines P, Wong F, Bernardi M, Boyer TD, Gerbes A, Moreau R, Jalan R, Sarin SK, Piano S, Moore K, Lee SS, Durand F, Salerno F, Caraceni P, Kim WR, Arroyo V, Garcia-Tsao G. Diagnosis and management of acute kidney injury in patients with cirrhosis: revised consensus recommendations of the International Club of Ascites. Int J Hepatol. 2015;62:968–74.

46. Arroyo V, Ginès P, Gerbes AL, Dudley FJ, Gentilini P, Laffi G, Reynolds TB, Ring-Larsen H, Schölmerich J. Definition and diagnostic criteria of refractory ascites and hepatorenal syndrome in cirrhosis. Hepatology. 1996;23:164–76.

47. Drolz A, Horvatits T, Roedl K, Rutter K, Staufer K, Haider DG, Zauner C, Heinz G, Schellongowski P, Kluge S, Trauner M, Fuhrmann V. Outcome and features of acute kidney injury complicating hypoxic hepatitis at the medical intensive care unit. Ann Intensive Care. 2016;6:61.

48. Dell'Anna AM, Sandroni C, Lamanna I, Belloni I, Donadello K, Creteur J, Vincent J-L, Taccone FS. Prognostic implications of blood lactate concentrations after cardiac arrest: a retrospective study. Ann Intensive Care. 2017;7:101.

49. Edmark C, McPhail MJW, Bell M, Whitehouse T, Wendon J, Christopher KB. LiFe: a liver injury score to predict outcome in critically ill patients. Intensive Care Med. 2016;42:361–9.

13

Cardiac function during weaning failure: the role of diastolic dysfunction

Ferran Roche-Campo[1,2], Alexandre Bedet[1,3*†] ⓘ, Emmanuel Vivier[1,4†], Laurent Brochard[1,5,6]
and Armand Mekontso Dessap[1,3]

Abstract

Background: Cardiac dysfunction is a common cause of weaning failure. Weaning shares some similarities with a cardiac stress test and may challenge active phases of the cardiac cycle-like ventricular contractility and relaxation. This study aimed at assessing systolic and diastolic function during the weaning process and scrutinizing their dynamics during weaning trials.

Methods: Echocardiography was performed during baseline ventilator settings to assess cardiac function at the initiation of the weaning process and at the start and the end of consecutive weaning trials (performed at day-1, day-2, and before extubation if applicable) to explore the evolution of left ventricle contractility and relaxation in a subset of patients.

Results: Among 67 patients included, weaning was prolonged ($\geq$ 7 days) in 18 (27%) patients and short (< 7 days) in 49 (73%). Prevalence of systolic dysfunction and isolated diastolic dysfunction before the initiation of weaning process were 37 and 17%, respectively. Isolated diastolic dysfunction was more frequent in patients with prolonged weaning as compared to their counterparts. Thirty-one patients were explored by echocardiography during consecutive weaning trials. An increase in filling pressures with an alteration of ventricular relaxation (as assessed by a decrease in tissue Doppler early mitral diastolic wave velocity) was found during failed weaning trials.

Conclusions: Isolated diastolic dysfunction was associated with a prolongation of weaning. Increased filling pressures with left ventricle relaxation impairment may be a key mechanism of weaning trial failure.

Keywords: Weaning, Diastolic function, Relaxation, Diastolic reserve

Background

Weaning from mechanical ventilation is an essential step in the care of critically ill intubated patients, accounting for approximately 40% of the total duration of mechanical ventilation [1]. Given that increased time on mechanical ventilation is associated with higher mortality rates [2], it is crucial to safely wean the patient from the ventilator as soon as possible. Pulmonary edema is one of the main causes of weaning failure [3], and cardiovascular dysfunction during weaning may involve systolic [4] and/or diastolic alterations [5, 6].

In healthy subjects, relaxation enhancement during exercise blunts the increase in venous return to maintain normal filling pressures [7]. However, an impaired relaxation may be unmasked during exercise in patients with mild symptoms of heart failure, irrespective of the presence of diastolic dysfunction at rest [8, 9]. Because weaning shares some similarities with a cardiorespiratory stress test [10, 11], the same pathophysiology is conceivable to explain the increase in filling pressures during weaning failure of cardiac origin. We hypothesized that diastolic dysfunction at baseline or impaired diastolic relaxation during weaning trials may mediate weaning failure.

*Correspondence: alexandre.bedet@aphp.fr
†Alexandre Bedet and Emmanuel Vivier contributed equally to this work
[1] Service de Réanimation Médicale, DHU A-TVB, Hôpitaux Universitaires Henri Mondor, Assistance Publique – Hôpitaux de Paris, 51 Avenue du Maréchal de Lattre de Tassigny, 94010 Créteil Cedex, France

The present study had two primary aims: first, to assess cardiac function at initiation of the weaning process and evaluate its association with weaning outcomes; second, to assess the dynamics of left ventricle (LV) contractility and relaxation in a subgroup of patients during consecutive weaning trials.

Methods

Study population

This ancillary study, planned a priori, was performed in one (Henri Mondor University hospital, Creteil, France) of the nine centers participating in the B-type natriuretic peptide (BNP) for the fluid Management of Weaning (BMW) trial [12]. The BMW study was a randomized, controlled trial comparing a biomarker-guided depletive fluid management strategy to usual care during ventilator weaning. A detailed description of the BMW study design (NCT00473148) has been published previously [12]. Inclusion criteria of the BMW study were those allowing early initiation of ventilator weaning in patients receiving mechanical ventilation for at least 24 h. Permanent non-inclusion criteria were: pregnancy or lactation, age < 18 years, known allergy to furosemide or sulfonamides, tracheostomy at inclusion, hepatic encephalopathy, cerebral edema, acute hydrocephalus, myasthenia gravis, acute idiopathic polyradiculoneuropathy, decision to withdraw life support, and prolonged cardiac arrest with a poor neurological prognosis. The protocol was approved by our institution's local ethics committee (Comité de Protection des Personnes Ile-de-France IX, approval number 06–035), and informed consent was signed by the patient or a close relative. The main result of the BMW trial was to show that a BNP-driven depletive fluid management strategy decreased the duration of weaning without increasing adverse events [12].

Study protocol

To standardize the weaning process, patients were ventilated using a computer-driven automated weaning system (AWS, Evita Smart Care System, Dräger Medical, Lubeck, Germany), which gradually decreased the pressure support level (while maintaining the patient within a zone of respiratory comfort), as previously described [13]. When the AWS declared the patient ready for separation, extubation was performed as soon as possible (including during the night), provided the patient met the other criteria required for extubation [12].

In a subgroup of 31 patients for whom echocardiography availability allowed consecutive examinations, a daily weaning trial was performed if the patient was still ventilated with the AWS and not ready for separation. The weaning trial lasted one hour and consisted of a low-pressure support trial (10 cm H_2O in case of moisture humidifier or 7 cm H_2O in case of heated humidifier) with zero-PEEP [11]. Criteria for weaning trial failure were: respiratory rate > 35 breaths/min and/or increased accessory muscle activity, SpO_2 < 90%, heart rate > 140 beats/min, systolic blood pressure > 200 or < 80 mmHg, diaphoresis and clinical signs of distress. More information about the study protocol is available in the data supplement (Additional file 1: ESM Study protocol).

Classification of weaning

Successful extubation was defined as patient alive and without reintubation 72 h after extubation. We adapted the WIND study classification of weaning process [2] to the use of the AWS and further summarized this classification into two groups as follows: short weaning (patients successfully extubated within 6 days of AWS) and prolonged weaning (patients still ventilated after 7 days of AWS or more). Patients who died between 1 to 6 days and after 6 days of AWS were classified as short and prolonged weaning, respectively. This dichotomization was driven by the need for parsimony as per the limited sample size, and the fact that prolonged weaning identifies a subgroup of patients at increased risk of mortality, as compared to their counterparts [14].

Echocardiography

In all included patients ($n = 67$), echocardiography was performed to assess cardiac function during baseline ventilator settings (in pressure support ventilation), just before starting the weaning process with the AWS. In addition, we examined in a subset of patients ($n = 31$) whether weaning trials (low-pressure support with zero-PEEP) could induce an alteration of systolic or diastolic function, independently from their baseline function. In this subgroup, echocardiography was performed at the beginning and end of consecutive weaning trials performed at day-1, day-2, and before extubation. All echocardiographic examinations were performed by a single trained operator (FRC, with competence in advanced critical care echocardiography) not involved in patient care, using a transthoracic ultrasound device (EnVisor, Philips ultrasound, Bothell, WA). Briefly, the following echocardiographic views were examined with the patient in the semi-recumbent position: four-chamber and two-chamber long-axis views to assess left ventricle ejection fraction (LVEF), computed from LV volumes using the bi-plane Simpson method when image quality was suitable, or visually estimated when poor image quality did not allow sufficient identification of the endocardium; tissue Doppler peak systolic (s') wave at the lateral mitral valve annulus; right ventricle size (a dilated right ventricle was defined by an end-diastolic right ventricle/left ventricle area ratio > 0.6) and function (using the tricuspid annular plane systolic excursion); diastolic function [using pulsed-wave Doppler early (E) and late (A) diastolic wave velocities at the mitral valve, and tissue Doppler early (e') and late (a') diastolic wave velocities at the lateral mitral valve annulus]. Systolic dysfunction was defined as LVEF < 50%. Isolated diastolic dysfunction (with preserved LVEF) was defined using the 2016 European Society of Cardiology guidelines (LVEF ≥ 50% with plasma BNP concentration > 35 pg/mL and [E/e' ratio ≥ 13 or e' < 9]) [15]. Because there is no single widely accepted definition for diastolic dysfunction, we also assessed, as a sensitivity analysis (available in Additional file 2: Table 1), other definitions proposed by scientific societies and experts, as follows: (1) LVEF ≥ 50% and e' < 8 cm/s [16]; (2) LVEF ≥ 50% and (E/e' ratio > 8 or e'/a' ratio < 1) [17]; or (3) LVEF ≥ 50%, E/e' ratio > 8 and plasma BNP concentration > 200 pg/mL [18]. Dynamics of LV contractility and relaxation during weaning trials were assessed using the s' and e' waves, respectively [19–22]. Pulsed-wave Doppler flows were obtained below the aortic valve to assess LV outflow tract for cardiac output computation. Mitral and aortic regurgitation were measured semi-quantitatively using color-flow Doppler and

were considered severe at grades III–IV [23]. Echocardiographic images were digitally stored, and a computer-assisted evaluation was performed off-line by two trained operators (EV, AMD). All measures were averaged over a minimum of three cardiac cycles (five to ten in case of non-sinus rhythm).

Statistical analysis

The data were analyzed using SPSS Base 20 (IBM-SPSS Inc, Chicago, IL, USA). Categorical variables were expressed as numbers (percentage) and continuous data as medians (25th–75th percentiles), unless otherwise specified. We used the Chi-squared or Fisher exact test to compare categorical variables between groups and the Student's T test, Mann–Whitney test or Wilcoxon paired test to compare continuous variables, as appropriate. A p value of < 0.05 was considered statistically significant.

Results

Patient population, cardiac function and weaning outcome

Among the 75 participants enrolled, we have explored cardiac function in 67. Eight patients were excluded because of echocardiography unavailability (Fig. 1). Weaning was prolonged in 18 (27%) patients and short

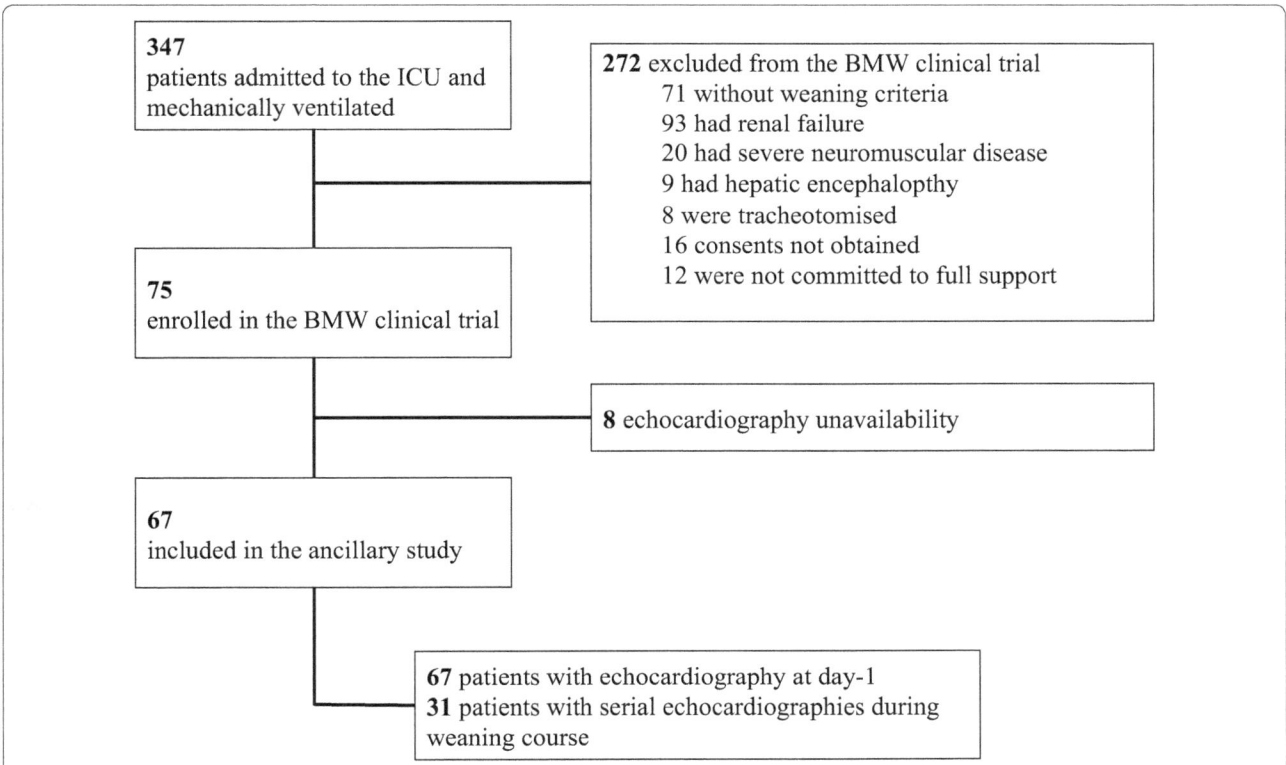

Fig. 1 Study flow chart. *BMW* B-type natriuretic peptide for the fluid management of weaning

Table 1 Patient characteristics and echocardiographic variables just before the weaning process, according to weaning category ($n = 67$)

	All patients ($n = 67$)	Weaning		p
		Short ($n = 49$)	Prolonged ($n = 18$)	
Patient characteristics				
Age, year	64 (47–76)	61 (49–75)	69 (44–81)	0.50
Male sex	44 (66)	31 (63)	13 (72)	0.49
SAPS II at ICU admission	46 (34–53)	44 (34–58)	46 (34–50)	0.50
Comorbidities				
Hypertension	33 (49)	23 (47)	10 (56)	0.52
Diabetes	17 (26)	9 (19)	8 (44)	0.05
Chronic obstructive pulmonary disease	17 (25)	13 (27)	4 (22)	> 0.99
History of ischemic heart disease	13 (19)	11 (22)	2 (11)	0.48
Atrial fibrillation	22 (33)	13 (27)	9 (50)	0.07
Reason for intubation				0.67
Coma	13 (19)	9 (18)	4 (22)	
Septic shock	8 (12)	5 (10)	3 (17)	
Cardiogenic pulmonary edema	17 (25)	14 (29)	3 (17)	
Pneumonia	18 (27)	12 (25)	6 (33)	
Cardiac arrest	4 (6)	4 (8)	0 (0)	
Surgery	7 (10)	5 (10)	2 (11)	
Events between ICU admission and inclusion				
Septic shock	33 (49)	25 (51)	8 (44)	0.63
Ventilator-associated pneumonia	15 (22)	9 (18)	6 (33)	0.21
Acute respiratory distress syndrome	26 (39)	18 (37)	8 (44)	0.56
Use of neuromuscular blockers	11 (16)	9 (18)	2 (11)	0.71
Cumulative fluid balance before inclusion, mL	4322 (949–7898)	4322 (175–7253)	4228 (1757–17,957)	0.27
Duration of invasive MV before inclusion, days	3 (2–6)	3 (2–6)	5 (3–13)	0.08
Clinical and biological data at inclusion				
SOFA score	4 (3–6)	4 (3–6)	5 (4–6)	0.25
Systolic arterial pressure, mmHg	129 (122–144)	132 (113–146)	127 (108–136)	0.44
Heart rate, beats/min	93 (82–105)	93 (83–106)	91 (79–104)	0.60
Respiratory rate, beats/min	25 (19–30)	23 (18–29)	29 (27–33)	0.06
RPP, beats/min·mmHg	12,500 (11,288–15,346)	12,576 (10,744–15,520)	12,423 (12,245–13,035)	> 0.99
Arterial blood gases				
pH, units	7.44 (7.40–7.47)	7.44 (7.40–7.47)	7.44 (7.41–7.47)	0.77
PaO_2/FiO_2 ratio, mmHg	210 (182–270)	222 (188–277)	186 (153–226)	< 0.01
$PaCO_2$, mmHg	41 (35–46)	40 (35–46)	42 (37–49)	0.42
BNP, pg/ml	331 (114–602)	302 (108–588)	415 (114–842)	0.51
Protidemia, g/L	58 (51–66)	58 (54–66)	54 (49–66)	0.39
Creatinine, micromol/L	79 (57–101)	81 (59–98)	73 (55–107)	0.96
Randomization in the interventional group	34 (51)	25 (51)	9 (50)	0.94
Echocardiographic variables				
LVEF, %	55 (40–60)	50 (37–60)	60 (50–62)	0.26
Cardiac index, L/min/m2	3.0 (2.2–3.6)	3.1 (2.3–3.6)	2.7 (2.1–3.7)	0.52
Systolic dysfunction				
LVEF < 50%	25 (37)	21 (43)	4 (22)	0.12
Diastolic dysfunction[a]				
LVEF $\geq$ 50% and BNP > 35 pg/mL and (*E/e′* ratio $\geq$ 13 or *e′* < 9)	11 (17)	4 (8)	7 (39)	0.01
Heart valve disease[b]	23 (34)	14 (29)	9 (50)	0.10

Table 1 continued

	All patients (n = 67)	Weaning		p
		Short (n = 49)	Prolonged (n = 18)	
RV/LV area ratio	0.6 (0.5–0.7)	0.6 (0.4–0.7)	0.6 (0.5–0.7)	0.67
Tricuspid annular plane systolic excursion, cm	1.9 (1.5–2.6)	2.1 (1.7–2.7)	1.5 (1.3–1.9)	0.03
Systolic pulmonary artery pressure, mmHg	38 (25–51)	37 (25–49)	46 (25–66)	0.16

SAPS Simplified Acute Physiologic Score, *ICU* intensive care unit, *MV* mechanical ventilation, *SOFA* sequential organ failure assessment, *RPP* product of heart rate and systolic arterial pressure, *FiO$_2$* fraction of inspired oxygen, *BNP* B-type natriuretic peptide, *LVEF* left ventricle ejection fraction, *E* early diastolic velocity measured using Doppler transmitral flow, *A* late diastolic velocity measured using Doppler transmitral flow, *e'* early peak diastolic velocity of mitral annulus, *a'* late peak diastolic velocity of mitral annulus, *RV* right ventricular end-diastolic area, *LV* left ventricular end-diastolic area

[a] Diastolic function could not be assessed in one patient for *e'* and in two patients for *E/e'* ratio

[b] Heart valve disease is defined as a severe aortic or mitral regurgitation (grade III/IV). Data are presented as *n* (%) or median (1st quartile–3rd quartile)

in 49 (73%) patients. All patient characteristics were similar between groups, except for a lower PaO_2/FiO_2 ratio at inclusion in patients with prolonged weaning as compared to their counterparts (Table 1). Before starting the weaning process, the majority of patients had an impaired cardiac function; overall, the prevalence of systolic dysfunction and isolated diastolic function were 37 and 17%, respectively. Isolated diastolic dysfunction was more frequent in patients with prolonged weaning ($\geq$ 7 days) as compared to their counterparts (Table 1). Tricuspid annular plane systolic excursion was also lower in patients with prolonged weaning as compared to others, while other echocardiographic variables were similar

between groups (Table 1). End-diastolic right ventricle/left ventricle area ratio and pulmonary artery systolic pressure were similar in patients with or without isolated diastolic dysfunction: 0.59 [0.58–0.66] versus 0.56 [0.44–0.67], $p = 0.46$ and 43 [25–61] versus 37 [25–50] mmHg, $p = 0.41$, respectively. Cardiovascular treatments and weaning outcomes are reported in Table 2. Most patients received diuretics, including all those with prolonged weaning, but the latter group had a more positive fluid balance during weaning as compared to the short weaning group. In comparison with the short weaning group, fewer patients in the prolonged weaning group received vasodilators. Weaning duration, ICU length of stay and

Table 2 Cardiovascular treatments and outcomes according to weaning category (n = 67)

	All patients (n = 67)	Weaning		p
		Short (n = 49)	Prolonged (n = 18)	
Cardiovascular treatments during weaning				
Diuretics	56 (84)	38 (78)	18 (100)	0.03
Dobutamine	19 (28)	15 (31)	4 (22)	0.50
Vasodilator	30 (45)	26 (53)	4 (22)	0.02
Amiodarone	19 (28)	13 (27)	6 (33)	0.58
Any cardiovascular treatment	62 (93)	44 (90)	18 (100)	0.31
Average daily furosemide dose during weaning, mg	25 (4–59)	30 (1–59)	22 (6–56)	0.94
Average daily fluid balance during weaning, mL	− 757 (− 2016 to − 81)	− 1202 (− 2342 to − 477)	51 (− 638 to 449)	< 0.01
Average daily urine output during weaning, mL	2588 (1971 to 3863)	2950 (2205 to 4167)	1967 (1649 to 2912)	0.02
Outcomes				
Time to first successful extubation, days	2 (1–6)	1 (1–2)	13 (10–32)	< 0.01
Ventilator free days at day-28, days	24 (18–27)	27 (25–27)	0 (0–16)	< 0.01
Time to discharge from ICU, days	9 (5–18)	7 (4–10)	31 (15–53)	< 0.01
Time to discharge from hospital, days	28 (15–53)	22 (13–32)	39 (22–53)	0.07
ICU mortality	9 (13)	2 (4)	7 (39)	< 0.01
Hospital mortality	10 (15)	3 (6)	7 (39)	< 0.01

Data are presented as *n* (%) or median (1st quartile–3rd quartile). Patient who died before day-28 had 0 ventilator free days

ICU intensive care unit

mortality were significantly greater in the prolonged weaning group (Table 2).

Dynamics of LV contractility and relaxation during weaning trials

Among the 67 patients included, 31 were explored during consecutive weaning trials (Additional file 2: Table 2). Sixteen of these patients (52%) successfully passed the first weaning trial (day-1), whereas 15 (48%) failed. The evolution of cardiac clinical parameters and echocardiographic parameters during consecutive weaning trials (day-1, day-2, and before extubation) are displayed in Figs. 2 and 3, respectively. Failure of weaning trial was more often associated with an increase in systolic arterial pressure, heart rate and their product (pressure-rate product), as compared with weaning trial successes (Fig. 2). A marked increase in LV filling pressures (as assessed by E/e' ratio) concomitant with an alteration of diastolic relaxation (as assessed by e' velocity) were found in failed weaning trials (Fig. 3, Table 3). The e' velocity increased in fewer (6.7%) and decreased in greater (93.3%) number of patients who failed weaning trials, as compared to successes ($p < 0.001$).

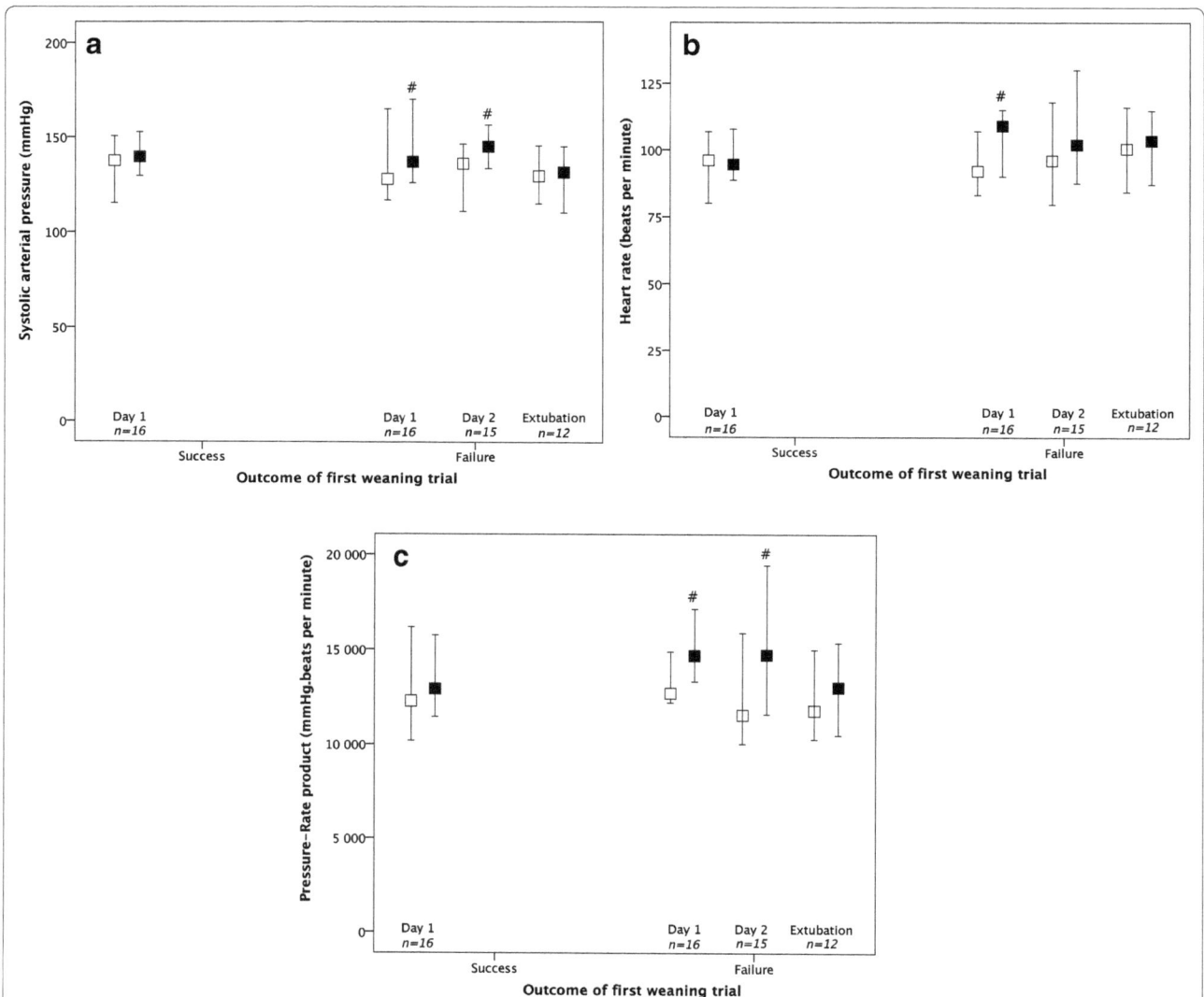

Fig. 2 Systolic arterial pressure (**a**), heart rate (**b**) and pressure-rate product (**c**) at the start (white square) and the end (black square) of consecutive weaning trials during the weaning process ($n = 31$), according to first trial outcome (success or failure). #p value < 0.05 as compared to the start of weaning trial (Wilcoxon test)

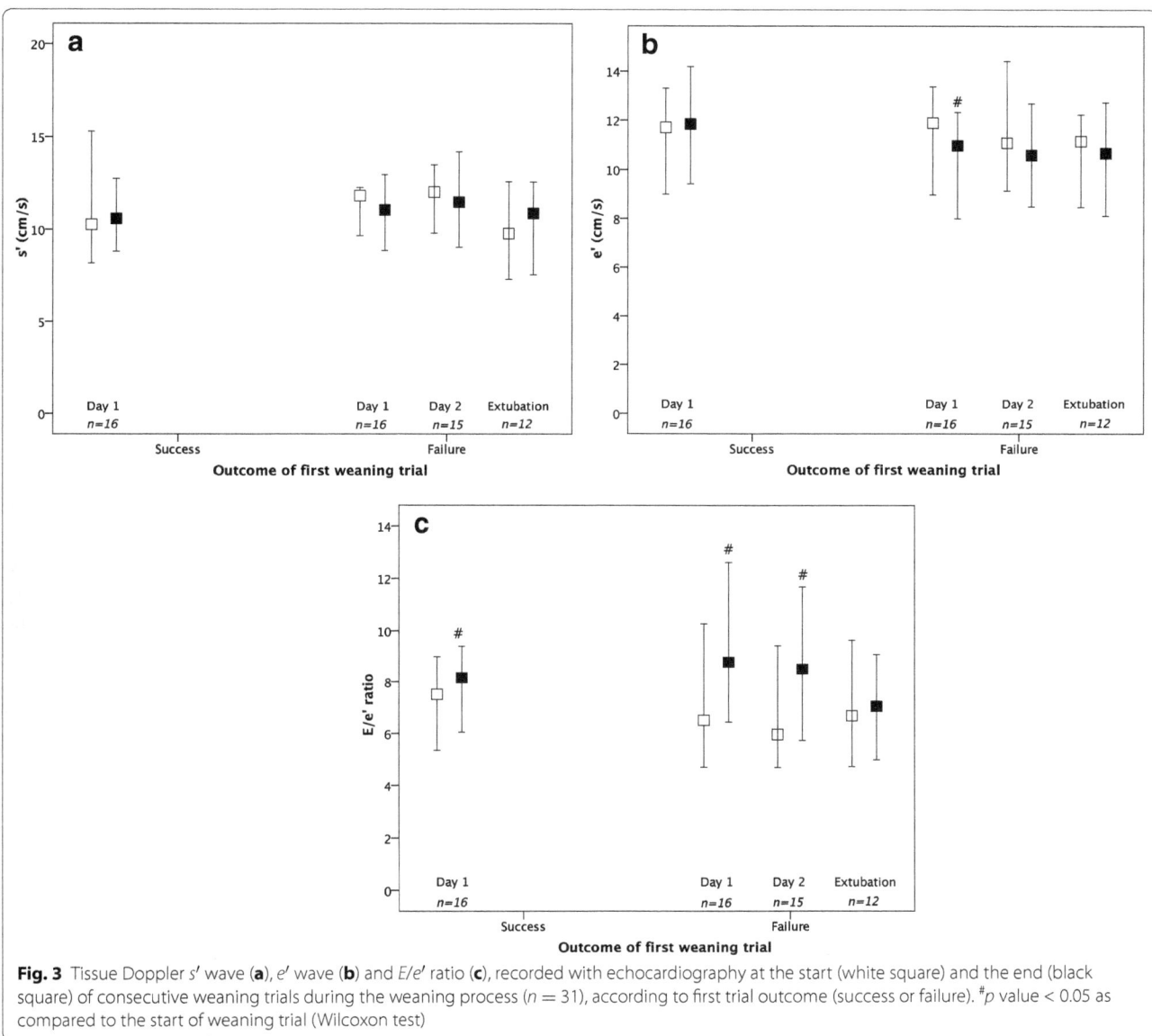

Fig. 3 Tissue Doppler *s'* wave (**a**), *e'* wave (**b**) and *E/e'* ratio (**c**), recorded with echocardiography at the start (white square) and the end (black square) of consecutive weaning trials during the weaning process ($n = 31$), according to first trial outcome (success or failure). #*p* value < 0.05 as compared to the start of weaning trial (Wilcoxon test)

Discussion

We herein report a high prevalence of cardiac dysfunction at initiation of weaning. Prolonged weaning was associated with a predominantly isolated diastolic rather than systolic dysfunction in our cohort. Echocardiographic exploration suggested that LV relaxation impairment with increased filling pressures may be a key mechanism of failed weaning trials.

Cardiac dysfunction before the initiation of weaning

Cardiac dysfunction plays a critical role in weaning outcome. In patients with prolonged weaning (≥ 7 days) in our series, systolic and isolated diastolic dysfunction were found in 22 and 39% of patients, respectively. Systolic dysfunction is a known risk factor for extubation failure [4]. However, in patients with preserved LVEF, increase in preload (volume status) and afterload (arterial stiffness) during weaning may also impair LV compliance and provoke pulmonary edema, especially in case of pre-existing diastolic dysfunction [24]. Our results are consistent with some previous reports describing diastolic dysfunction as a risk factor for weaning failure [5, 6, 25]. The heterogeneity of diastolic dysfunction definitions may explain the variability of its incidence and prevalence in critically ill patients [26].

Table 3 Percent change in echocardiographic variables between the start and the end of the first weaning trial ($n = 31$), according to outcome (success or failure)

	All $n = 31$	Success $n = 16$	Failure $n = 15$	p
Delta s'^a	− 3% (− 12%; 9%)	− 3% (− 7%; 5%)	− 2% (− 15%; 9%)	0.872
Delta e'	− 3% (− 12%; − 4%)	3% (− 9%; 6%)	− 6% (− 18%; − 3%)	0.02
Delta E	13% (8%; 19%)	12% (7%; 16%)	14% (11%; 23%)	0.20
Delta E/e'	16% (9%; 25%)	10% (4%; 14%)	26% (20%; 28%)	< 0.01

Data are presented as median (1st quartile; 3rd quartile)

s' peak systolic velocity at the lateral mitral valve annulus, e' early peak diastolic velocity of mitral annulus, E early diastolic velocity measured using Doppler transmitral flow

[a] s' could not be assessed in three patients

Cardiac dynamics during weaning

During weaning, removal of positive-pressure ventilation increases LV preload and afterload, inducing some physiologic changes similar to those observed during a cardiovascular stress test. Tachycardia and hypertension are two major determinants of diastolic dysfunction. They were more pronounced during weaning failure in our series and have been reported as frequent features of weaning-induced cardiac dysfunction [27]. Pressure-rate product was significantly increased during failed weaning trials, as compared to successes. Tachycardia could participate in the alteration of diastolic function by reducing diastolic filling time and/or decreasing coronary perfusion [28]. In addition, LV diastolic performance has been shown to be strongly influenced by the hypertensive response to exercise. Hypertension is well known to exacerbate heart failure in patients with preserved ejection fraction [29].

The fall in LV pressure during relaxation is a key determinant of diastolic function, and depends on intrinsic (contractility, LV stiffness) and extrinsic (preload, afterload) factors [30, 31]. The E wave velocity of mitral inflow assesses the early diastolic filling of LV, primarily reflecting the driving pressure between the left atrium and the left ventricle, and is therefore affected by preload and relaxation. The e' velocity, measured with tissue Doppler at the lateral mitral valve annulus, is usually used to correct for the effect of LV relaxation on E wave [21, 22, 32]. Thus, the E/e' ratio is considered a reliable measure of LV filling pressure, with minimal influence of intrinsic relaxation or age [33]. Although the assessment of diastolic function with these validated Doppler indices is usually highly reproducible [21, 32, 34], the detection of small changes may be challenging for non-experts in routine practice.

We found an increase in E/e' ratio during weaning trial, which is compatible with an elevation of filling pressures, as previously demonstrated [25, 35]. Several studies have found an independent association between e' and LV relaxation [22, 33, 36]. As compared to the E wave velocity, preload may have a minimal effect on e' [21, 22, 37], especially in patients with diastolic dysfunction [38]. Our finding that e' velocity tends to reduce during failed weaning trials is therefore compatible with an impaired diastolic relaxation in these patients, although a causality cannot be ascertained. This phenomenon is compatible with a lack of diastolic reserve, which may prevent the ability of LV to improve diastolic function and maintain normal filling pressures during stress [39–41]. Several studies evaluated the diastolic reserve with echocardiography in patients with heart failure and preserved ejection fraction [8, 9]. A decrease in e' wave, together with a concomitant increase in E/e' ratio, was the strongest markers of impaired diastolic reserve in these patients. Similar results were found in our study during failed weaning trials. A dynamic alteration of diastolic function during weaning stress in patients lacking diastolic reserve could be a possible mechanism of weaning failure, independently from the cardiac function at baseline. This hypothesis is in accordance with a previous work by Moschietto et al., who suggested the evolution of the LV relaxation rate during a spontaneous breathing trial (SBT) as the key factor in weaning outcome. However, the decrease in e' velocity during failed weaning trials is in contrast with this former study which found no significant variation during SBT. This discrepancy may be explained by the timing of the second echocardiography. These authors repeated echocardiographic examination only 10 min after starting the weaning trial, whatever its total duration [25], whereas we rather assessed dynamic changes at the end of the weaning trial. The modality of weaning trial may also play a critical role [11].

Therapeutic implications

The key mechanism of weaning failure did not seem to involve systolic dysfunction in our study, as also suggested by others [5, 25, 35]. Inotropic support could hypothetically exacerbate stress-induced diastolic dysfunction by increasing heart rate and/or myocardial oxygen demand. Dobutamine was even used as a stress test to diagnose heart failure with preserved ejection fraction [42]. Isolated diastolic dysfunction is frequent in ICU patients, especially in the elderly [43], and its diagnosis may deserve a specific therapeutic management in case of complicated weaning. Conservative and depletive fluid management are known to decrease the duration of ventilator support [44] and weaning [12], respectively. In our series, we could not assess the specific role of diuretics on SBT-induced cardiovascular burden because the vast majority of patients in the entire cohort received diuretics. Despite the use of diuretics in all patients with prolonged weaning, the urine output was lower and the fluid balance was higher in this group. The control of volume overload during diastolic heart failure may require higher doses of furosemide and/or the association of thiazide-like diuretics [29]; these strategies should be tested in future trials of fluid management during weaning. Fewer patients with prolonged weaning were treated with vasodilators as compared to those with short weaning. Vasodilators may be used to blunt the hypertensive response to weaning and expedite separation from the ventilator [45]. Future trials are needed to determine the optimal blood pressure target during ventilator weaning. Whether aerobic exercise training in ventilated patients could improve the diastolic reserve [46], ameliorate the tolerance of weaning trials and fasten the weaning process also needs to be explored in future studies.

Strengths and limitations

Strengths of our study include its prospective design and the detailed cardiac assessment using echocardiography. In particular, our study comprehensively assessed diastolic function at weaning start and its dynamics during consecutive weaning trials. Limitations include the monocentric setting and the limited sample size, which precluded any multivariable analysis of factors associated with prolonged weaning. Also, only a minority of patients explored consecutively fulfilled our definition of diastolic dysfunction, preventing any evaluation of the relationship between diastolic dysfunction at baseline and relaxation dynamics during weaning trials. The lack of a single gold standard definition of diastolic dysfunction complicated the analysis of our data, inasmuch as there was some patient heterogeneity concerning the changes in diastolic indices. Last, the characterization of the cardiac origin of weaning failure with tools like the pulmonary artery catheter or cardiac biomarkers would have strengthened our findings.

Conclusions

Isolated diastolic dysfunction is more frequent in patients with prolonged weaning ($\geq$ 7 days), as compared to those with a shorter weaning. In addition, failure of weaning trial seems associated with an elevation of filling pressures mediated by a stress-induced impairment of diastolic relaxation, which is compatible with a lack of diastolic reserve. Documentation of diastolic dysfunction as a cause of weaning failure is critical, as it may require specific management (especially vasodilators to blunt the hypertensive response to the weaning cardiovascular stress).

Abbreviations
A: late diastolic velocity measured using pulsed-wave Doppler transmitral flow; a': tissue Doppler late diastolic wave velocities at the lateral mitral valve annulus; AWS: automated weaning system; BNP: B-type natriuretic peptide; E: early diastolic velocity measured using pulsed-wave Doppler transmitral flow; e': tissue Doppler early diastolic wave velocities at the lateral mitral valve annulus; ICU: intensive care unit; LV: left ventricle; LVEF: left ventricle ejection fraction; PEEP: positive end-expiratory pressure; s': tissue Doppler peak systolic wave velocity at the lateral mitral valve annulus; SpO_2: peripheral oxygen saturation; SBT: spontaneous breathing trial.

Authors' contributions
AMD have full access to all data and take responsibility for the integrity of the data and the accuracy of the data analysis. FRC, EV, LB and AMD contributed to initial study design, data analysis and interpretation, drafting of the manuscript, critical revisions for intellectual content, and final approval of the version to be published. AB contributed to data analysis and interpretation, drafting and critical revisions of the manuscript, and final approval of the version to be published. All authors read and approved the final manuscript

Author details
[1] Service de Réanimation Médicale, DHU A-TVB, Hôpitaux Universitaires Henri Mondor, Assistance Publique – Hôpitaux de Paris, 51 Avenue du Maréchal de Lattre de Tassigny, 94010 Créteil Cedex, France. [2] Servei de Medicina Intensiva, Hospital Verge de la Cinta, Tortosa, Tarragona, Spain. [3] Groupe de Recherche Clinique CARMAS, Institut Mondor de Recherche Biomédicale, Faculté de Médecine de Créteil, Université Paris Est Créteil, 94010 Créteil, France. [4] Service de Réanimation Polyvalente, Centre hospitalier Saint-Joseph Saint-Luc, Lyon, France. [5] Keenan Research Centre and Critical Care Department, St Michael's Hospital, Toronto, Canada. [6] Interdepartmental Division of Critical Care Medicine, University of Toronto, Toronto, Canada.

Competing interests
The authors declare that they have no competing interests.

References
1. Esteban A, Alia I, Ibañez J, Benito S, Tobin MJ. Modes of mechanical ventilation and weaning: a National Survey of Spanish Hospitals. Chest. 1994;106(4):1188–93.
2. Béduneau G, Pham T, Schortgen F, Piquilloud L, Zogheib E, Jonas M, et al. Epidemiology of weaning outcome according to a new definition. The WIND study. Am J Respir Crit Care Med. 2016;195(6):772–83.
3. Liu J, Shen F, Teboul J-L, Anguel N, Beurton A, Bezaz N, et al. Cardiac dysfunction induced by weaning from mechanical ventilation: incidence, risk factors, and effects of fluid removal. Crit Care. 2016;20(1):369.

4. Thille AW, Boissier F, Ben Ghezala H, Razazi K, Mekontso-Dessap A, Brun-Buisson C. Risk factors for and prediction by caregivers of extubation failure in ICU patients: a prospective study*. Crit Care Med. 2015;43(3):613–20.

5. Papanikolaou J, Makris D, Saranteas T, Karakitsos D, Zintzaras E, Karabinis A, et al. New insights into weaning from mechanical ventilation: left ventricular diastolic dysfunction is a key player. Intensive Care Med. 2011;37(12):1976–85.

6. Konomi I, Tasoulis A, Kaltsi I, Karatzanos E, Vasileiadis I, Temperikidis P, et al. Left ventricular diastolic dysfunction–an independent risk factor for weaning failure from mechanical ventilation. Anaesth Intensive Care. 2016;44(4):466–73.

7. Ha J-W, Lulic F, Bailey KR, Pellikka PA, Seward JB, Tajik AJ, et al. Effects of treadmill exercise on mitral inflow and annular velocities in healthy adults. Am J Cardiol. 2003;91(1):114–5.

8. Burgess MI, Jenkins C, Sharman JE, Marwick TH. Diastolic stress echocardiography: hemodynamic validation and clinical significance of estimation of ventricular filling pressure with exercise. J Am Coll Cardiol. 2006;47(9):1891–900.

9. Chattopadhyay S, Alamgir MF, Nikitin NP, Rigby AS, Clark AL, Cleland JGF. Lack of diastolic reserve in patients with heart failure and normal ejection fractionclinical perspective. Circ Heart Fail. 2010;3(1):35–43.

10. Pinsky MR. Breathing as exercise: the cardiovascular response to weaning from mechanical ventilation. Intensive Care Med. 2000;26(9):1164–6.

11. Cabello B, Thille AW, Roche-Campo F, Brochard L, Gómez FJ, Mancebo J. Physiological comparison of three spontaneous breathing trials in difficult-to-wean patients. Intensive Care Med. 2010;36(7):1171–9.

12. Mekontso Dessap A, Roche-Campo F, Kouatchet A, Tomicic V, Beduneau G, Sonneville R, et al. Natriuretic peptide–driven fluid management during ventilator weaning. Am J Respir Crit Care Med. 2012;186(12):1256–63.

13. Lellouche F, Mancebo J, Jolliet P, Roeseler J, Schortgen F, Dojat M, et al. A multicenter randomized trial of computer-driven protocolized weaning from mechanical ventilation. Am J Respir Crit Care Med. 2006;174(8):894–900.

14. Peñuelas O, Frutos-Vivar F, Fernández C, Anzueto A, Epstein SK, Apezteguía C, et al. Characteristics and outcomes of ventilated patients according to time to liberation from mechanical ventilation. Am J Respir Crit Care Med. 2011;184(4):430–7.

15. Ponikowski P, Voors AA, Anker SD, Bueno H, Cleland JGF, Coats AJS, et al. 2016 ESC Guidelines for the diagnosis and treatment of acute and chronic heart failure The Task Force for the diagnosis and treatment of acute and chronic heart failure of the European Society of Cardiology (ESC) Developed with the special contribution of the Heart Failure Association (HFA) of the ESC. Eur Heart J. 2016;37(27):2129–200.

16. Garcia MJ, Thomas JD, Klein AL. New Doppler echocardiographic applications for the study of diastolic function. J Am Coll Cardiol. 1998;32(4):865–75.

17. Kasner M, Westermann D, Steendijk P, Gaub R, Wilkenshoff U, Weitmann K, et al. Utility of Doppler Echocardiography And Tissue Doppler imaging in the estimation of diastolic function in heart failure with normal ejection fraction. Circulation. 2007;116(6):637–47.

18. Paulus WJ, Tschöpe C, Sanderson JE, Rusconi C, Flachskampf FA, Rademakers FE, et al. How to diagnose diastolic heart failure: a consensus statement on the diagnosis of heart failure with normal left ventricular ejection fraction by the Heart Failure and Echocardiography Associations of the European Society of Cardiology. Eur Heart J. 2007;28(20):2539–50.

19. Nikitin NP, Loh PH, de Silva R, Ghosh J, Khaleva OY, Goode K, et al. Prognostic value of systolic mitral annular velocity measured with Doppler tissue imaging in patients with chronic heart failure caused by left ventricular systolic dysfunction. Heart. 2006;92(6):775–9.

20. Seo J-S, Kim D-H, Kim W-J, Song J-M, Kang D-H, Song J-K. Peak systolic velocity of mitral annular longitudinal movement measured by pulsed tissue Doppler imaging as an index of global left ventricular contractility. Am J Physiol Heart Circ Physiol. 2010;298(5):H1608–15.

21. Nagueh SF, Middleton KJ, Kopelen HA, Zoghbi WA, Quiñones MA. Doppler tissue imaging: a noninvasive technique for evaluation of left ventricular relaxation and estimation of filling pressures. J Am Coll Cardiol. 1997;30(6):1527–33.

22. Sohn D-W, Chai I-H, Lee D-J, Kim H-C, Kim H-S, Oh B-H, et al. Assessment of mitral annulus velocity by Doppler tissue imaging in the evaluation of left ventricular diastolic function. J Am Coll Cardiol. 1997;30(2):474–80.

23. Dujardin KS, Enriquez-Sarano M, Bailey KR, Nishimura RA, Seward JB, Tajik AJ. Grading of mitral regurgitation by quantitative Doppler echocardiography: calibration by left ventricular angiography in routine clinical practice. Circulation. 1997;96(10):3409–15.

24. Zapata L, Vera P, Roglan A, Gich I, Ordonez-Llanos J, Betbesé AJ. B-type natriuretic peptides for prediction and diagnosis of weaning failure from cardiac origin. Intensive Care Med. 2011;37(3):477–85.

25. Moschietto S, Doyen D, Grech L, Dellamonica J, Hyvernat H, Bernardin G. Transthoracic echocardiography with Doppler tissue imaging predicts weaning failure from mechanical ventilation: evolution of the left ventricle relaxation rate during a spontaneous breathing trial is the key factor in weaning outcome. Crit Care. 2012;16(3):R81.

26. De Meirelles Almeida CA, Nedel WL, Morais VD, Boniatti MM, de Almeida-Filho OC (2016) Diastolic dysfunction as a predictor of weaning failure: a systematic review and meta-analysis. J Crit Care [Internet]. 2016 Apr 18 [cited 2016 Apr 18]. http://www.sciencedirect.com/science/article/pii/S0883944116000897.

27. Grasso S, Leone A, De Michele M, Anaclerio R, Cafarelli A, Ancona G, et al. Use of N-terminal pro-brain natriuretic peptide to detect acute cardiac dysfunction during weaning failure in difficult-to-wean patients with chronic obstructive pulmonary disease *. Crit Care Med. 2007;35(1):96–105.

28. Selby DE, Palmer BM, LeWinter MM, Meyer M. Tachycardia-induced diastolic dysfunction and resting tone in myocardium from patients with normal ejection fraction. J Am Coll Cardiol. 2011;58(2):147–54.

29. Redfield MM. Heart failure with preserved ejection fraction. N Engl J Med. 2016;375(19):1868–77.

30. Buda AJ, Pinsky MR, Ingels NBJ, Daughters GTI, Stinson EB, Alderman EL. Effect of intrathoracic pressure on left ventricular performance. N Engl J Med. 1979;301(9):453–9.

31. Westermann D, Kasner M, Steendijk P, Spillmann F, Riad A, Weitmann K, et al. Role of left ventricular stiffness in heart failure with normal ejection fraction. Circulation. 2008;117(16):2051–60.

32. Nagueh SF, Smiseth OA, Appleton CP, Byrd BF III, Dokainish H, Edvardsen T, et al. Recommendations for the evaluation of left ventricular diastolic function by echocardiography: an update from the American Society of Echocardiography and the European Association of Cardiovascular Imaging. J Am Soc Echocardiogr. 2016;29(4):277–314.

33. Ommen SR, Nishimura RA, Appleton CP, Miller FA, Oh JK, Redfield MM, et al. Clinical utility of Doppler echocardiography and tissue Doppler imaging in the estimation of left ventricular filling pressures: a comparative simultaneous Doppler-catheterization study. Circulation. 2000;102(15):1788–94.

34. Frikha Z, Girerd N, Huttin O, Courand PY, Bozec E, Olivier A, et al (2015) Reproducibility in echocardiographic assessment of diastolic function in a population based study (The STANISLAS Cohort Study). PLoS ONE [Internet] 8:10(4). https://www.ncbi.nlm.nih.gov/pmc/articles/PMC4390157/.

35. Lamia B, Maizel J, Ochagavia A, Chemla D, Osman D, Richard C, et al. Echocardiographic diagnosis of pulmonary artery occlusion pressure elevation during weaning from mechanical ventilation*. Crit Care Med. 2009;37(5):1696–701.

36. Hasegawa H, Little WC, Ohno M, Brucks S, Morimoto A, Cheng H-J, et al. Diastolic mitral annular velocity during the development of heart failure. J Am Coll Cardiol. 2003;41(9):1590–7.

37. Graham RJ, Gelman JS, Donelan L, Mottram PM, Peverill RE. Effect of preload reduction by haemodialysis on new indices of diastolic function 1979. Clin Sci Lond Engl. 2003;105(4):499–506.

38. Nagueh SF, Sun H, Kopelen HA, Middleton KJ, Khoury DS. Hemodynamic determinants of the mitral annulus diastolic velocities by tissue Doppler. J Am Coll Cardiol. 2001;37(1):278–85.

39. Borlaug BA, Nishimura RA, Sorajja P, Lam CSP, Redfield MM. Exercise hemodynamics enhance diagnosis of early heart failure with preserved ejection fractionclinical perspective. Circ Heart Fail. 2010;3(5):588–95.

40. Borlaug BA, Jaber WA, Ommen SR, Lam CSP, Redfield MM, Nishimura RA. Diastolic relaxation and compliance reserve during dynamic exercise

in heart failure with preserved ejection fraction. Heart Br Card Soc. 2011;97(12):964–9.

41. Holland DJ, Prasad SB, Marwick TH. Contribution of exercise echocardiography to the diagnosis of heart failure with preserved ejection fraction (HFpEF). Heart. 2010;96(13):1024–8.

42. Erdei T, Smiseth OA, Marino P, Fraser AG. A systematic review of diastolic stress tests in heart failure with preserved ejection fraction, with proposals from the EU-FP7 MEDIA study group. Eur J Heart Fail. 2014;16(12):1345–61.

43. Kitzman DW, Gardin JM, Gottdiener JS, Arnold A, Boineau R, Aurigemma G, et al. Importance of heart failure with preserved systolic function in patients ≥ 65 years of age. Am J Cardiol. 2001;87(4):413–9.

44. The National Heart Lung, Network BIARDS (ARDS) CT. Comparison of two fluid-management strategies in acute lung injury. N Engl J Med. 2006;354(24):2564–75.

45. Routsi C, Stanopoulos I, Zakynthinos E, Politis P, Papas V, Zervakis D, et al. Nitroglycerin can facilitate weaning of difficult-to-wean chronic obstructive pulmonary disease patients: a prospective interventional non-randomized study. Crit Care Lond Engl. 2010;14(6):R204.

46. Edelmann F, Gelbrich G, Düngen H-D, Fröhling S, Wachter R, Stahrenberg R, et al. Exercise training improves exercise capacity and diastolic function in patients with heart failure with preserved ejection fraction. J Am Coll Cardiol. 2011;58(17):1780–91.

Incidence of airway complications in patients using endotracheal tubes with continuous aspiration of subglottic secretions

Jordi Vallés[1,2,3]*, Susana Millán[1], Emili Díaz[1,3], Eva Castanyer[4], Xavier Gallardo[4], Ignacio Martín-Loeches[1,3], Marta Andreu[4], Mario Prenafeta[4], Paula Saludes[1], Jorge Lema[1], Montse Batlle[1], Néstor Bacelar[1] and Antoni Artigas[1,2,3]

Abstract

Background: Continuous aspiration of subglottic secretions is effective in preventing ventilator-associated pneumonia, but it involves a risk of mucosal damage. The main objective of our study was to determine the incidence of airway complications related to continuous aspiration of subglottic secretions.

Methods: In consecutive adult patients with continuous aspiration of subglottic secretions, we prospectively recorded clinical airway complications during the period after extubation. A multidetector computed tomography of the neck was performed during the period of 5 days following extubation to classify subglottic and tracheal lesions as mucosal thickening, cartilage thickening or deep ulceration.

Results: In the 86 patients included in the study, 6 (6.9%) had transient dyspnea, 7 (8.1%) had upper airway obstruction and 18 (20.9%) had dysphonia at extubation. Univariate analysis identified more attempts required for intubation (2.3 ± 1.1 vs. 1.2 ± 0.5; $p = 0.001$), difficult intubation (71.4 vs. 10.1%, $p = 0.001$) and Cormack score III–IV (71.4 vs. 8.8%; $p < 0.001$) as risk factors for having an upper airway obstruction at extubation. The incidence of failed extubation among patients after planned extubation was 18.9% and 11 patients (12.7%) required tracheostomy. A multidetector computed tomography was performed in 37 patients following extubation, and injuries were observed in 9 patients (24.3%) and classified as tracheal injuries in 2 patients (1 cartilage thickening and 1 mild stenosis with cartilage thickening) and as subglottic mucosal thickenings in 7 patients.

Conclusions: The incidence of upper airway obstruction after extubation in patients with continuous aspiration of subglottic secretions was 8.1%, and the injuries observed by computed tomography were not severe and located mostly in subglottic space.

Keywords: Mechanical ventilation, Ventilator-associated pneumonia, Continuous aspiration of subglottic secretions

Background

More than 500,000 patients with acute respiratory failure receive invasive mechanical ventilation in the USA each year [1, 2]. The most frequent complications that develop during mechanical ventilation are ventilator-associated infections, especially ventilator-associated pneumonia (VAP). VAP is associated with increased morbidity and mortality [3, 4].

VAP is mainly due to the use of an artificial airway and repeated microaspirations of secretions from the oropharynx containing microorganisms through the space between the endotracheal tube and the tracheal wall.

*Correspondence: jvalles@tauli.cat
[1] Critical Care Department, Hospital-Sabadell, Corporació Sanitària Universitària Parc Taulí, ParcTaulí s/n, 08208 Sabadell, Spain

In recent decades, multiple pharmacological and non-pharmacological prevention strategies administered individually or in bundles have lowered the incidence of VAP [5].

One recommended non-pharmacological measure reduces microaspirations by using an endotracheal tube with an accessory channel that allows subglottic secretions accumulated above the endotracheal cuff to be removed. These tubes allow secretions to be aspirated intermittently or continuously [6–8].

Although continuous aspiration of subglottic secretions (CASS) is effective in preventing VAP, it involves a risk of mucosal damage secondary to aspiration because the external diameter is higher than conventional tubes. One experimental study [9] and some clinical reports suggest that CASS can cause subglottic injuries around the point in the endotracheal tube where secretions are suctioned with the possibility of secondary laryngeal edema and upper airway obstruction [10–12]. However, clinical studies focusing on subglottic and tracheal damage associated with CASS are lacking.

Thus, we aimed to analyze the incidence of significant clinical complications and tracheal damage level in patients intubated with an endotracheal tube with CASS as a method to prevent VAP.

Methods

Study population

This was a prospective observational study of patients admitted to the intensive care unit (ICU) of a university hospital (between December 1, 2013, and November 30, 2014).

All patients aged > 18 years intubated with endotracheal tubes with CASS and who were expected to require mechanical ventilation for at least 48 h were eligible. In our hospital, all patients admitted to the ICU who require mechanical ventilation are intubated with endotracheal tubes that allow subglottic aspiration. We excluded patients transferred from hospitals who were intubated with endotracheal tubes without accessory channel that allows subglottic aspiration, those with a history of tracheostomy or tracheal lesions (including laryngeal surgery), those intubated > 48 h in the 30 days prior to the current admission and those enrolled in other trials.

Tracheal tube size was 7.5 and 8 in women and men, respectively, as used in the study of Touat et al. [13] with conventional tubes. All patients included in the study were intubated with tracheal tubes with an accessory channel for subglottic aspiration (Mallinckrodt™ TaperGuard™ Evac; Covidien Healthcare; Mansfield, MA, USA). The aspiration pressure was continuously monitored and maintained at 20 mmHg with a continuous vacuum regulator (Push-To-Set™;Ohio Medical;

Gurnee, IL, USA). By protocol in our ICU, cuff pressure is checked intermittently every 4 h with a hand pressure gauge (Mallinckrodt™; Covidien Healthcare; Mansfield, MA, USA) to maintain it between 20 cm H_2O and 30 cm H_2O. Systemic corticosteroids were not used to prevent post-extubation laryngeal edema.

Data collection

The following data were prospectively recorded at ICU admission: age, sex, Acute Physiology and Chronic Health Evaluation II (APACHE II) score at admission, reason for ICU admission, comorbidities (diabetes, chronic obstructive pulmonary disease (COPD), chronic liver failure, chronic heart failure, chronic kidney disease requiring dialysis, cancer, previous surgery and immunosuppression) and information related to tracheal intubation (date, whether urgent or scheduled, place (outpatient or inpatient), size of tracheal tube, Cormack–Lehane score, number of attempts and need for auxiliary devices, such as laryngeal mask or video laryngoscopy. We defined a difficult airway as the clinical situation in which a conventionally trained physician experiences difficulty with facemask ventilation of the upper airway, difficulty with tracheal intubation or both [14]; specific criteria for difficult intubation were Cormack–Lehane score grade III or IV, more than two attempts and need for auxiliary devices for intubation.

The following data were recorded during the ICU stay: self-extubations, reintubations and cause of reintubation, tracheostomy, mean daily aspiration pressure of the subglottic space, post-extubation complications (upper airway obstruction, dysphagia, dyspnea or dysphonia), days intubated, VAP, length of ICU stay and ICU mortality. Upper airway obstruction was considered when the patient presented stridor secondary to laryngeal edema after the extubation. The patients with planned extubation were extubated following a spontaneous breathing trial with a standard test for extubation using the T-piece for 30 min.

Diagnosis of tracheal lesions

To detect damage of the larynx and trachea, patients' airways were studied within 5 days of extubation using a 128-row multidetector computed tomography (MDCT) scanner (Somaton Definition AS plus; Siemens Healthcare; Erlangen, Germany) which obtained 1 mm slices with a 0.75-mm interslice gap from the vocal cords to 2 cm below the carina focused on the airway. No MDCT studies were carried out in patients aged < 50 years or pregnant women (to avoid possible adverse effects secondary to radiation), in patients with tracheostomies or previously known tracheal lesions (including laryngeal surgery), in patients mechanically ventilated < 72 h or in terminal patients extubated in order to withdraw life support or in patients without consent.

Four independent radiologists blinded to clinical information analyzed the MDCT images and classified the site (the arytenoid region, the subglottic region or the trachea to 2 cm below the carina) and severity of injuries (from mildest to most severe: mucosal thickening, cartilage thickening or deep ulceration) and evaluated whether tracheal stenosis was present. The group reached a consensus on discrepant readings.

Statistical analysis

Categorical variables are reported as frequencies (%), and normally distributed continuous variables are reported as mean ± SD. We used the Chi-square test or Fischer's exact test to compare qualitative variables and Student's *t* test or the Mann–Whitney *U* test to compare continuous variables. All tests were two-tailed, and significance was set at $p < 0.05$. SPSS software (SPSS Inc.; Chicago, IL, USA) was used for data all analysis.

Results

During the study period, 386 patients admitted to the ICU were mechanically ventilated. Of these, 266 were excluded: 216 because they were ventilated < 48 h and 50 for other reasons (Fig. 1). Thus, a total of 120 patients were enrolled in the study; however, 34 of these were excluded: 19 because they died before extubation and 15

because they were tracheostomized before extubation was attempted.

The study population consisted of the remaining 86 patients (mean age, 61 ± 14 years; 55 (64%) male; mean Apache II at admission, 18 ± 2). Table 1 reports the

Table 1 Patient characteristics at ICU admission

Characteristics	N:86
Age, mean ± SD	61 ± 14
Male (%)	55 (64)
Apache II, mean ± SD	18 ± 2
Reason for admission (%)	
Acute respiratory failure	22 (25.5)
Neurological illness	18 (21.0)
Severe sepsis or septic shock	14 (16.3)
Shock	11 (12.7)
Other[a]	21 (24.4)
Comorbidities (%)	
Diabetes	24 (28.0)
Cardiovascular	21 (24.4)
COPD	17 (19.7)
Cancer	17 (19.7)
Immunosuppression	13 (15.0)
Chronic liver failure	8 (9.3)
Chronic renal failure	5 (5.8)

COPD chronic obstructive pulmonary disease

[a] Intoxications, trauma, cardiac arrest, gastrointestinal bleeding

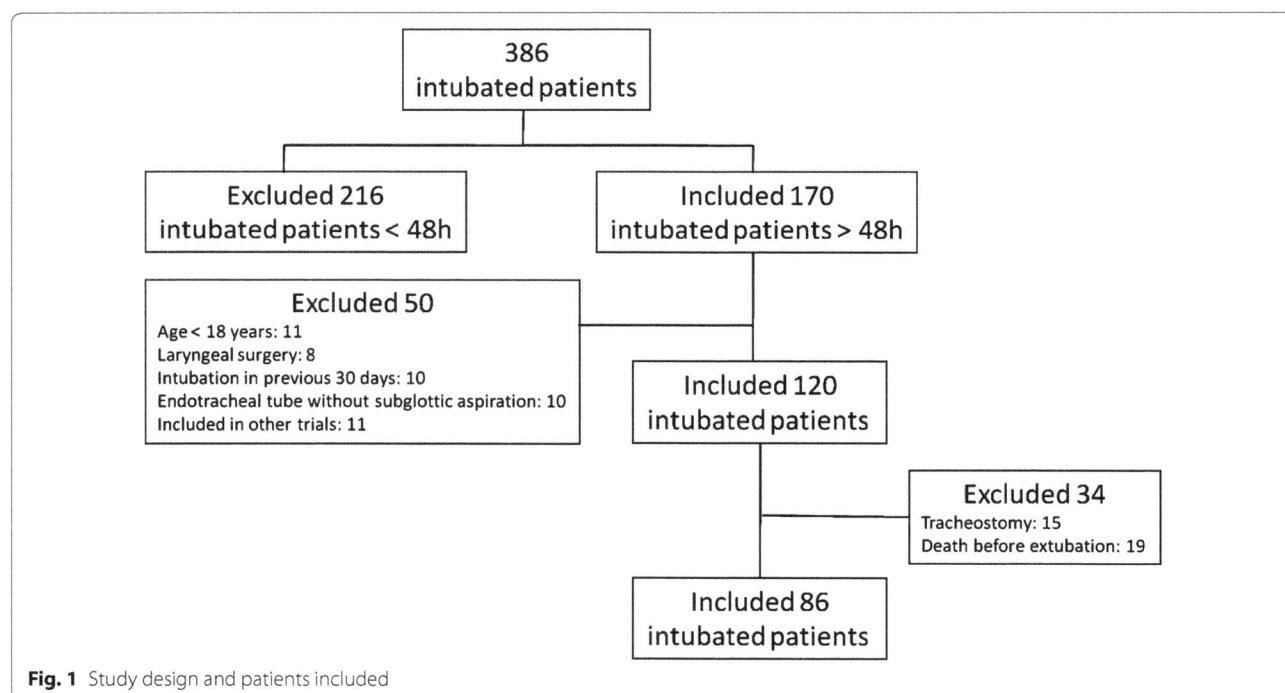

Fig. 1 Study design and patients included

characteristics of these patients. Table 2 reports the variables recorded during the intubation procedure and the ICU stay. Nearly all patients (95.4%) were intubated

Table 2 Patient characteristics during intubation and during ICU stay

Characteristics	N:86
During intubation procedure	
Number of attempts required for intubation, mean ± SD	1.3 ± 0.6
Diameter of endotracheal tube (mm), mean ± SD	7.8 ± 0.3
Difficult intubation (%)	13 (15)
Urgent intubation (%)	77 (89.5)
Intubation outside the hospital (%)	4 (4.6)
During ICU stay	
Subglottic aspiration pressure (mmHg), mean ± SD	19.7 ± 2.5
Length of intubation (days), mean ± SD	6.1 ± 4.8
Accidental or self-extubation (%)	7 (8.1)
Planned extubation (%)	79 (91.8)
Reintubation (%)	18 (20.9)
Tracheostomy (%)	11 (12.7)
Post-extubation complications (%)	
Dyspnea	6 (6.9)
Upper airway obstruction (Stridor)	7 (8.1)
Severe dysphagia > 24 h[a]	0
Dysphonia	18 (20.9)
Length of ICU stay (days), mean ± SD	16.4 ± 23.3
Crude mortality (%)	7 (8.1)

[a] Excluded patients with tracheostomy or with neurological disorders

inside the hospital, and most intubations (89.5%) were urgent. A total of 15.1% of patients fulfilled the criteria of difficult intubation. The incidence rate of VAP during the study period was 4.7 episodes per 1000 days of mechanical ventilation. ICU mortality of 120 patients initially included was 21.6%, and the mortality of 86 extubated patients was 8.1%.

Of the 86 extubated patients, 79 (91.8%) underwent a planned extubation and 7 (8.1%) had accidental or self-extubation (Fig. 2). Among patients with accidental or self-extubation, 3 (42.8%) required reintubation (2 for ineffective cough with airway secretion buildup and 1 for upper airway obstruction), and 2 of these required tracheostomy. Among patients extubated after planned extubation, 15 (18.9%) required reintubation (9 for ineffective cough with airway secretion buildup, 5 for upper airway obstruction and 1 for hypoxemia), and 9 of these required tracheostomy. Among the 15 patients extubated after planned extubation who needed reintubation, 7 (46.6%) were neurocritical patients. Compared with patients without reintubation, ICU mortality in patients who required reintubation was 33.3 versus 1.5% ($p < 0.001$).

Post-extubation complications included dysphonia in 18 (20.9%) patients, upper airway obstruction in 7 (8.1%) patients and transient dyspnea in 6 (6.9%). Excepting patients with tracheostomy or neurological disorders, none of the extubated patients had severe dysphagia impeding swallowing > 24 h after extubation. Univariate analysis showed that the significant risk factors for upper

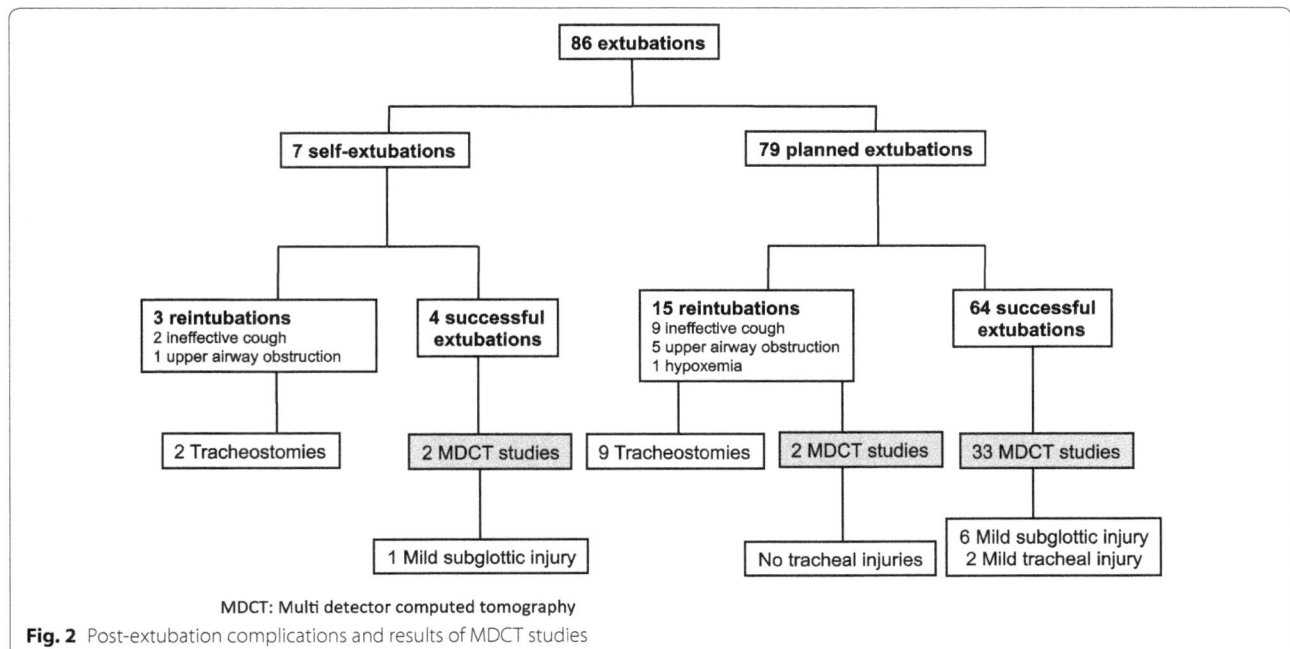

MDCT: Multi detector computed tomography

Fig. 2 Post-extubation complications and results of MDCT studies

airway obstruction were higher attempts for intubation, the presence of difficult intubation and a higher Cormack score (Table 3).

Thirty-seven patients (43.02%) underwent MDCT study. The remaining 49 patients were excluded by protocol. (Sixteen were intubated < 72 h, 12 were aged < 50 years, 11 were tracheostomized, 6 did not consent and 4 were extubated to withdraw life support.) The mean time between the MDCT study and extubation was 5 ± 2 days. There were no significant differences between patients who underwent MDCT and extubated patients who did not. Mean age and APACHE II were higher in those undergoing MDCT because only patients > 50 years we included (Table 4).

MDCT showed lesions in 9 out of 37 patients (24.3%), 2 had tracheal lesions (1 cartilage thickening and 1 mild stenosis and cartilage thickening) and 7 had mucosal thickening in the subglottic space. There were no significant differences between patients with lesions on the MDCT and those without, except mean subglottic aspiration pressure was unexpectedly higher in the group without lesions ($p = 0.002$) (Table 5).

Discussion

The incidence of clinically significant tracheal lesions in our patients using CASS was not higher than that reported in intubated patients without CASS, and suggests that CASS to prevent VAP is safe, at least when the pressure of subglottic aspiration is maintained at a safe level (20 mmHg).

MDCT was performed in 43% of extubated patients and found structural subglottic or tracheal injuries in 23.4% of them. However, MDCT could have underdiagnosed the incidence of lesions compared with fiber optic tracheoscopy. Touat et al. [13] recently reported that tracheoscopy within 24 h after extubation found at least one ischemic lesion in the cuff contact area in 83% of patients. Most lesions were mild and classified as edema or hyperemia. In the early 1980s, a study using fiber optic tracheoscopy found an incidence of ischemic lesions in 31% [15], and another using postmortem analysis found an incidence of 95% [16].

However, several studies have demonstrated the usefulness of MDCT in the detection of moderate and severe subglottic and tracheal lesions (thickenings, ulcers, granulomas, stenosis), with a 90% sensitivity compared

Table 3 Characteristics of patients with upper airway obstruction

Characteristics	Upper airway obstruction (N:7)	Non-upper airway obstruction (N:79)	p value
Length of intubation (days), mean ± SD	5.9 ± 2.8	6.0 ± 5.0	0.90
Attempts at intubation, mean ± SD	2.3 ± 1.1	1.2 ± 0.5	0.001
Cormack–Lehane score II–IV (%)	5 (71.4)	7 (8.8)	< 0.001
Difficult intubation (%)	5 (71.4)	8 (10.1)	0.001
Intubation outside the hospital (%)	0	4 (5.1)	0.70
Crude mortality (%)	1 (14.3)	6 (7.6)	0.53

Table 4 Characteristics of patients included in the multidetector computed tomography study

Characteristics	MDCT (N:37)	No MDCT (N:49)	p value
Age, mean ± SD	64.7 ± 8.9	58.7 ± 16.2	0.04
Apache II, mean ± SD	18.8 ± 1.6	17.7 ± 1.9	0.005
Airway and intubation			
Cormack–Lehane score III–IV (%)	5 (13.5)	7 (14.2)	0.91
Number of attempts required for intubation, mean ± SD	1.3 ± 0.6	1.3 ± 0.4	0.40
Diameter of endotracheal tube (mm), mean ± SD	7.8 ± 0.2	7.8 ± 0.3	0.49
Subglottic aspiration pressure (mmHg), mean ± SD	19.4 ± 3.4	19.9 ± 1.6	0.34
Difficult intubation (%)	6 (16.2)	7 (14.3)	0.80
Urgent intubation (%)	34 (91.8)	43 (87.8)	0.53
Stridor (%)	2 (5.4)	5 (10.2)	0.69
Dysphonia (%)	7 (18.9)	9 (18.3)	0.77
Length of ICU stay (days), mean ± SD	6.5 ± 3.9	5.8 ± 5.6	0.67

MDCT multidetector computed tomography

Table 5 Characteristics of patients with injuries detected at multidetector computed tomography

Characteristics	Airway injury (N:9)	No airway injury (N:28)	p value
Age, mean ± SD	62.4 ± 10.8	65.5 ± 8.2	0.20
Apache II, mean ± SD	19 ± 1	19 ± 2	0.08
Airway and intubation			
Cormack–Lehane score III–IV (%)	1 (11.1)	4 (14.2)	1.00
Number of attempts required for intubation, mean ± SD	1.4 ± 0.8	1.4 ± 0.7	0.60
Diameter of endotracheal tube (mm), mean ± SD	7.7 ± 0.3	7.8 ± 0.2	0.12
Subglottic aspiration pressure (mmHg), mean ± SD	17.8 ± 6.6	19.9 ± 1	0.002
Difficult intubation (%)	2 (22)	4 (14)	0.62
Urgent intubation (%)	9 (100)	25 (89.3)	0.56
Length of ICU stay (days), mean ± SD	7.4 ± 3.7	6.2 ± 2.0	0.80

to fiber optic tracheoscopy studies [17–20]. Although MDCT probably detected the most severe injuries, it probably failed to detect clinically insignificant injuries such as those reported in Touat et al.'s [14] study, where most lesions were mild and described as edema or hyperemia.

In their experimental study in sheep, Berra et al. [9] studied the tracheal injuries caused by CASS and classified most injuries as erythemic or hemorrhagic. The incidence of more severe lesions such as necrosis and cartilage thickening was less common. The objective of our study was to detect severe injuries related to CASS. Although MDCT is able to detect the majority of these severe injuries, the sensitivity of MDCT to detect mild injuries without significant clinical repercussion may be less than in tracheoscopy studies.

In our study, the group with injuries had a significantly lower mean subglottic aspiration pressure than in the group without lesions. This finding was unexpected because our hypothesis stated that more injuries should have occurred with a higher subglottic aspiration pressure. However, it is possible that the level of subglottic aspiration is not directly related to the tracheal injuries if the level of aspiration is maintained < 20 mmHg. On the other hand, other variables such as the difficult or urgent intubation were higher in the group of patients with injuries detected by MDCT and could therefore be responsible for the lesions. However, these differences were not statistically significant which could be due to the small number of patients included in the study.

One of the most severe complications related to endotracheal intubation is laryngeal edema, which may present as upper airway obstruction that can lead to respiratory failure requiring reintubation. The incidence of post-extubation laryngeal edema reported in the last 25 years with conventional endotracheal tubes ranges from 5 to 54.4%, depending on the definitions and method of diagnosis, and the incidence of stridor varies

widely, ranging from 1.6 to 26.3% [21]. Little information is available about the incidence of complications with the use of endotracheal tubes with CASS. In 2004, analyzing the utility of CASS and the semi-recumbent position as methods of VAP prevention, Girou et al. [10] found laryngeal edema in two out of five patients, suggesting that this method of prevention might be unsafe. However, it is important to note that the aspiration pressure applied in that study was 30 mmHg. Moreover, some recent clinical reports suggest that device malfunctioning may cause tracheal mucosa to be drawn into the hole of the aspiration channel, obstructing the system and subsequently injuring the mucosa [11, 12].

In our prospective study, the incidence of upper airway obstruction was 8.1%. Previous studies reported that the upper airway obstruction was more common in women and in patients with larger endotracheal tubes, longer mechanical ventilation and traumatic or difficult intubation [22, 23]. Our findings partially corroborate these results as we found that intubation-related factors associated with upper airway obstruction were the number of attempts required for intubation ($p = 0.001$), difficult intubation ($p = 0.001$) and a higher Cormack score ($p = 0.003$). The size of the endotracheal tube in our study was not identified as a risk factor for upper airway obstruction despite the fact that the accessory channel for subglottic aspiration increases the external diameter in these tubes.

Reintubation is necessary in 10–100% of patients with post-extubation laryngeal edema or stridor [21]. In our study, the rate of reintubation due to upper airway obstruction was 87.5%, representing a third of all patients who required reintubation. The mortality in patients who required reintubation was 33.3%, but the crude mortality in the group of patients with upper airway obstruction who required reintubation was 14.2% and suggests that, unlike reintubation for other reasons, reintubation for transitory upper airway obstruction is probably not associated with increased mortality.

Extubation failure occurs in about 10–20% of patients who meet weaning criteria and pass a spontaneous breathing trial [24]. In our study, the overall incidence of extubation failure requiring reintubation was 20.9%. However, the incidence in the group with accidental or self-extubation (42.8%) was higher than in the group with planned extubation (18.9%). In addition, it is important to highlight that a large proportion (46.6%) of the patients needing reintubation in the group with planned extubation had neurological disorders. In several studies, neurological disorders or impaired neurological status is independently associated with extubation failure [25–27].

About 10% of critically ill patients who require mechanical ventilation undergo tracheostomy [28–30]. The incidence of tracheostomy in our study was 12.7%. This incidence is similar to the 13% reported in a recent study in 31 ICUs throughout Spain [31].

Some limitations of our study should be taken into account: It was carried out in a single medical surgical ICU with extensive experience in the use of endotracheal tubes with CASS and aspiration pressure was strictly controlled. Caution is therefore warranted if our results are extrapolated to other contexts. A substantial limitation is that the study was observational and not randomized versus conventional endotracheal tubes. However, in our ICU all patients use CASS to prevent VAP, and we considered it unethical to increase the risk of pneumonia in a group without CASS. Another potential limitation is that MDCT might underestimate the incidence of structural lesions of the upper airway. However, MDCT's sensitivity in the diagnosis of severe and significant tracheal lesions is higher than 90% [17–20]. Another limitation is due to the fact that MDCT was only performed in 43% of cases for safety reasons, and we cannot be sure that the incidence of lesions in the entire group was not higher. However, the absence of significant clinical manifestations makes this unlikely. And finally, the mean time from extubation to evaluation to tracheal lesions was 5 ± 2 days. Moderate lesions could have been missed, and thus, the incidence might have been underestimated.

Conclusion

The risk of clinically significant complications such as extubation failure related to upper airway obstruction in patients with CASS was 8.1% and the subglottic and tracheal lesions observed by computed tomography were not severe and located mostly in subglottic space.

Abbreviations

ICU: Intensive care unit; VAP: Ventilator-associated pneumonia; CASS: Continuous aspiration subglottic secretions; APACHE II: Acute Physiology and Chronic

Health Evaluation II; COPD: Chronic obstructive pulmonary disease; MDCT: Multidetector computed tomography.

Authors' contributions

JV had full access to all of the data in the study and takes responsibility for the integrity of the data and the accuracy of the data analysis. He also contributed to the design of the study, coordinated patient recruitment, analyzed and interpreted the data, assisted in writing and revising the paper, and served as principle author. SM contributed to the design of the study, coordinated patient recruitment, analyzed and interpreted the data, and assisted in writing the paper. ED contributed to the acquisition and analysis of data. EC, XG, MA, MP analyzed the MDCT images and classified the site and severity of injuries and contributed to the analysis of data. IM-L contributed to the design of the study, coordinated patient recruitment, analyzed and interpreted the data, and assisted in writing the paper. JL, PS, MB, NB contributed to the acquisition and analysis of data. AA contributed to the design of the study and assisted in writing the paper. All authors read and approved the final manuscript.

Author details

[1] Critical Care Department, Hospital-Sabadell, Corporació Sanitària Universitària Parc Tauli, ParcTauli s/n, 08208 Sabadell, Spain. [2] Universitat Autonoma Barcelona, Sabadell, Spain. [3] CIBERES Enfermedades Respiratorias, Valladolid, Spain. [4] UDIAT, Hospital Universitari Parc Tauli, Sabadell, Spain.

Acknowledgements

The authors acknowledge the nursing staff of the Critical Care Department of Hospital Universitari Parc Tauli. Sabadell. English language editing assistance was provided by John Giba, independent medical writer.

Competing interests

The authors declare that they have no competing interests.

Funding

The authors declare that they have not received funding for the work from any organization.

References

1. Wunsch H, Linde-Zwirble WT, Angus DC, Hartman ME, Milbrandt EB, Kahn JM. The epidemiology of mechanical ventilation use in the United States. Crit Care Med. 2010;38:1947–53.
2. Stefan MS, Shieh MS, Pekow PS, Rothberg MB, Steingrub JS, Lagu T, Lindenauer PK. Epidemiology and outcomes of acute respiratory failure in the United States, 2001 to 2009: a national survey. J Hosp Med. 2013;8:76–82.
3. Magill SS, Klompas M, Balk R, Burns SM, Deutschman CS, Diekema D, Fridkin S, Greene L, Guh A, Gutterman D, Hammer B, Henderson D, Hess D, Hill NS, Horan T, Kollef M, Levy M, Septimus E, Vanantwerpen C, Wright D, Lipsett P. Developing a new, national approach to surveillance for ventilator-associated events. Crit Care Med. 2013;41:2467–75.
4. Safdar N, Defzulian C, Collard HR, Saint S. Clinical and economic consequences of ventilator-associated pneumonia: a systematic review. Crit Care Med. 2005;33:2184–93.
5. Lorente L, Blot S, Rello J. Evidence on measures for the prevention of ventilator-associated pneumonia. EurRespir J. 2007;30:1193–207.
6. Muscedere J, Rewa O, McKechnie K, Jiang X, Laporta D, Heyland DK. Subglottic secretion drainage for the prevention of ventilator-associated pneumonia: a systematic review and meta-analysis. Crit Care Med. 2011;39:1985–91.
7. Dezfulian C, Shojania K, Collard HR, Kim HM, Matthay MA, Saint S. Subglottic secretion drainage for preventing ventilator-associated pneumonia: a meta-analysis. Am J Med. 2005;118:11–8.
8. Vallés J, Artigas A, Rello J, Bonsoms N, Fontanals D, Blanch L, Fernández

R, Baigorri F, Mestre J. Continuous aspiration of subglottic secretions in preventing ventilator-associated pneumonia. Ann Intern Med. 1995;122:179–86.

9. Berra L, De Marchi L, Panigada M, Yu ZX, Baccarelli A, Kolobow T. Evaluation of continuous aspiration of subglottic secretion in an in vivo study. Crit Care Med. 2004;32:2071–8.

10. Girou E, Buu-Hoi A, Stephan F, Novara A, Gutmann L, Safar M, Fagon JY. Airwaycolonisation in long-term mechanically ventilated patients. Effect of semi-recumbent position and continuous subglottic suctioning. Intensive Care Med. 2004;30:225–33.

11. Harvey RC, Miller P, Lee JA, Bowton DL, MacGregor DA. Potential mucosal injury related to continuous aspiration of subglottic secretion device. Anesthesiology. 2007;107:666–9.

12. Dragoumanis CK, Vretzakis GI, Papaioannou VE, Didilis VN, Vogiatzaki TD, Pneumatikos IA. Investigating the failure to aspirate subglottic secretions with the Evac endotracheal tube. Anesth Analg. 2007;105:1083–5.

13. Touat L, Fournier C, Ramon P, Salleron J, Durocher A, Nseir S. Intubation-related tracheal ischemic lesions: incidence, risk factors, and outcome. Intensive Care Med. 2013;39:575–82.

14. Apfelbaum JL, Hagberg CA, Caplan RA, Blitt CD, Connis RT, Nickinovich DG, Hagberg CA, Caplan RA, Benumof JL, Berry FA, Blitt CD, Bode RH, Cheney FW, Connis RT, Guidry OF, Nickinovich DG, Ovassapian A. Practice guidelines for management of the difficult airway: an updated report by the American Society of Anesthesiologists Task Force on Management of the Difficult Airway. Anesthesiology. 2013;118:251–70.

15. Kastanos N, Estopá R, Marín A, Xaubet A, Agustí-Vidal A. Laryngotracheal injury due to endotracheal intubation: incidence, evolution, and predisposing factors. A prospective long-term study. Crit Care Med. 1983;11:362–7.

16. Stauffer JL, Olson DE, Petty TL. Complications and consequences of endotracheal intubation and tracheotomy.A prospective study of 150 critically ill adult patients. Am J Med. 1981;70:65–76.

17. Morshed K, Trojanowska A, Szymański M, Trojanowski P, Szymańska A, Smoleń A, Drop A. Evaluation of tracheal stenosis: comparison between computed tomography virtual tracheobronchoscopy with multiplanar reformatting, flexible tracheofiberoscopy and intra-operative findings. Eur Arch Otorhinolaryngol. 2011;268:591–7.

18. Hoppe H, Dinkel H-P, Walder B, von Allmen G, Gugger M, Vock P. Grading airway stenosis down to the segmental level using virtual bronchoscopy. Chest. 2004;125:704–11.

19. Taha MS, Mostafa BE, Fahmy M, Ghaffar MK, Ghany EA. Spiral CT virtual bronchoscopy with multiplanar reformatting in the evaluation of post-intubation tracheal stenosis: comparison between endoscopic, radiological and surgical findings. Eur Arch Otorhinolaryngol. 2009;266:863–6.

20. Sun M, Ernst A, Boiselle P. MDCT of the central airways. Comparison with bronchoscopy in the evaluation of complications of endotracheal and tracheostomy tubes. J Thorac Imaging. 2007;22:136–42.

21. Pluijms WA, van Mook W, Wittekamp BH, Bergmans D. Postextubation laryngeal edema and stridor resulting in respiratory failure in critically ill patients: updated review. Crit Care. 2015;19:295.

22. Darmon JY, Rauss A, Dreyfuss D, Bleichner G, Elkharrat D, Schlemmer B, Tenaillon A, Brun-Buisson C, Huet Y. Evaluation of risk factors for laryngeal edema after tracheal extubation in adults and its prevention by dexamethasone: a placebo-controlled, double-blind, multicenter study. Anesthesiology. 1992;77:245–51.

23. François B, Bellissant E, Gissot V, Desachy A, Normand S, Boulain T, Brenet O, Preux PM, Vignon P, Association des Réanimateurs du Centre-Ouest (ARCO). 12-h pretreatment with methylprednisolone versus placebo for prevention of postextubation laryngeal oedema: a randomised double-blind trial. Lancet. 2007;369:1083–9.

24. Thille AW, Richard J-CM, Brochard L. The decision of extubate in the intensive care unit. Am J Respir Crit Care Med. 2013;187:1294–302.

25. Vallverdú I, Calaf N, Subirana M, Net A, Benito S, Mancebo J. Clinical characterics, respiratory functional parameters, and outcome of a two-hour T-piece trial in patients weaning from mechanical ventilation. Am J Respir Crit Care Med. 1998;158:1855–62.

26. Namen AM, Ely EW, Tatter SB, Case LD, Lucia MA, Smith A, Landry S, Wilson JA, Glazier SS, Branch CL, Kelly DL, Bowton DL, Haponik EF. Predictors of successful extubation in neurosurgical patients. Am J Respir Crit Care Med. 2001;163:658–64.

27. Mokhlesi B, Tulaimat A, Gluckman TJ, Wang Y, Evans AT, Corbridge TC. Predicting extubation failure after successful completion of spontaneous breathing trial. Respir Care. 2007;52:1710–7.

28. Kollef MH, Ahrens TS, Shannon W. Clinical predictors and outcomes for patients requiring tracheostomy in ten intensive care unit. Crit Care Med. 1999;27:1714–20.

29. Esteban A, Anzueto A, Alía I, Gordo F, Apezteguía C, Pálizas F, Cide D, Goldwaser R, Soto L, Bugedo G, Rodrigo C, Pimentel J, Raimondi G, Tobin MJ. How is mechanical ventilation employed in the intensive care unit? An international utilization review. Am J Respir Crit Care Med. 2000;161:1450–8.

30. Fischler L, Erhart S, Kleger GR, Frutiger A. Prevalence of tracheostomy in ICU patients: a nation-wide survey in Switzerland. Intensive Care Med. 2000;26:1428–33.

31. Fernández R, Tizón AI, González J, Monedero P, Garcia-Sanchez M, de-la-Torre MV, Ibañez P, Frutos F, del-Nogal F, Gomez MJ, Marcos A, Hernández G, Sabadell Score Group. Intensive care unit discharge to the ward with a tracheostomy cannula as a risk factor for mortality: a prospective, multicenter propensity analysis. Crit Care Med. 2011;39:2240–5.

15

Duration of acute kidney injury in critically ill patients

Christine K. Federspiel[1,2], Theis S. Itenov[2], Kala Mehta[3], Raymond K. Hsu[4], Morten H. Bestle[2] and Kathleen D. Liu[5]* [iD]

Abstract

Background: Duration of acute kidney injury (AKI) has been recognized a risk factor for adverse outcomes following AKI. We sought to examine the relationship of AKI duration and recurrent AKI with short-term outcomes in critically ill patients who were mechanically ventilated and met criteria for the acute respiratory distress syndrome.

Methods: Participants in the NHLBI ARDS Network SAILS multicenter trial who developed AKI were included in this analysis and divided into groups based on AKI duration. Differences in outcomes were evaluated using t test and Chi-square test. Competing risks regression and Cox regression were used to evaluate factors associated with resolving AKI and recurrent AKI.

Results: In total, 238 patients were included in the study. Seventy-seven patients had short duration AKI (1–2 days), 47 medium duration AKI (3–7 days), 87 persistent AKI (> 7 days) and 38 died during their AKI episode. Persistent AKI was associated with worse outcomes including increased ICU length of stay, time on the ventilator and days with cardiovascular failure. We found no clinical differences between patients with short and medium duration AKI, even when accounting for AKI severity and recurrent AKI. Patients with resolving AKI were less likely to have oliguria or moderate/severe ARDS on the day AKI criteria were met. Recurrent AKI was associated with poorer clinical outcomes. No baseline clinical factors were found to predict development of recurrent AKI.

Conclusions: In critically ill patients with sepsis-associated ARDS and AKI, the impact of short and medium duration AKI on clinical outcomes was modest. Persistent and recurrent AKI were both associated with worse clinical outcomes, emphasizing the importance of identifying these patients, who may benefit from novel interventions.

Keywords: Acute kidney injury, Intensive care, Acute respiratory distress syndrome, Sepsis

Background

Acute kidney injury (AKI) is a common illness in critically ill patients that is associated with increased morbidity and mortality [1–3]. The severity of AKI is typically graded by the magnitude of the serum creatinine rise and/or fall in urine output, and more severe AKI is associated with poorer outcomes [4]. Recently, the duration of AKI has been recognized as an important risk factor for adverse outcomes, where short duration AKI (also

*Correspondence: Kathleen.Liu@ucsf.edu
[5] Divisions of Nephrology and Critical Care Medicine, Departments of Medicine and Anesthesia, University of California, San Francisco, Box 0532, San Francisco, CA 94143-0532, USA

called rapid reversal or transient AKI), typically defined as less than 48–72 h, has been associated with a lower risk of chronic kidney disease (CKD), end-stage renal disease (ESRD) and mortality compared to AKI of longer duration [4–7]. However, a recent ICU-based study demonstrated that although persistent AKI was associated with an increased risk of in-hospital death, this relationship was attenuated after accounting for AKI severity [8].

The main aim of the current study was to further examine the relationship of AKI duration with clinical outcomes in a cohort of critically ill patients, accounting for AKI severity as well as for subsequent recurrent AKI. Given the lack of pharmacologic therapies for AKI and the urgent need to identify relevant patient populations for clinical trials, we sought to identify factors associated with resolving AKI as well as risk factors for development of recurrent AKI. For this analysis, we focused on patients with sepsis-associated acute respiratory distress syndrome (ARDS) who were enrolled in a clinical trial of rosuvastatin for ARDS [9].

Methods

Patient population

The Statins for Acutely Injured Lungs from Sepsis (SAILS) study was a randomized clinical trial conducted from March 2010 to September 2013 at 44 hospitals in the USA as part of the National Heart, Lung, and Blood Institute (NHLBI) ARDS Network (ClinicalTrials.gov NCT00979121) [9]. The trial tested the potential benefit of rosuvastatin on mortality in patients with sepsis-associated ARDS. Specific inclusion and exclusion criteria are described elsewhere [9]. Ventilator management and weaning along with fluid management after shock resolution were protocolized; specifically, ventilator management included a lung protective, low tidal volume ventilation strategy [9]. The trial was stopped early for futility; in the final analysis, there was no relationship of rosuvastatin therapy with mortality. For the SAILS study, the IRB at each site approved the study. The current study used de-identified data from the trial and was therefore exempt from IRB review.

Patients with known ESRD or who were on dialysis for AKI at study enrollment were excluded. Daily serum creatinine measurements were available for days 1–14 after study enrollment along with the maximum serum creatinine value from days 14 to 28 and all measurements from the 48 h prior to enrollment. AKI was defined according to the KDIGO serum creatinine criteria [10]. Baseline serum creatinine was defined as the lowest serum creatinine within the 48 h prior to randomization. AKI was defined as either a $\geq$ 1.5 times increase from baseline, or $\geq$ 0.3 mg/dL increase during a 48-h rolling window [10]. We included all study participants who developed AKI during the first 5 days of study enrollment, to allow for sufficient follow-up time to ascertain AKI duration.

Duration of AKI

AKI duration was defined as the number of consecutive days where KDIGO AKI serum creatinine criteria were met over the first 7 days from the day AKI criteria were met.

We classified patients into four categories based on AKI duration: (1) resolving AKI which lasted 1–2 days (short duration AKI), (2) resolving AKI which lasted 3–7 days (medium duration AKI), (3) persistent AKI, where AKI lasted more than 7 days and (4) death during the current AKI episode. Relevant cutoffs were chosen to allow comparison with previous studies [4, 7].

Recurrent AKI

The incidence of recurrent AKI was only examined in patients who had an initial episode of resolving AKI (e.g., short or medium duration AKI). Recurrent AKI was defined by KDIGO serum creatinine criteria using a rolling baseline. Patients were censored at hospital discharge.

Study outcomes

Study outcomes were analyzed from the first day of AKI. Mortality was defined as death before hospital discharge up to day 30. Ventilator-free days were defined as patients being alive and breathing without ventilator assistance up to day 28. ICU-free days were defined as patients being alive and discharged from the ICU to up day 28. Patients who died before day 28 were assigned zero ventilator days and zero ICU-free days. To examine the effects of AKI duration on other organ systems, we evaluated Brussels cardiovascular failure-free days up to day 7 [11]. Patients were considered to be free from organ failure after hospital discharge. For outcome analyses, we did not include patients who died during their AKI episode, since their outcome is already well known.

Statistical analysis

Categorical variables are presented as counts (%) and continuous variables as either median [interquartile range (IQR)] or mean $\pm$ standard deviation (SD) and compared by Chi-square test and t test, respectively.

We evaluated factors associated with resolving AKI versus persistent AKI using the proportional subdistribution hazards model proposed by Fine and Gray, with death as a competing risk [12]. Values were missing for a small number of subjects in the urine output or platelet count variables ($n = 16$ and $n = 3$, respectively). These were carried forward from the prior study day. PaO_2/FiO_2 was missing in 58 subjects on the day of AKI; 57 values were imputed using a validated nonlinear imputation of PaO_2/FiO_2 from SpO_2/FiO_2 that was developed for patients with ARDS [13]. Two patients were excluded from the multivariate analysis due to missing data in PaO_2/FiO_2 and vasopressor use.

In patients with an initial episode of resolving AKI ($n = 123$), we also examined the association of recurrent AKI with outcomes. Patients were stratified according to the presence or absence of recurrent AKI. Risk factors for recurrent AKI were examined using standard Cox regression and hazard ratios with 95% confidence intervals for this analysis, and the assumption of proportional hazards was tested using Schoenfeld residuals (data not shown).

A p value < 0.05 was considered statistically significant. All analyses were conducted using R software (http://www.R-project.org/) including the "cmprsk" R-package.

Results

Patients and outcomes

Of the 745 SAILS participants, we excluded 34 patients with end-stage renal disease or who were on acute dialysis at ICU admission. Of the 711 remaining patients, 254 developed AKI between study days 1 and 5, but 16 were excluded due to critical missing data (serum creatinine or use of dialysis) to form our final cohort of 238 patients (Fig. 1).

In the overall SAILS trial, 30-day mortality was 23.9%. The patients who developed AKI were in general more severely ill, with a higher APACHE III score at enrollment, and greater use of vasopressors. In our study population (who developed AKI within the first 5 days of enrollment), 30-day mortality was 31.5%, significantly higher than those who were excluded from our analysis ($p < 0.001$). The median age was 54 (25–75% interquartile range [IQR] 40–66); 181 (76.1%) were white and 53 (22.3%) had diabetes (Table 1). The median number of days in the ICU before study enrollment was 1 (25–75% IQR 1–2), and the median day of AKI development was day 1 after study enrollment (25–75% IQR 1–3). The median baseline serum creatinine was 1.0 mg/dL (25–75% IQR 0.7–1.4), and the median serum creatinine on the day of AKI development was 1.7 mg/dL (25–75% IQR 1.2–2.6). One hundred and seventy-two (72.3%) subjects

presented with KDIGO AKI stage 1, but during follow-up 56 (23.5%) progressed to either stage 2 or 3 AKI.

Duration of acute kidney injury

Of the 238 study subjects, 76 (31.9%) experienced short duration AKI (1–2 days), 47 (19.7%) had medium duration AKI (3–7 days), 77 (32.4%) had persistent AKI on day 7, and 38 (16.0%) died during AKI. A histogram of patients' AKI duration is presented in Fig. 2.

Table 1 presents baseline and AKI characteristics stratified by AKI duration. The groups with short and medium duration AKI had similar distributions of comorbidities, APACHE III score at enrollment, as well as measures of general disease severity including platelet count, use of vasopressors and PaO_2/FiO_2 ratio on the day of AKI development ($p > 0.05$ for listed characteristics for short duration vs. medium duration, data not shown). Patients who experienced persistent AKI or who died were sicker, with higher APACHE III at enrollment, greater use of vasopressors, lower platelet counts, and lower PaO_2/FiO_2 ratio on the day of AKI development. Patients with short duration or medium duration AKI presented with less severe AKI and had a lower maximum AKI stage, compared to patients with persistent AKI.

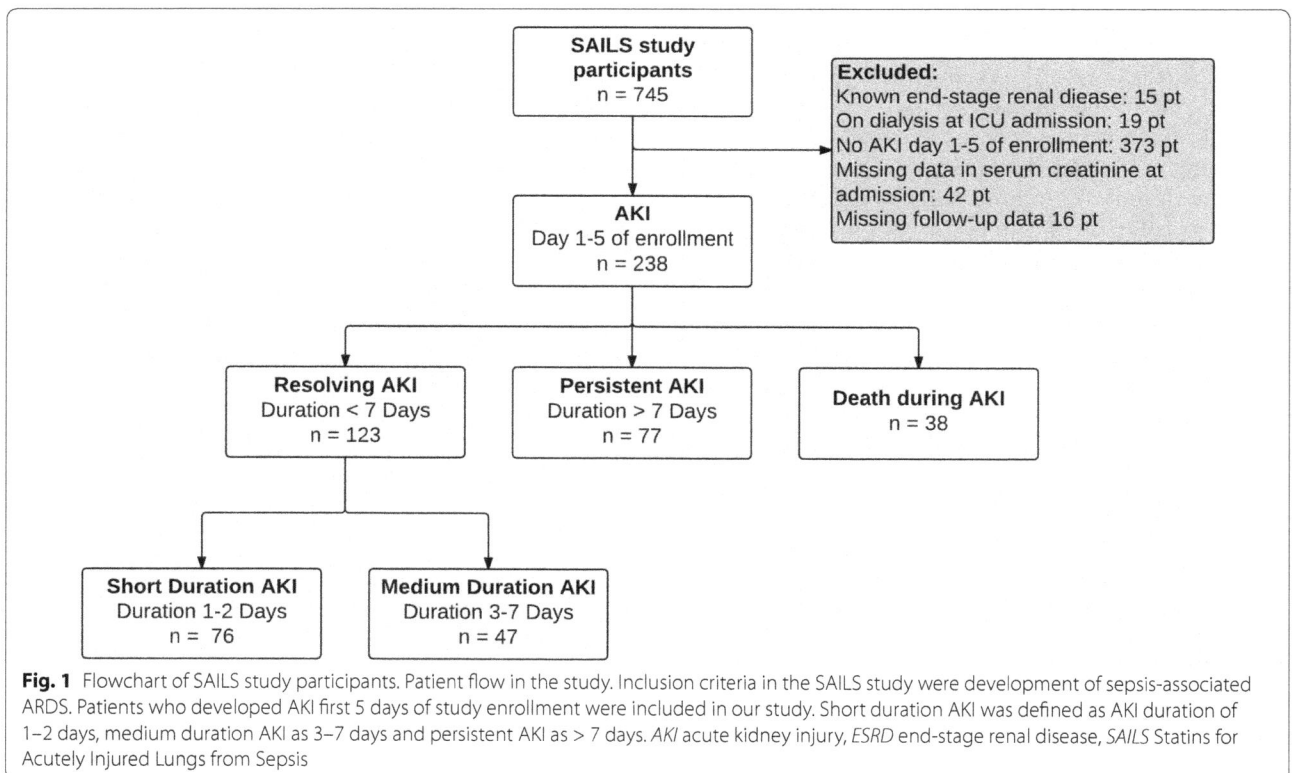

Fig. 1 Flowchart of SAILS study participants. Patient flow in the study. Inclusion criteria in the SAILS study were development of sepsis-associated ARDS. Patients who developed AKI first 5 days of study enrollment were included in our study. Short duration AKI was defined as AKI duration of 1–2 days, medium duration AKI as 3–7 days and persistent AKI as > 7 days. *AKI* acute kidney injury, *ESRD* end-stage renal disease, *SAILS* Statins for Acutely Injured Lungs from Sepsis

Table 1 Baseline characteristics of study population stratified by AKI duration

	SAILS patients AKI n = 238	Short duration AKI n = 76	Medium duration AKI n = 47	Persistent AKI n = 77	Death during AKI n = 38
Baseline characteristics					
Age in years	54 [40, 66]	50 [40, 65]	53 [39, 65]	54 [40, 66]	58 [47, 68]
Female gender, n (%)	114 (47.9)	32 (42.1)	23 (48.9)	40 (51.9)	19 (50.0)
White race, n (%)	181 (76.1)	58 (76.3)	36 (76.6)	58 (75.3)	29 (76.3)
Hispanic or Latino, n (%)	32 (13.4)	14 (18.4)	7 (14.9)	8 (10.4)	3 (7.9)
BMI (kg/m^2)	28.6 [23.6, 34.2]	28.0 [22.5, 33.3]	26.4 [22.8, 32.1]	30.5 [25.7, 34.6]	27.9 [24.0, 34.7]
Medical admission, n (%)	218 (91.6)	70 (92.1)	41 (87.2)	70 (90.9)	37 (97.4)
ICU days before study enrollment n (%)	1 [1, 2]	1 [1, 2]	2 [1, 3]	1 [1, 2]	2 [1, 2]
Rosuvastatin therapy, n (%)	120 (50.4)	33 (43.4)	19 (40.4)	46 (59.7)	22 (57.9)
Day of randomization APACHE III	98 [81, 121]	92 [78, 107]	91 [73, 112]	105 [89, 123]	121 [95, 139]
Comorbidities					
Diabetes mellitus, n (%)	53 (22.3)	16 (21.1)	10 (21.3)	17 (22.1)	10 (26.3)
Hypertension, n (%)	112 (47.1)	35 (46.1)	20 (42.6)	35 (45.5)	22 (57.9)
Congestive heart failure, n (%)	16 (6.7)	2 (2.6)	5 (10.6)	8 (10.4)	1 (2.6)
Peripheral vascular disease, n (%)	12 (5.0)	4 (5.3)	3 (6.4)	4 (5.2)	1 (2.6)
Chronic pulmonary disease, n (%)	35 (14.7)	13 (17.1)	7 (14.9)	10 (13.0)	5 (13.2)
Cancer, n (%)	38 (16.0)	14 (18.4)	4 (8.5)	8 (10.4)	12 (31.6)
Day of AKI development					
Study day that AKI developed	1 [1, 3]	2 [1, 3]	1 [1, 3]	1 [1, 2]	1 [1, 2]
Urine output (mL/kg/h)	0.78 [0.28, 1.48]	1.05 [0.70, 1.81]	1.36 [0.58, 2.87]	0.43 [0.06, 0.86]	0.31 [0.12, 0.88]
Platelets × 10^6/L	168 [74, 256]	204 [120, 292]	185 [115, 272]	143 [67, 220]	68 [26, 184]
Vasopressor use, n (%)	105 (44.3)	22 (28.9)	13 (27.7)	39 (51.3)	31 (81.6)
Systolic BP (mm Hg)	90 [80, 100]	94 [85, 105]	92 [82, 107]	86 [79, 98]	78 [70, 89]
PaO$_2$/FiO$_2$ ratio	155 [110, 220]	184 [129, 257]	192 [133, 272]	147 [106, 190]	123 [87, 151]
AKI characteristics					
Baseline creatinine (mg/dL)	1.0 [0.7, 1.4]	0.9 [0.7, 1.4]	0.9 [0.6, 1.3]	1.2 [0.7, 1.9]	1.0 [0.7, 1.2]
Creatinine at AKI diagnosis (mg/dL)	1.7 [1.2, 2.6]	1.4 [1.0, 2.0]	1.4 [1.1, 2.0]	2.4 [1.6, 3.8]	1.8 [1.4, 2.4]
On dialysis, n (%)	25 (10.5)	1 (1.3)	0 (0.0)	18 (23.4)	6 (15.8)
KDIGO AKI stage at presentation					
Stage 1, n (%)	172 (72.3)	72 (94.7)	40 (85.1)	35 (45.5)	25 (65.8)
Stage 2, n (%)	25 (10.5)	1 (1.3)	5 (10.6)	14 (18.2)	5 (13.2)
Stage 3, n (%)	41 (17.2)	3 (3.9)	2 (4.3)	28 (36.4)	8 (21.1)
KDIGO AKI maximum severity stage day 1–7					
Stage 1, n (%)	116 (48.7)	63 (82.9)	31 (66.0)	13 (16.9)	9 (23.7)
Stage 2, n (%)	36 (15.1)	5 (6.6)	12 (25.5)	11 (14.3)	8 (21.1)
Stage 3, n (%)	86 (36.1)	8 (10.5)	4 (8.5)	53 (68.8)	21 (55.3)

Continuous variables are presented as median and interquartile range

AKI acute kidney injury, *SAILS* Statins for Acutely Injured Lungs from Sepsis, *BMI* body mass index, *APACHE III* acute physiologic and chronic health evaluation III, *ICU* intensive care unit, *BP* blood pressure, *KDIGO* kidney disease: improving global outcomes, *PaO$_2$/FiO$_2$ ratio* partial pressure arterial oxygen/fraction of inspired oxygen

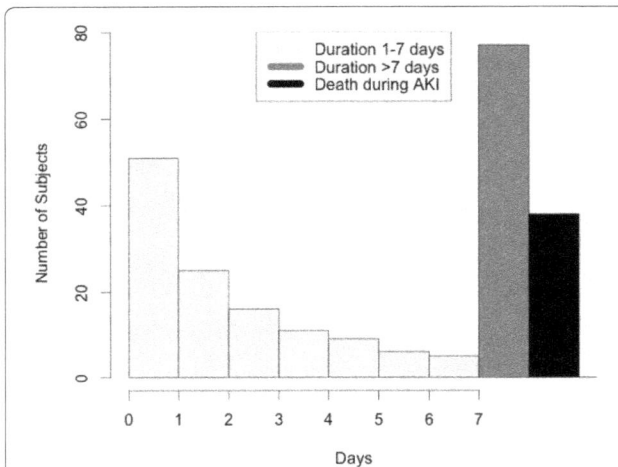

Fig. 2 Histogram of AKI duration. Histogram of AKI duration in patients included on our study (n = 238) with a 7-day follow-up. One hundred and eighteen patients had an AKI duration lasting less than 7 days. Seventy-seven patients experienced AKI duration > 7 days, while 43 patients died during an AKI episode

Effect of AKI duration of outcomes

Table 2 presents outcomes stratified according to AKI duration. There were no significant differences or observable trends between the groups with short and medium duration AKI with regard to cardiovascular failure-free days, ventilator-free days, ICU-free days or 30-day mortality. Compared to patients with persistent AKI, patients with short duration AKI had more cardiovascular failure-free days (4.8 ± 2.3 vs. 3.2 ± 2.4, $p < 0.001$), ventilator-free days (17.6 ± 10.8 vs. 13.2 ± 10.0, $p < 0.01$) and ICU-free days (16.6 ± 10.7 vs. 10.8 ± 9.3, $p < 0.01$),

but there was no difference in 30-day mortality (18.4 vs. 20.8%, $p = 0.87$). Further, patients with medium duration AKI had more cardiovascular failure-free days (4.8 ± 2.2 vs. 3.2 ± 2.4, $p < 0.01$), ventilator-free days (17.5 ± 10.7 vs. 13.2 ± 10.0, $p = 0.02$) and ICU-free days (16.9 ± 9.9 vs. 10.8 ± 9.3, p < 0.01) when compared to patients with persistent AKI. No difference in 30-day mortality (14.9 vs. 20.8%, $p = 0.56$) was found between patients with medium duration AKI and persistent AKI. There were no differences in duration of AKI or mortality based on treatment assignment to rosuvastatin or placebo (data not shown).

In the sensitivity analysis where only those with maximum KDIGO AKI severity stage 1 (Additional file 1: Table 1) were analyzed, cardiovascular failure-free days, ventilator-free days, ICU-free days and 30-day mortality were virtually the same in those with short and medium duration AKI, as observed in the main analysis. A very small number of individuals had persistent AKI that remained Stage 1 ($n = 13$), so we had very limited power to detect differences in outcomes between those with persistent AKI and those with short or medium duration AKI among those with Stage 1 AKI.

Factors associated with resolving AKI

We next examined factors associated with resolving AKI to day 7 (Table 3). In univariate analyses, higher systolic blood pressure was associated with higher rates of resolving AKI while oliguria, moderate/severe ARDS and higher serum creatinine on the day of AKI were associated with lower rates of resolving AKI and remained significant predictors in multivariate analysis.

Table 2 Association of AKI duration with outcomes

	Short duration AKI n = 76	Medium duration AKI n = 47	Persistent AKI n = 77	p value (short vs. medium duration AKI)	p value (short duration vs. persistent AKI)	p value (medium duration vs. persistent AKI)
Cardiovascular failure-free days to day 7 (mean ± SD)	4.8 ± 2.3	4.8 ± 2.2	3.2 ± 2.4	0.98	< 0.001	0.001
Ventilator-free days to day 28 (mean ± SD)	17.6 ± 10.8	17.5 ± 10.7	13.2 ± 10.0	0.97	0.009	0.02
ICU-free days to day 28 (mean ± SD)	16.6 ± 10.7	16.9 ± 9.9	10.8 ± 9.3	0.85	0.001	0.001
Death in health care facility to day 30, n (%)	14 (18.4)	7 (14.9)	16 (20.8)	0.80	0.87	0.56

Cardiovascular failure was defined as the need for vasopressor or a systolic blood pressure of 90 mmHg or less. Patients who died before day 28 were assigned zero ventilator days and zero ICU-free days

AKI acute kidney injury, ICU intensive care unit, SD standard deviation, NS nonsignificant

Table 3 Factors associated with resolving AKI

$n = 236$	Univariate Cox regression (hazard ratio)		p value	Multivariate Cox regression (hazard ratio)		p value
	HR	(95% CI)		HR	(95% CI)	
Age, per 10 year increase	0.94	0.86–1.03	0.19			
Female gender	0.85	0.61–1.17	0.31			
White race	1.03	0.70–1.51	0.88			
Hispanic or Latino ethnic group	1.50	0.98–2.30	0.06			
BMI	1.00	0.98–1.02	0.88			
Diabetes mellitus	0.91	0.61–1.34	0.63			
History of hypertension	0.91	0.65–1.26	0.55			
Platelet count			< 0.001			0.27
> 150×10^9/L	1			1		
< 150×10^9/L	0.54	0.38–0.78		0.80	0.53–1.19	
Urine output			< 0.0001			0.01
> 0.5 mL/kg/h	1			1		
< 0.5 mL/kg/h	0.31	0.20–0.47		0.53	0.32–0.87	
PaO_2/FiO_2 ratio			< 0.0001			0.001
> 200	1			1		
< 200	0.52	0.38–0.71		0.59	0.44–0.81	
Creatinine mg/dl, per unit increase	0.59	0.48–0.74	< 0.0001	0.71	0.57–0.89	0.003
Systolic BP, per 10 mm Hg increase	1.15	1.05–1.25	0.002	1.09	0.99–1.20	0.07
Vasopressor use	0.46	0.32–0.67	< 0.0001	0.91	0.59–1.41	0.68

Factors associated with resolving AKI, defined as an AKI duration of less than 7 days, analyzed by the proportional subdistribution hazards model proposed by Fine and Gray, with death as a competing risk. Two patients were excluded from the original population ($n = 238$) due to missing values

AKI acute kidney injury, BMI body mass index, BP blood pressure, PaO_2/FiO_2 ratio partial pressure arterial oxygen/fraction of inspired oxygen

Impact of recurrent AKI on outcomes and risk factors for recurrent AKI

We examined the incidence of recurrent AKI in those with an initial episode of resolving AKI. Of the 123 subjects, 43 subjects (35.0%) met criteria for AKI again during in the hospital admission. When outcomes were examined in patients with or without recurrent AKI (Table 4), there were still no differences or trends in outcomes between those short versus medium duration AKI, similar to our main analysis. However, those with an

Table 4 Association of recurrent AKI with outcomes

$n = 123$	No recurrent AKI		p value*	Recurrent AKI	p value§
	Short duration AKI $n = 46$	Medium duration AKI $n = 34$		Short and medium duration AKI $n = 43$	
Cardiovascular failure-free days to day 7 (mean ± SD)	5.1 ± 2.3	4.8 ± 2.3	0.47	4.4 ± 2.3	0.06
Ventilator-free days to day 28 (mean ± SD)	20.4 ± 10.0	20.0 ± 9.8	0.89	12.7 ± 10.6	0.003
ICU-free days to day 28 (mean ± SD)	19.7 ± 9.5	19.4 ± 8.7	0.89	11.4 ± 10.7	0.001
Death in health care facility to day 30, n (%)	5 (10.9)	4 (11.8)	1.00	12 (27.9)	0.04

Cardiovascular failure was defined as the need for vasopressor or a systolic blood pressure of 90 mmHg or less. Patients who died before day 28 were assigned zero ventilator days and zero ICU-free days

AKI acute kidney injury, ICU intensive care unit, SD standard deviation, NS nonsignificant

*Short duration AKI without recurrent AKI vs. medium duration AKI without recurrent AKI

§ Short and medium duration AKI without recurrent AKI versus short and medium duration AKI with recurrent AKI

initial episode of short and medium duration AKI *without* recurrent AKI had better outcomes than those who experienced an episode of recurrent AKI, with more ventilator-free days (mean ± SD, 20.2 ± 9.8 vs. 12.7 ± 10.6, $p = 0.003$), ICU-free days (mean ± SD, 19.5 ± 9.1 vs. 11.4 ± 10.7, $p = 0.001$), and lower 30-day mortality (11.2 vs. 27.9%, $p = 0.039$). Similar results were observed when the analysis was restricted to patients with a maximum of stage 1 AKI and stratified according to the presence or absence of recurrent AKI (data not shown). However, no baseline factors were found to be significantly associated with development of recurrent AKI in the univariate Cox regression analysis (Additional file 2: Table 2).

Discussion

AKI remains a disease with poor outcomes for which there are no treatments, apart from supportive care. Duration of AKI has been recognized as an important factor associated with outcomes following AKI. It has been implied that differences in AKI duration may represent distinct phenotypes of AKI due to etiology of injury, but these views are still to be confirmed at a mechanistic level [6, 8, 14]. In this study, we explored the effect of AKI duration on outcomes in a cohort of critically ill patients with sepsis-associated ARDS.

We found that 31.9% of the patients had an AKI duration of less than 48 h, demonstrating that short duration AKI is very common. Consequently, to further examine the effect of short duration AKI on outcomes, we divided those with resolving AKI into two subgroups of short and medium duration AKI. Although we expected the patients with short AKI to have lower severity of illness than patients with medium duration AKI, there were no differences between the groups with regard to comorbidities, AKI severity or general disease severity measurements. Patients with short duration AKI had similar outcomes compared to the patients with medium duration AKI, and these results were confirmed in two subsequent analyses. First, to examine whether the results were due to differences in AKI severity, we restricted our analysis to those whose maximum AKI severity was Stage 1. Second, we hypothesized that those with short duration AKI might have an increased risk of adverse outcomes due to recurrent AKI episodes and therefore stratified our analysis by the presence or absence of recurrent AKI. Again, there were no differences in outcomes, suggesting that short duration AKI is not associated with better outcomes than medium duration AKI in critically ill patients.

A significant proportion of patients (32.4%) had persistent kidney failure lasting 7 or more days, and these patients experienced poorer clinical outcomes including increased length of ICU stay, time on the ventilator and days with cardiovascular failure. This emphasizes the importance of identifying high-risk patients who may benefit the most from early interventions and novel treatments. Along the same lines, those with quick and spontaneous resolving AKI may dilute trials and perhaps should not be the target of new treatment trials. Here, we found that lack of oliguria, lower serum creatinine on the day of AKI and having mild ARDS were associated with increased likelihood of resolving AKI.

Patients with recurrent AKI were found to have worse short-term outcomes. It has previously been reported that recurrent AKI episodes are associated with an increased risk of CKD progression and other adverse long-term outcomes [14], but, to the best of our knowledge, this is one of the first studies to examine the effect of recurrent AKI in critically ill patients and during a single hospitalization. We went on to examine risk factors for recurrent AKI and were not able to identify any, other than a trend for gender and ethnicity. This may reflect the fact that we only studied risk factors at baseline and upon development of the first AKI episode, whereas future or time-updated risk factors (e.g., new or recurrent sepsis, repeated exposures to nephrotoxins) are likely the strongest drivers of recurrent AKI. Alternatively, this may have been due to a lack of power given our relatively small sample size or the exclusion of certain very high-risk populations (e.g., those with advanced heart failure or liver failure) from the overall population. A similar study examined predictors of recurrent AKI after renal transplantation [15] and was unable to identify any risk factors, while other studies have mostly focused on predictors of a second hospitalization with AKI, rather than a second episode during a single hospitalization [16].

Our overall results differ somewhat from other studies, which have highlighted the importance of AKI duration and especially transient AKI. Many of these studies have focused on less severely ill patients or have only included patients who survive hospitalization [17]. In contrast, our population of critically ill patients had multi-organ failure with sepsis and ARDS in addition to AKI, and the in-hospital mortality rate of this patient group was very high. While other studies have only focused on mortality as primary endpoint, we here report the influence of AKI duration on other relevant outcomes along with mortality while accounting for AKI severity and recurrent AKI status.

Potential limitations of our study include the very specific nature of our population, all of whom were critically ill adults with sepsis-associated ARDS who developed AKI. However, this is an extremely well-characterized population from a large randomized clinical trial, where a number of aspects of care including mechanical ventilation and fluid management were protocolized, resulting in less concern about variations in clinical care and the effect of these variations on outcomes. Furthermore, there has been much interest in the interplay of ARDS and AKI, which thought to be closely connected as part of multi-organ dysfunction, with the presence of both diseases associated with worse clinical outcomes [18]. Although more studies are needed to determine the direct effects of ARDS on AKI, our study focuses on a well-recognized and important clinical population. Outpatient creatinine measurements were unfortunately not unavailable, but this is often the case the clinical settings, where many patients lack an outpatient baseline creatinine. As part of the study protocol, serum creatinine values were recorded for up to 48 h before study enrollment, which allowed us to use these serum creatinine values as baseline values and to calculate a rolling 48-h window for AKI ascertainment, rather than using an imputed baseline or nadir serum creatinine as baseline. Our study is greatly strengthened by its richness and completeness in clinical variables obtained as part of a multicenter clinical trial as well as the racial/ethnic diversity of the study population.

Conclusions

In summary, we evaluated the association of AKI duration on outcomes in a cohort of critically ill patients with sepsis-associated ARDS. We found no differences in outcomes in patients with short duration AKI compared to those with medium duration AKI, while persistent AKI was associated with worse outcomes. Compared to patients with persistent AKI or who died during AKI, patients with resolving AKI were less likely to have oliguria, moderate/severe ARDS or higher serum creatinine on the day of AKI. We found that recurrent AKI was associated with poorer clinical outcomes, but no clinical factors at baseline could predict the development of recurrent AKI. Our findings suggest that the ideal population for AKI clinical trials in patients with ARDS may be those with persistent AKI or at increased risk of persistent AKI, since the impact of short and medium duration AKI on clinical outcomes is modest.

Abbreviations
AKI: acute kidney injury; ARDS: acute respiratory distress syndrome; CKD: chronic kidney disease; ICU: intensive care unit; IQR: interquartile range; KDIGO: kidney disease: improving global outcomes (KDIGO), guidelines form 2012.

Authors' contributions
CF, TS, MB, KL contributed to study design. CF, KM, RH, KL helped with analysis and data interpretation. CF, KM involved in statistical analysis. CF, TS, KM, RH, MB, KL helped in drafting manuscript and revision. All authors read and approved the final manuscript.

Author details
[1] Division of Nephrology, Department of Medicine, University of California, San Francisco, Box 0532, San Francisco, CA 94143-0532, USA. [2] Department of Anesthesiology, Nordsjællands Hospital, University of Copenhagen, Copenhagen, Denmark. [3] Department of Epidemiology and Biostatistics, University of California, San Francisco, San Francisco, USA. [4] Division of Nephrology, Department of Medicine, University of California, San Francisco, San Francisco, USA. [5] Divisions of Nephrology and Critical Care Medicine, Departments of Medicine and Anesthesia, University of California, San Francisco, Box 0532, San Francisco, CA 94143-0532, USA.

Acknowledgements
We thank the SAILS Study investigators and the National Heart, Lung, and Blood Institute ARDS Clinical Trials Network for the data used in this study.

Competing interests
The authors declare that they have no competing interests.

Funding
This work was supported by a research grant from the Lundbeck Foundation Clinical Research Fellowship Program. RKH was supported by NIH Grant DK100468. KDL was supported by NIH Grant DK113381.

References
1. Uchino S, Kellum JA, Bellomo R, Doig GS, Morimatsu H, Morgera S, et al. Acute renal failure in critically ill patients: a multinational, multicenter study. JAMA. 2005;294:813–8.
2. Pannu N, James M, Hemmelgarn B, Klarenbach S. Association between AKI, recovery of renal function, and long-term outcomes after hospital discharge. Clin J Am Soc Nephrol. 2013;8:194–202.
3. Wald R, Quinn RR, Luo J, Li P, Scales DC, Mamdani MM, et al. Chronic dialysis and death among survivors of acute kidney injury requiring dialysis. JAMA. 2009;302:1179–85.
4. Coca SG, King JT, Rosenthal RA, Perkal MF, Parikh CR. The duration of postoperative acute kidney injury is an additional parameter predicting long-term survival in diabetic veterans. Kidney Int. 2010;78:926–33.
5. Bellomo R, Ronco C, Mehta RL, Asfar P, Boisramé-Helms J, Darmon M, et al. Acute kidney injury in the ICU: from injury to recovery: reports from the 5th Paris international conference. Ann Intensive Care. 2017;7:49.
6. Uchino S, Bellomo R, Bagshaw SM, Goldsmith D. Transient azotaemia is associated with a high risk of death in hospitalized patients. Nephrol Dial Transplant. 2010;25:1833–9.
7. Brown JR, Kramer RS, Coca SG, Parikh CR. Duration of acute kidney injury impacts long-term survival after cardiac surgery. Ann Thorac Surg. 2010;90:1142–8.
8. Perinel S, Vincent F, Lautrette A, Dellamonica J, Mariat C, Zeni F, et al. Transient and persistent acute kidney injury and the risk of hospital mortality in critically ill patients: results of a multicenter cohort study. Crit Care Med. 2015;43:e269–75.
9. Truwit JD, Bernard GR, Steingrub J, Matthay MA, Liu KD, Albertson TE, et al. Rosuvastatin for sepsis-associated acute respiratory distress syndrome. N Engl J Med. 2014;370:2191–200.
10. KDIGO Acute Kidney Injury Workgroup. KDIGO clinical practice guideline for acute kidney injury. Kidney Int Suppl. 2012;2:1–138.
11. Bernard GRDG, Hudson LD, Lemeshow S, Marshall JC, Russell J, Sibbald W, Sprung CL, Vincent JLWA. Quantification of organ failure for clinical trials and clinical practice. Am J Respir Crit Care Med. 1995;151:A323.
12. Fine JP, Gray RJ. A proportional hazards model for the subdistribution of a competing risk. J Am Stat Assoc. 1999;94:496.

13. Brown SM, Grissom CK, Moss M, Rice TW, Schoenfeld D, Hou P, et al. Non-linear imputation of PaO_2/FIO_2 from SpO_2/FIO_2 among patients with acute respiratory distress syndrome. Chest. 2016;150:307–13.

14. Thakar CV, Christianson A, Himmelfarb J, Leonard AC. Acute kidney injury episodes and chronic kidney disease risk in diabetes mellitus. Clin J Am Soc Nephrol. 2011;6:2567–72.

15. Bardak S, Turgutalp K, Türkegün M, Demir S, Kıykım A. Recurrent acute kidney injury in renal transplant patients: a single-center study.

16. Siew ED, Parr SK, Abdel-Kader K, Eden SK, Peterson JF, Bansal N, et al. Predictors of recurrent AKI. J Am Soc Nephrol. 2016;27:1190–200.

17. Kellum JA, Sileanu FE, Murugan R, Lucko N, Shaw AD, Clermont G. Classifying AKI by urine output versus serum creatinine level. J Am Soc Nephrol. 2015;26:2231–8.

18. Darmon M, Clec'h C, Adrie C, Argaud L, Allaouchiche B, Azoulay E, et al. Acute respiratory distress syndrome and risk of AKI among critically ill patients. Clin J Am Soc Nephrol. 2014;9:1347–53.

16

Piperacillin–tazobactam as alternative to carbapenems for ICU patients

Benoit Pilmis[1,2], Vincent Jullien[3,4], Alexis Tabah[5,6], Jean-Ralph Zahar[7,8*] and Christian Brun-Buisson[9]

Abstract

Several studies suggest that alternatives to carbapenems, and particulary beta-lactam/beta-lactamase inhibitor combinations, can be used for therapy of extended-spectrum beta-lactamase-producing Enterobacteriaceae (ESBL-PE)-related infections in non-ICU patients. Little is known concerning ICU patients in whom achieving the desired plasmatic pharmacokinetic/pharmacodynamic (PK/PD) target may be difficult. Also, in vitro susceptibility to beta-lactamase inhibitors might not translate into clinical efficacy. We reviewed the recent clinical studies examining the use of BL/BLI as alternatives to carbapenems for therapy of bloodstream infection, PK/PD data and discuss potential ecological benefit from avoiding the use of carbapenems. With the lack of prospective randomized studies, treating ICU patients with ESBL-PE-related infections using piperacillin–tazobactam should be done with caution. Current data suggest that BL/BLI empirical use should be avoided for therapy of ESBL-PE-related infection. Also, definitive therapy should be reserved to patients in clinical stable condition, after microbial documentation and results of susceptibility tests. Optimization of administration and higher dosage should be used in order to reach pharmacological targets.

Keywords: Carbapenems, ESBL, Alternatives, Ecological consequences, Outcome

Introduction

Since the 1980s, extended-spectrum beta-lactamase (ESBL)-producing Enterobacteriaceae (ESBL-PE) have been spreading worldwide [1, 2]. Several reports underline the concomitant increasing use of carbapenems [3, 4]. Indeed, the recently published 2015 ESAC report noted a threefold increased use of carbapenems between 2010 and 2014 [5]. This induces a selective pressure for carbapenem-resistant isolates, and recent data suggest that even a brief exposure to carbapenems increases the risk of colonization with carbapenem-resistant bacteria (CRB) in intensive care unit patients [6].

To reduce the ecological risk associated with the increased consumption of last-line antibiotics, two main strategies are available: (1) searching for alternative treatments for ESBL-PE-related infections and (2) antimicrobial de-escalation (ADE). Therefore, the use of alternatives to carbapenems such as cephamycins, piperacillin–tazobactam and others for the treatment of ESBL-PE infections should be investigated. A recent systematic review, including two randomized controlled trials and 12 cohort studies, highlighted that the effects of ADE on antimicrobial resistance have not been properly studied [7]. However, this strategy is largely promoted by several scientific societies and specifically in critically ill patients [8, 9]. Indeed, for severely ill patients, international guidelines recommend the use of broad-spectrum antibiotics as first-line therapy to minimize the risk of inadequate initial antimicrobial treatment, and suggest streamlining initial antibiotic therapy and narrowing the spectrum whenever possible once the pathogen(s) are identified [10].

Until recently, the common rule is to treat infections caused by ESBL-producing organism with carbapenems. However, ESBLs are inhibited in vitro by beta-lactamase inhibitors and several studies have suggested the use of β-lactam/β-lactamase inhibitor combinations (BL/BLIs) such as piperacillin–tazobactam as a carbapenem-sparing strategy for the treatment of ESBL-PE-related infections [11–13]. The recent EUCAST and CLSI [14,

*Correspondence: jeanralph.zahar@aphp.fr
[7] Département de Microbiologie Clinique, Unité de Contrôle et de Prévention du risque Infectieux, Groupe Hospitalier Paris Seine Saint-Denis, AP-HP, CHU Avicenne, 125 rue de Stalingrad, 9300 Bobigny, France

15] guidelines include BL/BLIs and other beta-lactams (cefepime, third generation cephalosporins, temocillin, cefoxitin) as treatment options for infections caused by ESBL-producing organisms. For a long time, AST categorization was based not only on MIC and zone diameter measurements but also on the detection of individual resistance mechanisms, i.e., interpretative reading. Even if in vitro results indicated susceptibility to a drug, the reported category was edited to "resistant" if the presence of a resistance mechanism was confirmed, e.g., in the case of extended-spectrum beta-lactamases (ESBLs). To limit the consumption of carbapenems, CLSI and EUCAST recently abandoned editing of AST reports based on the detection of ESBLs.

While several studies are conducted in ICU, data remain scarce concerning other beta-lactams in non-ICU- [16, 17] and ICU-infected [18–21] patients. Therefore, only BL/BLIs such as piperacillin–tazobactam (Pip–Taz) could be used in ICU patients, but there are concerns that: (1) no randomized controlled trials compared specifically carbapenems to Pip–Taz for the treatment of ESBL-PE-related infections [22]; (2) in vitro susceptibility to β-lactamase inhibitors might not predict clinical efficacy; and (3) the success of BL/BLIs depends on pharmacokinetic–pharmacodynamic target attainment, which current dosing recommendations may not guarantee. Therefore, alternatives are seldom used in clinical practice for treating serious infections caused by ESBL-PE.

In critically ill patients, pharmacokinetics of beta-lactam antibiotics differs from healthy volunteers. Lower than expected concentrations have been reported for meropenem, piperacillin, amoxicillin, as well as for cephalosporins [23–26]. Besides, the risk of treatment failure may be exacerbated when using antibiotics exposed to the inoculum effect [27], as are most beta-lactams.

This narrative review, based on microbiological, pharmacodynamics, clinical and ecological data, describes the available evidence for the use of Pip–Taz as an alternative to carbapenems in critically ill patients and to provide some guidance to prescribers for using these drugs when treating infections caused by ESBL-PE.

Methods
Literature search
A literature search was performed via PubMed, including all records from 1990 through April 2016. The following search pattern was applied: (ESBL OR extended-spectrum β-lactamases) AND (infection) AND (cefepime OR cefoxitine OR cephamycins OR flomoxef OR BL/BLI OR Piperacillin–tazobactam OR Carbapenems OR temocillin OR alternatives). Reference lists were cross-checked to identify further publications for possible inclusion. We restricted inclusion to studies published in the English, Spanish and French languages.

Selection criteria
We screened and included studies in three categories according to the following criteria: (1) pharmacokinetics and pharmacodynamics studies, where all studies investigating the PK/PD of the potential alternatives to carbapenems in ICU patients were included. (2) For clinical studies, we restricted inclusion to studies reporting mortality of patients receiving empirical or definitive treatment with a non-carbapenem therapy for an ESBL bacteremia in adult patients. Patients with community-, hospital- and healthcare-associated bacteremia were eligible for inclusion. (3) Finally, considering ecological studies, we included any published article reporting carbapenem-resistant Enterobacteriaceae (CRE). Among the eligible articles, studies were included if they reported on exposure to any previous antibiotic class as a risk factor associated with CRE acquisition.

Results
Microbiological susceptibility
Several studies suggested that ESBL-PE were susceptible to non-carbapenem beta-lactams. However, the prevalence of susceptibility depends on the species concerned, the antibiotic class and local epidemiology. ESBL-producing E. coli is usually regarded as more susceptible to all beta-lactams than ESBL-producing K. pneumoniae, piperacillin–tazobactam (Pip–Taz) being the most effective antibiotic [28]. North American data from the 2010–2014 SMART programs find that 4, 10 and 46% of ESBL-producing E. coli were susceptible to ceftriaxone, cefepime and ceftazidime, respectively [28], whereas 96–98 and 69% of ESBL-producing E. coli isolates from urinary tract [29] and from patients with pneumonia [30] were found susceptible in vitro to Pip–Taz, respectively. Conversely, only 26.9% of ESBL-producing Klebsiella spp. isolates from patients with pneumonia were susceptible to Pip–Taz [30]. Asian data on ESBL-producing E. coli find similar susceptibilities, with 1.6, 9.5, 33.4 and 84.5% isolates susceptible to cefotaxime, cefepime, ceftazidime and Pip–Taz, respectively [29]. It is noteworthy that in silico PK/PD studies aiming to evaluate the use of alternatives to carbapenems for treatment of ESBL-PE infections suggest that ESBL-Kp susceptibility is overestimated by conventional methods in comparison with E-test susceptibility testing.

Pharmacokinetics and pharmacodynamics studies
According to epidemiological data, two main antibiotics could be used as an alternative to carbapenems: piperacillin and cefoxitin. Others antibiotics suggested in the

literature as temocillin, ceftolozane/tazobactam and/or ceftazidime/avibactam are less tested. Our goal was to define the optimal condition for using these antibiotics for ESBL-PE-related infections in ICU.

The pharmacokinetics of piperacillin in ICU patients was quite extensively investigated. There is, however, a lack of consensus on the pharmacokinetic/pharmacodynamic target to be achieved. Indeed targets as different as obtaining a free concentration > MIC (fT > MIC) or > 4 times the MIC (fT > 4xMIC) for 50 or 100% of a dose interval have been considered [31–36]. This is a crucial point as the dose to be administered will vary considerably according to the chosen target. There are, however, increasing data supporting a minimal efficacy criteria of fT > MIC = 100% in ICU patients, while a total trough concentration/MIC ratio of at least three was found to prevent the emergence of resistance in vitro [37–40]. Therefore, based on these more drastic PK/PD endpoints, it seems a dose of 4.5 g TID given as intermittent infusions should not be considered any more in ICU patients with normal renal functions [32, 36]. A 4.5-g × 4 daily dose appears more convenient, provided it is administered as prolonged infusion of at least 3 h [32, 34]. Indeed, for an intermittent bolus administration, a 4gx4 dose is associated with a very low probability of target attainment, even for the lowest PK/PD target of T > MIC = 50% [32]. However, even with a 4.5-g x 4 dose given by extended 3-h infusions, around one-third of the patients may not achieve a fT > MIC = 100%, which supports the need for an individual dose adjustment using therapeutic drug monitoring [35]. Such a result strongly supports the use of continuous infusion, and since this administration mode provides a better outcome than intermittent infusion [24], we believe a 16-g daily dose given as a continuous infusion, following a 4.5-g loading dose, should be considered as a starting point in ICU patients with normal renal function. Such an approach was found relevant for the treatment of ventilator-associated pneumonia, as it allowed the achievement of alveolar concentrations > 16 mg/L (i.e., the clinical breakpoint for gram-negative bacteria).

Slightly different results were observed in morbidly obese ICU patients, for whom the elimination half-life of piperacillin seems to be increased, compared to non-obese patients, resulting in an increased fT > MIC for equivalent doses [33]. Consequently, a 4.5-g × 4 daily dose given as a 4-h extended infusion should provide satisfying trough concentrations [33].

The pharmacokinetics of piperacillin in ICU patients undergoing continuous renal replacement therapy (CRRT) was also investigated, and similar results were found in case of venovenous hemofiltration or hemodiafiltration. A 4.5-g TID dose given as 30-min infusion should provide a free concentration > MIC for the entire dosing interval in almost all patients. Extending the infusion duration to 4 h should allow the attainment of several times the MIC. However, dose requirements seem to importantly depend on the membrane used and the effluent rate that are major aspects of CRRT poorly investigated to date [41, 42]. An interesting point is that piperacillin concentration in the dialysate effluent is equal to the free plasma concentration and can therefore be used for the individual adaptation of the dose via therapeutic drug monitoring (TDM) [43]. To our knowledge, the PK of piperacillin in the context of intermittent hemodialysis was not investigated to date in ICU patients. Based on the results obtained in sepsis-free volunteers with chronic renal failure [44], a dose of 4.5 g bid could be used as a starting point, with a subsequent TDM-guided individual adjustment of the dose. Conflicting results are available about the percentage of the dose that is eliminated by a 4-h session of hemodialysis (i.e., from 10 to 50%) [45, 46]. However, because a supplemental elimination is likely to occur during hemodialysis, it seems preferable to administrate the drug just after the end of the hemodialysis session.

Cefoxitin PK in ICU patients was not investigated to date. By using the PK parameters obtained in healthy subjects, it was shown that for a 8-g daily dose of cefoxitin, only an administration by continuous infusion provided a high probability to achieve targets of fT > MIC = 100% and fT > 4 × MIC = 100% for ESBL-PE [47]. However, since PK differences are expected in ICU subjects, PK data in this population are obviously needed [48].

Concerning temocillin, a 2-g TID dose given as intermittent 30-min infusion, provides a high probability to attain fT > MIC = 100% in ICU patients with normal renal function, provided the MIC is ≤ 4 mg/L. For higher MIC, administration of the same daily dose by continuous infusion is preferable [49]. In summary, among the different antibiotics suggested as alternatives to carbapenems, Pip–Tz is the one with the most frequent published PK/PD data in ICU. High daily doses and prolonged infusion should be promoted for ESBL-PE-related infections in ICU patients.

Clinical studies

The article selection process is shown in Fig. 1. Of the 54 articles selected initially, 23 provided data among patients treated with BL/BLIs for ESBL-producing Enterobacteriaceae-related infections (Table 1). Most of the published studies were retrospective (17/23; 73.9%), and all others were observational. Community-acquired, healthcare-associated and nosocomial infections were included without distinction. Among these 23 studies, 9 (39.1%), 6 (26%) and 7 (30.4%) evaluated antibiotic therapy as

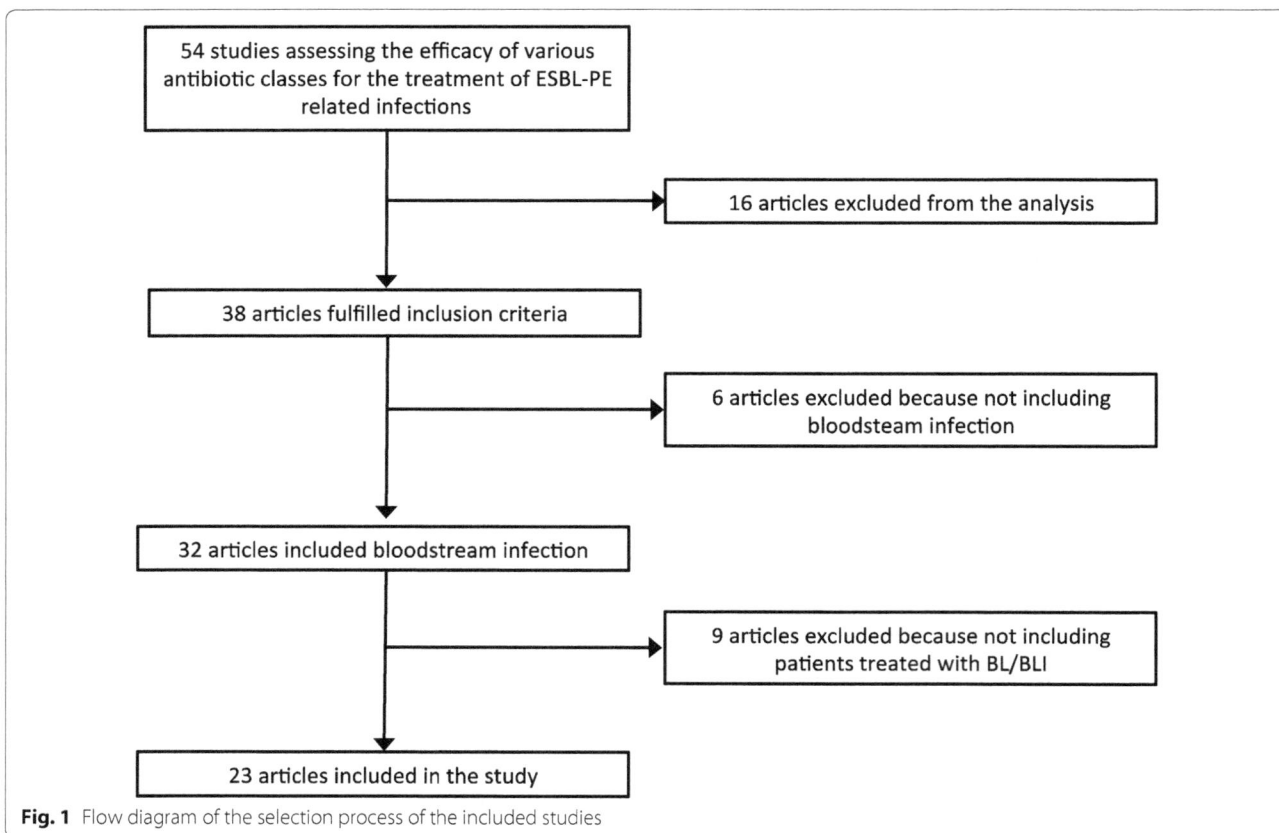

Fig. 1 Flow diagram of the selection process of the included studies

The flow diagram contains the following boxes:

- 54 studies assessing the efficacy of various antibiotic classes for the treatment of ESBL-PE related infections
- 16 articles excluded from the analysis
- 38 articles fulfilled inclusion criteria
- 6 articles excluded because not including bloodsteam infection
- 32 articles included bloodstream infection
- 9 articles excluded because not including patients treated with BL/BLI
- 23 articles included in the study

empirical therapy (ETC), definitive therapy or both, respectively. Among carbapenems, the selected molecule was available in 53% of included studies and imipenem–cilastatin was the most frequently used (45.7% of studies) followed by meropenem (35.2%) and ertapenem (19.1%).

Only 3 (13%) studies reported the doses of antibiotics [19, 20, 50] and none reported the modalities of antibiotic's administration. Indeed administered doses in patients without renal failure were variable; however, imipenem was used in most cases at an average dose of 0.5 g every 6 h, whereas 1 g every 8 h and 1 g every 24 h were used for meropenem and ertapenem, respectively. The two species most frequently involved were *E. coli* and *K. pneumoniae*. All patients included in these studies had bacteremia, and the two most frequent sites of infection were urinary tract and intra-abdominal infection. MIC was taken into account in adjusting antibiotic therapy in 11 (47.8%) of the 23 studies.

As mentioned above, 11 studies included between 6 and 131 ICU patients. In fact, some of the same patients were included in different cohorts [12, 51]. Only 4 studies [52–55] included patients with pneumonia caused by ESBL-PE, representing 8–50% of patients with ESBL-PE-related infections, indicating that less than 30 patients

with ESBL-related pneumonia could be evaluated. Data regarding outcome for patients treated with carbapenems versus alternatives were available from 20 (86.9%) of the 23 studies including bacteremic patients. Surprisingly, potential confounding factors, such as severity of underlying diseases or of infection, were seldom reported.

Among studies including ICU patients, 6 (56%) compared BL/BLIs to carbapenems as empirical therapy. However, BL/BLIs was the only alternative compared to carbapenems in only 3 studies [12, 20, 51]. In these studies, *E. coli* and *K. pneumoniae* represented more than two-third of the isolates and MICs were taken into account in only one study [20]. The difference of mortality didn't reach statistical significance in two studies [12, 51]. However, Ofer-friedman et al. [20] conducted a multicenter observational study including non-urinary BSI and comparing BL/BLI to carbapenem for the treatment of ESBL. In contrast to other studies, *E. coli* accounted for only half of the bloodstream infections; the median piperacillin MIC was 8 mg/L, and approximately half of patients required ICU care. In this study, the mortality was significantly higher in the piperacillin–tazobactam group [OR 7.9 (1.2–53)]. Thus, BL/BLIs may lead a poorer outcome than carbapenem therapy for critically

Table 1 Studies characteristics

Author/year of publication	Study design, region	No. of patients, ESBL/total	Type of infection (n, %)	Bacteria (n, %)	ICU (n, %)	ETC/DTC	Treatment (n, %)	MIC	Administration (CI, PI or II)	Posology
Apisarnthanarak et al. [52]	SC case–control, 2003–2007, Thailand	36/146	UK (36, 100%)	E. coli K. pneumoniae	UK	ETC (36, 100%)	Cephalosporins (17, 47.2%) BL/BLI (10, 27.8%) Carbapenem (5, 13.9%) Fluoroquinolones (4, 11.1%)	N	UK	UK
Balakrishnan et al. [94]	MC retrospective cohort, 2008–2010, United Kingdom	42/42	UK	UK	UK	DTC (42, 100%)	Temocillin (42, 100%)	Y	II	Y
Bin et al. [95]	SC prospective cohort, 2002–2005, China	22/22	IIA (11, 50%) Primary bacterae-mia (6, 27.2%) UTI (5, 22.7%)	E. coli (22, 100%)	UK	DTC (22, 100%)	Carbapenem (8, 36.4%) Cephalosporins (7, 31.8%) BL/BLI (7, 31.8%)	Y	Y	UK
Chaubey et al. [96]	MC prospective cohort, 2000–2007, Canada	79/79	Primary bacterae-mia (39, 49.3%) UTI (38, 48.1%) Pneumonia (2, 2.5%) IIA (1, 1.3%)	E. coli (72, 91.1%) K. pneumoniae (7, 8.9%)	UK	ETC (74, 93.7%) DTC (79, 100%)	Carbapenem (16, 20.2%) BL/BLI (16, 20.2%) Aminoglycosides (16, 20.2%) Fluoroquinolones (16, 20.2%) Cephalosporins (16, 20.2%) Carbapenem (16, 20.2%) BL/BLI (16, 20.2%) Fluoroquinolones (16, 20.2%) Sulfamides (16, 20.2%) Aminoglycosides (16, 20.2%)	N	UK	UK
Chopra et al. [50]	MC retrospective cohort, 2005–2007, USA	145/145	UK	E. coli (24, 16.6%) K. pneumoniae (121, 83.4%)	Y (37, 25,5%)	ETC (128, 88.2%) DTC (110)	Cephalosporins (85, 58.6%) Carbapenem (50, 34.4%) Fluoroquinolones (6, 3.9%) Aminoglycosides (4, 3.1%) Carbapenem (103, 70.9%) Cephalosporins (41, 28.2%) BL/BLI (24, 16.4%) Fluoroquinolones (17, 11.8%) Amikacin (17, 11.8%) Tigecycline (12, 8.2%)	Y	UK	UK

Table 1 continued

Author/year of publication	Study design, region	No. of patients, ESBL/total	Type of infection (n, %)	Bacteria (n, %)	ICU (n, %)	ETC/DTC	Treatment (n, %)	MIC	Administration (CI, PI or II)	Posology
Chung et al. [97]	SC retrospective cohort, 2005–2010, Taiwan	122/122	UTI (47, 38.5%), Primary bacteraemia (21, 17.2%), IIA (22, 18%), Pneumonia (6, 4.9%), CVC (6, 4.9%), Skin and soft tissue (4, 3.3%), Surgical site infection (3, 2.5%), Other (13, 10.7%)	E. coli (122, 100%)	UK	DTC (107 87.7%)	Carbapenem (71, 57.9%), Non-BL/BLI (48, 39.3%), BL/BLI (3, 2.8%)	N	UK	UK
De Rosa et al. [98]	SC retrospective cohort, 2000–2007, Italy	128/128	Primary bacteraemia (61, 47.6%), IIA (55, 43%), UTI (12, 9.4%)	E. coli (80, 62.5%), K. pneumoniae (28, 21.9%), P. mirabilis (20, 15.6%)	Y (8, 6.3%)	ETC (97 75.8%)	Carbapenem (101, 79.3%), BL/BLI (10, 8.2%), Fluoroquinolone (8, 6.2%), Trimethoprim/sulfamethoxazole (1, 1%), Aminoglycosides (8, 6.2%)	N	UK	UK
Du et al. [16]	SC retrospective cohort, 1997–1999, China	23/85	Primary bacteraemia (9, 39.1%), IIA (5, 21.7%), Pneumonia (4, 17.4%), UTI (2, 8.7%), CVC (2, 8.7%), Other (1, 4.4%)	E. coli (16, 69.5%), K. pneumoniae (7, 30.5%)	N	DTC (23, 100%)	Carbapenem (13, 56.5%), Cephalosporins (7, 30.4%), Fluoroquinolone (2, 8.7%), Aminoglycosides (1, 4.4%)	N	UK	UK
Endimiani et al. [99]	SC retrospective cohort, 1997–2004, Italy	9/23	Primary bacteraemia (5, 55.6%), UTI (4, 44.4%)	P. mirabilis (9, 100%)	UK	ETC (9, 100%), DTC (9, 100%)	Cephalosporins (5, 55.6%), BL/BLI (4, 44.4%), Cephalosporins (4, 44.4%), BL/BLI (3, 33.3%), Carbapenem (2, 22.3%)	Y	Y	UK
Ferrandez et al. [100]	Retrospective cohort, 2000–2006, Spain	53/53	UK	E. coli, K. pneumoniae	UK	–	Carbapenem (30, 56.6%), BL/BLI (5, 9.4%), Fluoroquinolone (4, 7.5%), Cephalosporins (2, 3.8%), Other (12, 22.7%)	Y	UK	UK
Gudiol et al. [101]	SC prospective observational study, 2006–2008, Spain	17/135	Primary bacteraemia (9, 52.9%), IIA (6, 35.3%), UTI (1, 5.9%), Other (1, 5.9%)	E. coli (17, 100%)	Y (2, 12%)	ETC (17, 100%), DTC (17, 100%)	BL/BLI (6, 35.3%), Carbapenem (5, 29.4%), Cephalosporins (5, 29.4%), Monobactam (1, 5.9%), Carbapenem (14, 82.3%), BL/BLI (2, 11.8%), Fluoroquinolone (1, 5.9%)	N	UK	UK

Table 1 continued

Author/year of publication	Study design, region	No. of patients, ESBL/total	Type of infection (n, %)	Bacteria (n, %)	ICU (n, %)	ETC/DTC	Treatment (n, %)	MIC	Administration (CI, PI or II)	Posology
Gutiérez-Gutiérez et al. [51]	MC, retrospective cohort study, 2004–2013, International	601/601	UTI (272, 45.2%) Other (258, 42.9%) IIA (71, 11.8%)	E. coli (439, 73%) K. pneumoniae (114, 19%) Other (48, 8%)	Y (64, 10.7%)	ETC (365, 60.7%) DTC (601, 100%)	Carbapenem (195, 53.5%) BL/BLI (169, 46.5%) Carbapenem (509, 84.7%) BL/BLI (92, 15.3%)	N	Y	II
Harris et al. [102]	SC retrospective cohort study, 2012–2013, China	92/92	UTI (43, 46.7%) Primary bacteramia (39, 42.2%) IIA (10, 11.1%)	E. coli (79, 85.9%) K. pneumoniae (13, 14.1%)	Y (11, 12.1%)	DTC (47, 51%)	Carbapenem (23, 48.9%) BL/BLI (24, 51.1%)	N	Y	II
Kang et al. [17]	SC retrospective cohort study, 1998–2002, South Korea	133/133	IIA (82, 61.6%) Primary bacterae-mia (33, 24.8%) UTI (14, 10.5%) Pneumonia (4, 3.1%)	E. coli (67, 50.4%) K. pneumoniae (66, 49.6%)	N	ETC (133, 100%) DTC (133, 100%)	Non cephalosporins (29, 21.8%) Cephalosporins (104, 78.2%) Non cephalosporins (101, 75.9%) Cephalosporins (32, 24.1%)	Y	UK	UK
Kang et al. [69]	MC retrospec-tive cohorts, 2008–2010, South Korea	114/114	UK	E. coli (78, 68.4%) K. pneumonia (36, 31.6%)	UK	ETC (114 100%)	Carbapenem (78, 68.4%) Piperacillin/tazobactam (36, 31.6%)	N	UK	UK
Lee et al. [53]	SC retrospective cohort, 2004–2005, Taiwan	27/27	Pneumonia (15, 55.5%) IIA (5, 18.5%) UTI (3, 11.1%) Primary bacterae-mia (3, 11.1%) Other (1, 3.8%)	K. pneumonia (27, 100%)	Y (13, 48.1%)	DTC (27, 100%)	Carbapenem (20, 74%) Flomoxef (7, 26%)	Y	UK	UK
Lee and al. [21]	SC retrospective cohort, 2001–2008, Taiwan	121/206	CVC (48, 39.6%) Primary bacterae-mia (32, 26.4%) Pneumonia (12, 9.9%) SSTI (9, 7.4%) UTI (9, 7.4%) IIA (6, 4.9%) Other (5, 4.3%)	E. cloacae (121, 100%)	Y (78, 64.4%)	ETC (114, 94.2%) DTC (114, 94.2%)	Cephalosporins (59, 49.1%) Carbapenem (26, 21%) BL/BLI (14, 11.4%) Other beta-lactam (13, 10.5%) Fluoroquinolones (3, 2.6%) Other Antibiotics (6, 5.4%) Carbapenem (53, 46.5%) Cephalosporins (38, 33.3%) Fluoroquinolones (16, 14%) BL/BLI (3, 2.6%) Other β-lactam (3, 2.6%) Other antibiotic therapy (1, 1%)	N	UK	UK

Table 1 continued

Author/year of publication	Study design, region	No. of patients, ESBL/total	Type of infection (n, %)	Bacteria (n, %)	ICU (n, %)	ETC/DTC	Treatment (n, %)	MIC	Administration (CI, PI or II)	Posology
Lee et al. [54]	MC retrospective cohort, 2002–2007, Taiwan	178/178	Pneumonia (43, 24.1%) UTI (39, 21.9%) CVC (37, 20.8%) IIA (28, 15.7%) Primary bacterae-mia (25, 14%) SSTI (11, 6.3%)	ND	UK	DTC (178, 100%)	Carbapenem (161, 90,4%) Cefepime (17, 9.6%)	Y	Y	II
Lee et al. [103]	MC retrospective cohort, 2007–2012, Taiwan	389/389	UTI (88, 22.6%) CVC (86, 22.1%) Pneumonia (80, 20.5%) IIA (61, 15.7%) Primary bacterae-mia (62, 16%) SSTI (12, 3.1%)	E. coli (156, 40.1%) K. pneumoniae (233, 59.9%)	UK	DTC (389, 100%)	Carbapenem (257, 66%) Flomoxef (132, 34%)	Y	UK	UK
Matsumura et al. [104]	MC retrospective cohort, 2005–2014, Japan	113/1440	UTI (57, 50.4%) IIA (32, 28.3%) Primary bacterae-mia (19, 16.8%) Other (5, 4.5%)	E. coli (113, 100%)	UK	ETC (71, 62.8%) DTC (113, 100%)	Carbapenem (45, 63.7%) Cefmetazole/flomoxef (26, 36.6%) Carbapenem (54, 47.8%) Cefmetazole/flomoxef (59, 52.2%)	Y	UK	UK
Ofer-Friedman et al. [20]	MC retrospective cohort, 2008–2012, International	79/79	Pneumonia (27, 34.2%) SSTI (22, 27.8%) IIA (20, 25.3%) Primary bacterae-mia (6, 7.6%) Undetermined (4, 5.1%)	E. coli (42, 53.1%) K. pneumoniae (22, 27.8%) P. mirabilis (15, 19.1%)	> 50%	ETC (33, 41.8%) DTC (79, 100%)	Carbapenem (24, 72.7%) Piperacillin/tazobactam (9, 27.3%) Carbapenem (69, 87.3%) Piperacillin/tazobactam (10, 12.7%)	Y	UK	UK
Qureshi et al. [105]	MC retrospective cohort, 2005–2008, USA	21/UK	UK	E. cloacae (21, 100%)	UK	ETC (21, 100%)	Cephalosporins (9, 42.8%) Carbapenem (8, 38%) BL/BLI (4, 19.2%)	Y	UK	UK
Paterson et al. [55]	Post hoc analysis MC prospective cohort, 1996–1997, International	85/455	UK	K. pneumoniae (85, 100%)	UK	ETC (71, 83.5%)	Monotherapy Carbapenem (27, 38%) Fluoroquinolones (11, 15.5%) Cephalosporins (5, 7%) BL/BLI (4, 5.6%) Aminoglycosides (2, 2.8%) Combination therapy (15, 21.1%) Sequential monotherapy (7, 10%)	N	UK	UK

Table 1 continued

Author/year of publication	Study design, region	No. of patients, ESBL/total	Type of infection (n, %)	Bacteria (n, %)	ICU (n, %)	ETC/DTC	Treatment (n, %)	MIC	Administration (CI, PI or II)	Posology
Pilmis et al. [106]	MC retrospective cohort, 2011, France	13/13	Primary bacterae-mia (11, 84.6%), UTI (2, 15.4%)	E. coli (5, 38.4%), K. pneumoniae (7, 53.8%), E. cloacae (1, 7.8%)	UK	ETC (13, 100%), DTC (13, 100%)	Carbapenem (12, 92.3%), Cefoxitin (1, 7.7%), Carbapenem (11, 84.6%), Cefoxitin (2, 15.4%)	N	UK	UK
Retamar et al. [107]	Post hoc analysis MC prospective cohort, 2001–2007, Spain	39/39	UTI (11, 28.2%), Other source (28, 71.8%)	E. coli (39, 100%)	UK	ETC (39, 100%)	BL/BLI (39, 100%)	Y	UK	UK
Rodriguez-Bano et al. [12]	Post hoc analysis MC prospective cohorts, 2001–2007, Spain	192/192	UTI or IIA (121, 63%), Other sources (71, 37%)	E. coli (192, 100%)	Y (24, 12.6%)	ETC (103, 53.6%), DTC (174, 90.6%)	Carbapenem (31, 30%), BL/BLI (72, 70%), Carbapenem (120, 68.9%), BL/BLI (53, 31.1%)	N	UK	UK
Tamma et al. [19]	MC, Prospective cohort, 2008–2015, USA	213/331	CVC (97, 45.5%), IIA (55, 25.8%), UTI (44, 20.6%), Pneumonia (17, 8.1%)	K. pneumoniae (145, 68%), E. coli (66, 31%), P. mirabilis (2, 1%)	Y (71, 33.3%)	ETC (213, 100%)	Carbapenem (110, 51.6%), BL/BLI (103, 48.4%)	Y	UK	UK
Tsai et al. [108]	MC retrospective cohort, 2005–2012, Taiwan	47/47	UTI (24, 51%), Pneumonia (9, 19.1%), SSTI (7, 14.9%), CVC (5, 10.6%), IIA (3, 6.4%), Primary bacterae-mia (2, 4.3%)	P. mirabilis (47, 100%)	UK	DTC (40, 85.1%)	Carbapenem (21, 52.5%), BL/BLI (13, 32.5%), Other antibiotic therapy (6, 15%)	Y	UK	
Tumbarello et al. [109]	SC retrospective cohort, 1999–2004, Italy	186/186	Primary bacterae-mia (86, 46.2%), UTI (53, 28.4%), IIA (24, 12.9%), SSTI (20, 10.7%), Pneumonia (6, 3.2%), CVC (5, 2.7%)	E. coli (104, 55.9%), K. pneumoniae (58, 31.2%), P. mirabilis (24, 12.9%)	UK	ETC (186 100%), DTC (171, 91.9%)	BL/BLI (45, 24.2%), Fluoroquinolones (45, 24.2%), Cephalosporins (38, 20.9%), Carbapenems (29, 15.4%), Aminoglycosides (29, 15.4%), Carbapenems (61, 35.7%), BL/BLI (55, 32.2%), Aminoglycosides (30, 17.5%), Fluoroquinolones (25, 14.6%)	Y	UK	UK
Tuon et al. [110]	SC retrospective cohort, 2006–2009, Brazil	28/58	UK	E. cloacae (28, 100%)	UK	DTC (25, 89.2%)	Carbapenems (15, 60%), BL/BLI (4, 16%), Non-BL/BLI (6, 24%)	N	UK	UK

Table 1 continued

Author/year of publication	Study design, region	No. of patients, ESBL/total	Type of infection (n, %)	Bacteria (n, %)	ICU (n, %)	ETC/DTC	Treatment (n, %)	MIC	Administration (CI, PI or II)	Posology
Tuon et al. [90]	SC retrospective cohort, 2006–2009, Brazil	63/104	UK	K. pneumoniae (63, 100%)	UK	DTC (62, 98.4%)	Carbapenems (43, 69.3%) Non-BL/BLI (17, 27.4%) BL/BLI (2, 3.1%)	N	UK	UK
Wang et al. [95]	MC, prospective cohort, 2006–2015, USA	68/68	CVC (30, 44.1%) UTI (21, 30.9%) IIA (15, 22.1%) Pneumonia (10, 14.7%) SSTI (2, 2.9%)	Klebsiella sp. (42, 62%) E. coli (24, 34%) P. mirabilis (2, 3%)	Y (20, 29%)	ETC (68, 100%)	Carbapenem (51, 75%) Cephalosporins (17, 25%)	N	UK	UK

BL/BLI beta-lactam/beta-lactamase inhibitor, CVC central venous catheter, DTC definitive therapy cohort, ETC empirical therapy cohort, ICU intensive care unit, IIA intra-abdominal infection, MC multicentric, SC single center, SSTI skin and soft tissue infection, UK unknown, UTI urinary tract infection

ill patients with ESBL-PE infection from non-urinary sources.

Finally 7/11 (63%) studies compared BL/BLIs to carbapenems as definitive therapy, of which 4 (36.3%) compared BL/BLIs as the only alternative to carbapenems [12, 19, 20, 22, 51]. It should be noted that only one of these studies took into account MICs [20], whereas none took into account dosages and modalities of administration for assessing the effectiveness of therapy [19].

Ecological studies

While initial research suggested the relative safety of imipenem–cilastatin on the intestinal microbiota [56], the recent analysis of rectal colonization of large number of ICU patients found that even a brief exposure to imipenem is a risk factor for carriage of resistant GNB in the intestinal flora [6].

The effect of non-carbapenem antibiotics on the emergence of multidrug-resistant bacteria and specifically carbapenem resistance is a major issue. In animal models, imipenem–cilastatin had no effect on the indigenous microflora [56]. In a mouse model, clindamycin and piperacillin–tazobactam promoted colonization, while ertapenem did not promote the establishment of intestinal colonization with KPC-Kp [57]. Also several authors highlighted the risk associated with the emergence/selection of resistant strains when using Pip–Taz. Firstly, in vitro/in vivo studies [27] suggested that Pip–Taz seems to be less resistant to the inoculum effect comparing to carbapenems. Secondly, several clinical studies [58] underlined the risk of promoting vancomycin-resistant enterococci (VRE) colonization. Finally the emergence of carbapenem-resistant PE has been documented for a variety of antibiotics in the clinical setting [59] (Table 2): Fluoroquinolones [60, 61], extended-spectrum cephalosporin [62], antipseudomonal penicillins [63] and β-lactams/β-lactamase inhibitors [64] have all been identified as risk factors for carbapenem resistance in *Klebsiella pneumoniae*.

Whether carbapenem is the only antibiotic class associated with the selection of carbapenem-resistant gram-negative isolates is an important issue, especially regarding the worldwide spread of carbapenemase-producing Enterobacteriaceae (CPE). These data suggest that antibiotics that disturb the intestinal anaerobic microflora and lack significant activity against KPC-Kp may promote colonization by this organism [65] (Table 3).

Discussion and conclusion

In our review of BL/BLI for the treatment of ESBL-PE, we found that they may be an alternative to carbapenems in a selected number of cases, based on antibiogram and CMI data, and always with pk/pd optimization.

The use of alternatives for empirical therapy in suspected ESBL-related infections is usually limited by the level of resistance [66], the risk of selecting resistant mutants [6] and clinical effectiveness [19]. We focused on BL/BLIs, chiefly piperacillin–tazobactam. Indeed, based on epidemiological data, the use of third- or fourth-generation cephalosporins such as cefepime is limited because of a high proportion of resistant isolates [66] that varies between 10 and 50% and concerns on their clinical efficacy with the associated risks of adverse patient outcomes [54]. The use of other alternatives such as temocillin is limited by unfavorable PK/PD parameters in critically ill patients [49].

The efficacy of Pip/Taz antibiotics on ESBL-PE depends on the variety and amount of enzyme produced by the isolates (Table 4). Overall, the rate of susceptibility of ESBL-PE to Pip/Taz is around 80% [28]. It may be reduced when the organisms produce multiple ESBLs, particularly if they also harbor an AmpC beta-lactamase [67]. Also it will vary within and between beta-lactamases classes [68]. The presence of additional resistance mechanisms may further decrease the activity of Pip/Taz against ESBL-producing organisms.

In the absence of a well-designed prospective randomized study comparing carbapenems to non-carbapenems in ICU patients infected with ESBL-PE, we must rely on the evidence provided by observational data. Observational studies considering the empirical treatment of ESBL-related infections with BL/BLIs have infrequently included ICU patients [12] and more often involved urinary or biliary tract infection caused by *E. coli* species [51]. Although several studies suggested no difference in mortality [12, 51, 69], 2 publications raise the warning of a potential negative impact of BL/BLI when used in patients with ESBL-PE [19, 20].

Furthermore, when analyzing those publications with a focus on the use of alternatives to carbapenems for definitive therapy, a number of limitations hamper the interpretation of studies comparing BL/BLI to carbapenems.

Firstly most of these studies were not designed to compare different antibiotic strategies. Secondly, the authors did not take into account the severity of underlying diseases, delays to antimicrobial treatment and effectiveness source control, which are all major predictors of outcome [70]. Thirdly, patients included differed largely across studies, with regard to sources of bacteremia, species involved and type of beta-lactamases; moreover, various antibiotics and different daily doses administered were included in the "alternative" group.

Fourthly, most of the studies included infections related to ESBL-producing *Escherichia coli* and did not account for the impact of MICs and pharmacodynamics data. The impact of MIC seems to be crucial for therapeutic

Table 2 Studies addressing the risk related to previous antibiotic therapy and emergence of carbapenem-resistant Enterobacteriaceae

	Year	Study design	Type of infection	Antibiotic concerned	OR, 95 % CI
Wang [62]	2016	Retrospective case–case–control	Nosocomial infection	Third–fourth-generation cephalosporins Carbapenems	4.557 (1.971–10.539) 4.058 (1.753–9.397)
Mittal G [80]	2016	Prospective	Colonization	Aminoglycosides	4.14 (1.14–14.99)
Ling [81]	2015	Retrospective case–control	Infection or colonization	Penicillins Glycopeptides	4.640 (1.529–14.079) 5.162 (1.377–19.346)
Jiao Y [82]	2015	Retrospective case–control	Infection or colonization	Glycopeptides Cefoperazone plus sulbactam	43.84 (1.73–1111.9) 49.56, (1.42–1726.72)
Candevir [83]	2015	Retrospective cohort	Infection	Meropenem Third-generation cephalosporins	3.244 (1.193–8.819) 3.590 (1.056–12.209)
Gómez Rueda [84]	2014	Retrospective case–case–control	Infection	Carbapenems	3.3 (1.2–9.3)
Ahn [85]	2014	Retrospective case–control	Colonization/infection	Fluoroquinolones Carbapenems	2.82 (1.14–6.99) 4.56 (1.44–14.46)
Mantzarlis [86]	2013	Prospective cohort	Pneumonia	Colistin*	1.156 per day (1.010–1.312)
Dizbay [87]	2013	Prospective cohort	Nosocomial infection	Imipenem	3.35 (1.675–6.726)
Orsi [88]	2013	Retrospective case control	BSI	Carbapenem	7.74 (1.70–35.2)
Chang [89]	2011	Retrospective case–control	BSI	Carbapenem	29.17 (1.76–484.70)
Falagas [63]	2007	Retrospective case control	KPC infection	Fluoroquinolones Antipseudomonal antibiotics	4.54 (1.18–11.54) 2.6 (1.00–6.71)
Schwaber [61]	2008	Retrospective case–case–control	CRKp colonization	Antibiotics Fluoroquinolones	4.4 (1–19.2) 7.2 (1.1–49.4)
Gasink [60]	2009	Retrospective case–control	KPC infection/colonization	Fluoroquinolones Third-generation cephalosporin	3.39 (1.5–7.66) 2.55 (1.18–5.22)
Papadimitriou [64]	2012	Prospective cohort	CRKp colonization	BL/BLI Carbapenems	6.7 (1–26.2) 5.2 (1–32.9)
Tuon [90]	2012	Retrospective case–control	KPC bacteremia	Fluoroquinolones	28.9 (1.85–454.6)
Papadimitriou [91]	2014	Prospective cohort	KPC bacteremia	Aminoglycosides	2.3 (1.1–4.7)
Gagliotti [79]	2014	Case–control	KPC colonization	Carbapenems Any antibiotic (other than carbapenems)	3.67 (1.37–9.83) 2.83 (1.10–7.31)
Maseda [92]	2016	Retrospective	CPE isolate colonization	Third–fourth-generation cephalosporins BL/BLI	27.96 (6.88–113.58) 11.71 (4.51–30.43)

KPC Klebsiella pneumoniae-producing carbapenemase, *CRKp* carbapenem-resistant *Klebsiella pneumoniae*, *BL/BLI* beta-lactams associated with beta-lactamase inhibitors, *BSI* bloodstream infection

efficacy when using alternatives to carbapenems as the cornerstone of treatment. Several studies [12] emphasize the risk of treatment failure when using a BL/BLI or third-generation cephalosporin for therapy of infection with isolates having MICs higher than the breakpoints. Indeed, as suggested by a recent pharmacological study, the efficacy of BL/BLI in the treatment of ESBL-related infections is related to the concentration reached in the plasma and at the site of infection [71]. However, as demonstrated by several authors [72] the probability of attaining therapeutic drug levels in ICU patients is low and variable depending on the antibiotic considered and dosing strategies [35]. Also it seems important to have MIC for piperacillin–tazobactam before using this class

of antibiotic. Considering several problems related to piperacillin–tazobactam gradient tests and differences noted between gradient tests and broth microdilution, it is recommended now to use broth microdilution.

There are now enough published data on the pk/pd of piperacillin/tazobactam to recommend the use of high daily doses and prolonged infusion ICU patients and in all cases of difficult to treat pathogens such as ESBL-PE.

The ecological consequences of a given antibiotic class depend on the amount of drug reaching the different microbiota. The net result depends on both the antibiotic concentrations achieved and the susceptibility of bacterial species in the microbiota. All antibiotics alter the composition, diversity and density of the microbiota

Table 3 (Adapted from [14, 15]) usual breakpoints and susceptibility of ESBL-producing Enterobacteriaceae

	Susceptibility (%)	Breakpoints (mg/L)	Ecological impact	Comments
Third-generation cephalosporins	*Escherichia coli*: < 10% *Klebsiella* species: 3%	EUCAST: S ≤ 1 CLSI: S ≤ 1	+++	Only for targeted therapy or de-escalation MIC required
Cefepime	*E. coli*: 5–30% *K. pneumoniae*: 5–60%	EUCAST: S < 1 CLSI: S ≤ 2	+++	Frequent failure if MICs > 1 mg/L MIC required
Cefoxitin	*E. coli*: 80%	EUCAST: NA	++	PK optimization
Ceftolozane–tazobactam	*E. coli*: 85–95% *K. pneumoniae*: 40–65%	EUCAST: S ≤ 1 CLSI: S ≤ 8	?	
Ceftazidime–avibactam	*E. coli*: 98–100% *K. pneumoniae*: 90–100%	EUCAST: S ≤ 8 CLSI: S ≤ 8	?	Probably as effective as carbapenems
Temocillin	*E. coli* 61% (CMI ≤ 8) *E. coli* 99% (CMI ≤ 32)	EUCAST: S ≤ 8 EUCAST: S ≤ 32 (urinary) CLSI: S ≤ 8 CLSI: S ≤ 32 (urinary)	±	PK optimization (high dosage and prolonged infusion)

CLSI Clinical and Laboratory Standard Institute, *EUCAST* European Committee on Antimicrobial Susceptibility Testing, *MIC* minimum inhibitory concentration, *NA* not applicable, *PK* pharmacokinetic, *VAP* ventilator-associated pneumonia

Table 4 (Adapted from Bonomo and Van Duin) Activity in clinical practice of different beta-lactamase inhibitors, according to type of enzymes [68, 111]

Enzymes	Class	Substrates	Clavulanic acid	Sulbactam	Tazobactam	Avibactam
TEM-1, TEM-2, SHV-1	A	Penicillins, early cephalosporins	+	–	+	+
TEM-3, SHV-2 CTX-M-14	A	Extended-spectrum cephalosporins, monobactams	–	–	+	+
KPC-2, KPC-3	A	Broad spectrum including carbapenems	–	–	–	+
IMP-1, NDM-1, VIM-1	B	Broad spectrum including carbapenems, but not monobactams	–	–	–	–
Escherichia coli AmpC	C	Cephalosporins	–	–	±	+
OXA-48	D	Carbapenem	–	–	–	+

and select for antibiotic resistance [73]. The "ecological consequences," however, may differ according to the antibiotic used. Increasing consumption of carbapenems raises concerns on the spread of carbapenem-resistant Enterobacteriaceae and specifically carbapenemase-producing Enterobacteriaceae (CPE) [74]. Also, there are some discrepancies between the first published studies [75, 76] and the more recent ones [6] regarding the ecological effect of carbapenems. There is a significant correlation between carbapenem consumption and rates of *Pseudomonas aeruginosa* resistance to imipenem and meropenem [6, 53]. However, this mechanism of resistance is not due to the effect of antibiotics on the microbiota, but the consequence of chromosomal mutation. Earlier human studies [77] and animal models [78] suggested a limited impact on the microbiota of this class of antibiotics. However, whatever the antibiotic used, selective antibiotic pressure is an important determinant of emergence and dissemination of antibiotic resistance [61, 62], and the increasing use of carbapenems will necessarily be associated with the increase in multidrug-resistant organisms [65]. Our review underlines the fact that the

administration of several other antibiotics can also be associated with the emergence of carbapenem-resistant organisms [60–64, 79–92]. Nevertheless, the heterogeneity of studies makes their comparison difficult. Indeed, all these studies are subject to several limitations, including inadequate adjustment for important confounding variables, control group selection, extent of prior antibiotic exposure and measurements of resistance outcomes.

One of the limitations of our study lies in the fact that we did not mentioned the two recent BL/BLIs approved by FDA and EMA, ceftolozane–tazobactam and ceftazidime–avibactam which are active in vitro against ESBL-producing Enterobacteriaceae. Several recent studies highlighted the in vitro efficacy of these two antibiotics on ESBL-producing Enterobacteriaceae [67, 93]. Also clinical data are scarce. Indeed for nosocomial pneumonia, a phase III study (MK-7625A-008) is currently leaded using ceftolozane–tazobactam.

A definitive answer to the question addressed in this review would need a randomized study conducted in ICU, including severe infections related to ESBL-PE. Cases should be selected according to the results of antibiotic susceptibility tests, and the trial should compare carbapenems to BL/BLI as definitive therapy. Pending such a trial, piperacillin–tazobactam should be used with caution for treatment of ESBL-PE-related infections. In ICU patients, empirical use should be avoided, and definitive therapy should be reserved to patients in clinical stable condition, after microbial documentation and results of susceptibility tests, together with adapting the administered dose and modalities of infusion to the MIC of the infecting microorganism in order to reach pharmacological targets.

Abbreviations
ADE: antimicrobial de-escalation; BL/BLI: beta-lactam/beta-lactamase inhibitor; CLSI: Clinical and Laboratory Standards Institute; CRB: carbapenem-resistant bacteria; CRE: carbapenem-resistant Enterobacteriaceae; EMA: European Medicine Agency; ESAC: European Surveillance of Antimicrobial Consumption; EUCAST: European Committee on Antimicrobial Susceptibility Testing; FDA: Food and Drug Administration; ICU: intensive care unit; KPC: *Klebsiella*-producing carbapenemase; MIC: minimal inhibitory concentration; OR: odds ratio; PD: pharmacodynamic; PK: pharmacokinetic; TDM: therapeutic drug monitoring; TID: three times in a day.

Authors' contributions
BP contributed to conception and design of the study, responsible for the "clinical studies" portion and gave final approval of the version to be published. VJ contributed to conception and design of the study, responsible for the "pharmacokinetics and pharmacodynamic studies" portion and gave final approval of the version to be published. AT revised the manuscript critically for important intellectual content and gave final approval of the version to be published. JRZ contributed to conception and design of the study, responsible for the "ecological studies" portion and gave final approval of the version to be published. CBB involved in design of the study, revised it critically for important intellectual content and gave final approval of the version to be published.

Author details
[1] Service de maladies infectieuses et tropicales, Hôpital Necker Enfants malades, Service de maladies infectieuses et tropicales, Université Paris Descartes, Paris, France. [2] Equipe mobile de microbiologie clinique, Groupe Hospitalier Paris Saint-Joseph, Paris, France. [3] Service de Pharmacologie, Hôpital Européen Georges Pompidou, Université Paris Descartes, Paris, France. [4] INSERM U1129, Paris, France. [5] Intensive Care Unit, The Redcliffe Hospital, Brisbane, Australia. [6] Burns, Trauma and Critical Care Research Centre, The University of Queensland, Brisbane, Australia. [7] Département de Microbiologie Clinique, Unité de Contrôle et de Prévention du risque Infectieux, Groupe Hospitalier Paris Seine Saint-Denis, AP-HP, CHU Avicenne, 125 rue de Stalingrad, 9300 Bobigny, France. [8] Infection Control Unit, IAME, UMR 1137, Université Paris 13, Sorbonne Paris Cité, Paris, France. [9] Réanimation médicale, Hôpital Henri Mondor, Université Paris Est Créteil (UPEC), Créteil, France.

Acknowledgements
Not applicable.

Competing interests
BP, AT and CBB declare that they have no competing interests. VJ has received research grants from Astellas, Sanofi-Aventis, Biocodex and travel Grants from MSD. JRZ has participated in an advisory board for MSD.

References
1. Arpin C, Quentin C, Grobost F, Cambau E, Robert J, Dubois V, et al. Nationwide survey of extended-spectrum {beta}-lactamase-producing enterobacteriaceae in the French community setting. J Antimicrob Chemother. 2009;63:1205–14.
2. Meier S, Weber R, Zbinden R, Ruef C, Hasse B. Extended-spectrum β-lactamase-producing Gram-negative pathogens in community-acquired urinary tract infections: an increasing challenge for antimicrobial therapy. Infection. 2011;39:333–40.
3. Prinapori R, Guinaud J, Khalil A, Lecuyer H, Gendrel D, Lortholary O, et al. Risk associated with a systematic search of extended-spectrum β-lactamase-producing Enterobacteriaceae. Am J Infect Control. 2013;41:259–60.
4. Barbier F, Pommier C, Essaied W, Garrouste-Orgeas M, Schwebel C, Ruckly S, et al. Colonization and infection with extended-spectrum β-lactamase-producing enterobacteriaceae in ICU patients: what impact on outcomes and carbapenem exposure? J Antimicrob Chemother. 2016;71:1088–97.
5. http://ecdc.europa.eu/en/eaad/antibiotics-news/Documents/antimicrobial-consumption-ESAC-Net-summary-2015.pdf.
6. Armand-Lefèvre L, Angebault C, Barbier F, Hamelet E, Defrance G, Ruppé E, et al. Emergence of imipenem-resistant gram-negative bacilli in intestinal flora of intensive care patients. Antimicrob Agents Chemother. 2013;57:1488–95.
7. Tabah A, Cotta MO, Garnacho-Montero J, Schouten J, Roberts JA, Lipman J, et al. A systematic review of the definitions, determinants, and clinical outcomes of antimicrobial de-escalation in the intensive care unit. Clin Infect Dis Off Publ Infect Dis Soc Am. 2016;62:1009–17.
8. Kalil AC, Metersky ML, Klompas M, Muscedere J, Sweeney DA, Palmer LB, et al. Management of adults with Hospital-acquired and ventilator-associated pneumonia: 2016 clinical practice guidelines by the infectious diseases society of America and the American thoracic society. Clin Infect Dis. 2016;63:e61–111.
9. Rhodes A, Evans LE, Alhazzani W, Levy MM, Antonelli M, Ferrer R, et al. Surviving sepsis campaign: international guidelines for management of sepsis and septic shock: 2016. Intensive Care Med. 2017;43:304–77.
10. Paterson DL. Recommendation for treatment of severe infections caused by Enterobacteriaceae producing extended-spectrum beta-lactamases (ESBLs). Clin Microbiol Infect Off Publ Eur Soc Clin Microbiol Infect Dis. 2000;6:460–3.
11. Piroth L, Aubé H, Doise JM, Vincent-Martin M. Spread of extended-spectrum beta-lactamase-producing *Klebsiella pneumoniae*: are beta-lactamase inhibitors of therapeutic value? Clin. Infect. Dis. Off. Publ. Infect. Dis. Soc. Am. 1998;27:76–80.
12. Rodríguez-Baño J, Navarro MD, Retamar P, Picón E, Pascual Á. Extended-Spectrum Beta-Lactamases—Red Española de Investigación en Patología Infecciosa/Grupo de Estudio de Infección Hospitalaria Group. β-Lactam/β-lactam inhibitor combinations for the treatment of bacteremia due to extended-spectrum β-lactamase-producing *Escherichia coli*: a post hoc analysis of prospective cohorts. Clin Infect Dis Off Publ Infect Dis Soc Am. 2012;54:167–74.
13. Ng TM, Khong WX, Harris PNA, De PP, Chow A, Tambyah PA, et al. Empiric piperacillin–tazobactam versus carbapenems in the treatment of bacteraemia due to extended-spectrum beta-lactamase-producing enterobacteriaceae. PLOS ONE. 2016;11:e0153696.
14. EUCAST: Clinical breakpoints [cited 2015 Aug 18]. http://www.eucast.org/clinical_breakpoints/.
15. CLSI Publishes New Antimicrobial Susceptibility Testing Standards—CLSI [cited 2016 Aug 5]. http://clsi.org/blog/2015/01/08/clsi-publishes-new-antimicrobial-susceptibility-testing-standards/.
16. Du B, Long Y, Liu H, Chen D, Liu D, Xu Y, et al. Extended-spectrum beta-lactamase-producing *Escherichia coli* and *Klebsiella pneumoniae* bloodstream infection: risk factors and clinical outcome. Intensive Care Med. 2002;28:1718–23.
17. Kang C-I, Kim S-H, Park WB, Lee K-D, Kim H-B, Kim E-C, et al. Bloodstream infections due to extended-spectrum beta-lactamase-producing *Escherichia coli* and *Klebsiella pneumoniae*: risk factors for mortality and

treatment outcome, with special emphasis on antimicrobial therapy. Antimicrob Agents Chemother. 2004;48:4574–81.

18. Wang R, Cosgrove SE, Tschudin-Sutter S, Han JH, Turnbull AE, Hsu AJ, et al. Cefepime therapy for cefepime-susceptible extended-spectrum β-lactamase-producing enterobacteriaceae bacteremia. Open Forum Infect Dis. 2016;3:ofw132.

19. Tamma PD, Han JH, Rock C, Harris AD, Lautenbach E, Hsu AJ, et al. Carbapenem therapy is associated with improved survival compared with piperacillin–tazobactam for patients with extended-spectrum β-lactamase bacteremia. Clin Infect Dis Off Publ Infect Dis Soc Am. 2015;60:1319–25.

20. Ofer-Friedman H, Shefler C, Sharma S, Tirosh A, Tal-Jasper R, Kandipalli D, et al. Carbapenems versus piperacillin–tazobactam for blood-stream infections of nonurinary source caused by extended-spectrum beta-lactamase-producing enterobacteriaceae. Infect Control Hosp Epidemiol. 2015;36:981–5.

21. Lee C-C, Lee N-Y, Yan J-J, Lee H-C, Chen P-L, Chang C-M, et al. Bacteremia due to extended-spectrum-beta-lactamase-producing *Enterobacter cloacae*: role of carbapenem therapy. Antimicrob Agents Chemother. 2010;54:3551–6.

22. Harris PN, Tambyah PA, Paterson DL. β-lactam and β-lactamase inhibitor combinations in the treatment of extended-spectrum β-lactamase producing *Enterobacteriaceae*: time for a reappraisal in the era of few antibiotic options? Lancet Infect Dis. 2015;15:475–85.

23. Roberts JA, Roberts MS, Robertson TA, Dalley AJ, Lipman J. Piperacillin penetration into tissue of critically ill patients with sepsis—bolus versus continuous administration? Crit Care Med. 2009;37:926–33.

24. Dulhunty JM, Roberts JA, Davis JS, Webb SAR, Bellomo R, Gomersall C, et al. Continuous infusion of beta-lactam antibiotics in severe sepsis: a multicenter double-blind, randomized controlled trial. Clin Infect Dis Off Publ Infect Dis Soc Am. 2013;56:236–44.

25. Roberts JA, Kirkpatrick CMJ, Roberts MS, Robertson TA, Dalley AJ, Lipman J. Meropenem dosing in critically ill patients with sepsis and without renal dysfunction: intermittent bolus versus continuous administration? Monte Carlo dosing simulations and subcutaneous tissue distribution. J Antimicrob Chemother. 2009;64:142–50.

26. Carlier M, Noë M, De Waele JJ, Stove V, Verstraete AG, Lipman J, et al. Population pharmacokinetics and dosing simulations of amoxicillin/clavulanic acid in critically ill patients. J Antimicrob Chemother. 2013;68:2600–8.

27. Wu N, Chen BY, Tian SF, Chu YZ. The inoculum effect of antibiotics against CTX-M-extended-spectrum β-lactamase-producing *Escherichia coli*. Ann Clin Microbiol Antimicrob. 2014;13:45.

28. Lob SH, Nicolle LE, Hoban DJ, Kazmierczak KM, Badal RE, Sahm DF. Susceptibility patterns and ESBL rates of *Escherichia coli* from urinary tract infections in Canada and the United States, SMART 2010–2014. Diagn Microbiol Infect Dis. 2016;85:459–65.

29. Jean S-S, Coombs G, Ling T, Balaji V, Rodrigues C, Mikamo H, et al. Epidemiology and antimicrobial susceptibility profiles of pathogens causing urinary tract infections in the Asia-Pacific region: results from the Study for Monitoring Antimicrobial Resistance Trends (SMART), 2010–2013. Int J Antimicrob Agents. 2016;47:328–34.

30. Sader HS, Farrell DJ, Flamm RK, Jones RN. Antimicrobial susceptibility of gram-negative organisms isolated from patients hospitalised with pneumonia in US and European hospitals: results from the SENTRY Antimicrobial Surveillance Program, 2009–2012. Int J Antimicrob Agents. 2014;43:328–34.

31. Lodise TP, Lomaestro B, Drusano GL. Piperacillin–tazobactam for *Pseudomonas aeruginosa* infection: clinical implications of an extended-infusion dosing strategy. Clin Infect Dis Off Publ Infect Dis Soc Am. 2007;44:357–63.

32. Roberts JA, Ulldemolins M, Roberts MS, McWhinney B, Ungerer J, Paterson DL, et al. Therapeutic drug monitoring of β-lactams in critically ill patients: proof of concept. Int J Antimicrob Agents. 2010;36:332–9.

33. Sturm AW, Allen N, Rafferty KD, Fish DN, Toschlog E, Newell M, et al. Pharmacokinetic analysis of piperacillin administered with tazobactam in critically ill, morbidly obese surgical patients. Pharmacotherapy. 2014;34:28–35.

34. De Waele JJ, De Neve N. Aminoglycosides for life-threatening infections: a plea for an individualized approach using intensive therapeutic drug monitoring. Minerva Anestesiol. 2014;80:1135–42.

35. De Waele JJ, Carrette S, Carlier M, Stove V, Boelens J, Claeys G, et al. Therapeutic drug monitoring-based dose optimisation of piperacillin and meropenem: a randomised controlled trial. Intensive Care Med. 2014;40:380–7.

36. Felton TW, McCalman K, Malagon I, Isalska B, Whalley S, Goodwin J, et al. Pulmonary penetration of piperacillin and tazobactam in critically ill patients. Clin Pharmacol Ther. 2014;96:438–48.

37. McKinnon PS, Paladino JA, Schentag JJ. Evaluation of area under the inhibitory curve (AUIC) and time above the minimum inhibitory concentration (T > MIC) as predictors of outcome for cefepime and ceftazidime in serious bacterial infections. Int J Antimicrob Agents. 2008;31:345–51.

38. Sádaba B, Azanza JR, Campanero MA, García-Quetglas E. Relationship between pharmacokinetics and pharmacodynamics of beta-lactams and outcome. Clin Microbiol Infect Off Publ Eur Soc Clin Microbiol Infect Dis. 2004;10:990–8.

39. Felton TW, Roberts JA, Lodise TP, Van Guilder M, Boselli E, Neely MN, et al. Individualization of piperacillin dosing for critically ill patients: dosing software to optimize antimicrobial therapy. Antimicrob Agents Chemother. 2014;58:4094–102.

40. Abdul-Aziz MH, Lipman J, Akova M, Bassetti M, De Waele JJ, Dimopoulos G, et al. Is prolonged infusion of piperacillin/tazobactam and meropenem in critically ill patients associated with improved pharmacokinetic/pharmacodynamic and patient outcomes? An observation from the Defining antibiotic levels in intensive care unit patients (DALI) cohort. J Antimicrob Chemother. 2016;71:196–207.

41. Ulldemolins M, Martín-Loeches I, Llauradó-Serra M, Fernández J, Vaquer S, Rodríguez A, et al. Piperacillin population pharmacokinetics in critically ill patients with multiple organ dysfunction syndrome receiving continuous venovenous haemodiafiltration: effect of type of dialysis membrane on dosing requirements. J Antimicrob Chemother. 2016;71:1651–9.

42. Shotwell MS, Nesbitt R, Madonia PN, Gould ER, Connor MJ, Salem C, et al. Pharmacokinetics and pharmacodynamics of extended infusion versus short infusion piperacillin–tazobactam in critically ill patients undergoing CRRT. CJASN. 2016;11:1377–83.

43. Connor MJ, Salem C, Bauer SR, Hofmann CL, Groszek J, Butler R, et al. Therapeutic drug monitoring of piperacillin–tazobactam using spent dialysate effluent in patients receiving continuous venovenous hemodialysis. Antimicrob Agents Chemother. 2011;55:557–60.

44. Thompson MI, Russo ME, Matsen JM, Atkin-Thor E. Piperacillin pharmacokinetics in subjects with chronic renal failure. Antimicrob Agents Chemother. 1981;19:450–3.

45. Giron JA, Meyers BR, Hirschman SZ, Srulevitch E. Pharmacokinetics of piperacillin in patients with moderate renal failure and in patients undergoing hemodialysis. Antimicrob Agents Chemother. 1981;19:279–83.

46. Francke EL, Appel GB, Neu HC. Pharmacokinetics of intravenous piperacillin in patients undergoing chronic hemodialysis. Antimicrob Agents Chemother. 1979;16:788–91.

47. Guet-Revillet H, Emirian A, Groh M, Nebbad-Lechani B, Weiss E, Join-Lambert O, et al. Pharmacological study of cefoxitin as an alternative antibiotic therapy to carbapenems in treatment of urinary tract infections due to extended-spectrum-β-lactamase-producing *Escherichia coli*. Antimicrob Agents Chemother. 2014;58:4899–901.

48. Vincent J-L, Bassetti M, François B, Karam G, Chastre J, Torres A, et al. Advances in antibiotic therapy in the critically ill. Crit Care Lond Engl. 2016;20:133.

49. Laterre P-F, Wittebole X, Van de Velde S, Muller AE, Mouton JW, Carryn S, et al. Temocillin (6 g daily) in critically ill patients: continuous infusion versus three times daily administration. J Antimicrob Chemother. 2015;70:891–8.

50. Chopra T, Marchaim D, Veltman J, Johnson P, Zhao JJ, Tansek R, et al. Impact of cefepime therapy on mortality among patients with bloodstream infections caused by extended-spectrum-β-lactamase-

producing *Klebsiella pneumoniae* and *Escherichia coli*. Antimicrob Agents Chemother. 2012;56:3936–42.

51. Gutiérrez-Gutiérrez B, Pérez-Galera S, Salamanca E, de Cueto M, Calbo E, Almirante B, et al. β-lactam/β-lactamase inhibitor combinations for the treatment of bloodstream infections due to extended-spectrum β-lactamase-producing enterobacteriaceae: a multinational, pre-registered cohort study. Antimicrob Agents Chemother. 2016;11:AAC-00365.

52. Apisarnthanarak A, Kiratisin P, Mundy LM. Predictors of mortality from community-onset bloodstream infections due to extended-spectrum beta-lactamase-producing *Escherichia coli* and *Klebsiella pneumoniae*. Infect Control Hosp Epidemiol. 2008;29:671–4.

53. Lee C-H, Su L-H, Tang Y-F, Liu J-W. Treatment of ESBL-producing *Klebsiella pneumoniae* bacteraemia with carbapenems or flomoxef: a retrospective study and laboratory analysis of the isolates. J Antimicrob Chemother. 2006;58:1074–7.

54. Lee N-Y, Lee C-C, Huang W-H, Tsui K-C, Hsueh P-R, Ko W-C. Cefepime therapy for monomicrobial bacteremia caused by cefepime-susceptible extended-spectrum beta-lactamase-producing enterobacteriaceae: MIC matters. Clin Infect Dis Off Publ Infect Dis Soc Am. 2013;56:488–95.

55. Paterson DL, Ko W-C, Von Gottberg A, Mohapatra S, Casellas JM, Goossens H, et al. Antibiotic therapy for *Klebsiella pneumoniae* bacteremia: implications of production of extended-spectrum beta-lactamases. Clin Infect Dis Off Publ Infect Dis Soc Am. 2004;39:31–7.

56. Nord CE, Heimdahl A, Kager L, Malmborg AS. The impact of different antimicrobial agents on the normal gastrointestinal microflora of humans. Rev Infect Dis. 1984;6(Suppl 1):S270–5.

57. Perez F, Pultz MJ, Endimiani A, Bonomo RA, Donskey CJ. Effect of antibiotic treatment on establishment and elimination of intestinal colonization by KPC-producing *Klebsiella pneumoniae* in mice. Antimicrob Agents Chemother. 2011;55:2585–9.

58. Efe Iris N, Sayıner H, Yildirmak T, Simsek F, Arat ME. Vancomycin-resistant Enterococcus carrier status in the reanimation units and related risk factors. Am J Infect Control. 2013;41:261–2.

59. Donskey CJ. Antibiotic regimens and intestinal colonization with antibiotic-resistant gram-negative bacilli. Clin Infect Dis Off Publ Infect Dis Soc Am. 2006;43(Suppl 2):S62–9.

60. Gasink LB, Edelstein PH, Lautenbach E, Synnestvedt M, Fishman NO. Risk factors and clinical impact of *Klebsiella pneumoniae* carbapenemase-producing K. pneumoniae. Infect Control Hosp Epidemiol. 2009;30:1180–5.

61. Schwaber MJ, Klarfeld-Lidji S, Navon-Venezia S, Schwartz D, Leavitt A, Carmeli Y. Predictors of carbapenem-resistant *Klebsiella pneumoniae* acquisition among hospitalized adults and effect of acquisition on mortality. Antimicrob Agents Chemother. 2008;52:1028–33.

62. Wang Q, Zhang Y, Yao X, Xian H, Liu Y, Li H, et al. Risk factors and clinical outcomes for carbapenem-resistant Enterobacteriaceae nosocomial infections. Eur J Clin Microbiol Infect Dis Off Publ Eur Soc Clin Microbiol. 2016;35:1679–89.

63. Falagas ME, Rafailidis PI, Kofteridis D, Virtzili S, Chelvatzoglou FC, Papaioannou V, et al. Risk factors of carbapenem-resistant *Klebsiella pneumoniae* infections: a matched case control study. J Antimicrob Chemother. 2007;60:1124–30.

64. Papadimitriou-Olivgeris M, Marangos M, Fligou F, Christofidou M, Bartzavali C, Anastassiou ED, et al. Risk factors for KPC-producing *Klebsiella pneumoniae* enteric colonization upon ICU admission. J Antimicrob Chemother. 2012;67:2976–81.

65. Stiefel U, Pultz NJ, Donskey CJ. Effect of carbapenem administration on establishment of intestinal colonization by vancomycin-resistant enterococci and *Klebsiella pneumoniae* in mice. Antimicrob Agents Chemother. 2007;51:372–5.

66. Antimicrobial resistance interactive database (EARS-Net) [cited 2016 Sep 20]. http://ecdc.europa.eu/en/healthtopics/antimicrobial-resistance-and-consumption/antimicrobial_resistance/database/Pages/table_reports.aspx.

67. Li H, Estabrook M, Jacoby GA, Nichols WW, Testa RT, Bush K. In vitro susceptibility of characterized β-lactamase-Producing strains tested with avibactam combinations. Antimicrob Agents Chemother. 2015;59:1789–93.

68. Drawz SM, Bonomo RA. Three decades of beta-lactamase inhibitors. Clin Microbiol Rev. 2010;23:160–201.

69. Kang C-I, Park SY, Chung DR, Peck KR, Song J-H. Piperacillin–tazobactam as an initial empirical therapy of bacteremia caused by extended-spectrum β-lactamase-producing *Escherichia coli* and *Klebsiella pneumoniae*. J Infect. 2012;64:533–4.

70. Bloos F, Rüddel H, Thomas-Rüddel D, Schwarzkopf D, Pausch C, Harbarth S, et al. Effect of a multifaceted educational intervention for anti-infectious measures on sepsis mortality: a cluster randomized trial. Intensive Care Med. 2017. http://doi.org/10.1007/s00134-017-4782-4

71. Guet-Revillet H, Tomini E, Emirian A, Join-Lambert O, Lécuyer H, Zahar J-R, et al. Piperacillin/tazobactam as an alternative antibiotic therapy to carbapenems in the treatment of urinary tract infections due to extended-spectrum β-lactamase-producing enterobacteriaceae: an in silico pharmacokinetic study. Int. J. Antimicrob Agents. 2016;49:62–6.

72. Roberts JA, Abdul-Aziz MH, Lipman J, Mouton JW, Vinks AA, Felton TW, et al. Individualised antibiotic dosing for patients who are critically ill: challenges and potential solutions. Lancet Infect Dis. 2014;14:498–509.

73. Pettigrew MM, Johnson JK, Harris AD. The human microbiota: novel targets for hospital-acquired infections and antibiotic resistance. Ann Epidemiol. 2016;26:342–7.

74. Gharbi M, Moore LSP, Gilchrist M, Thomas CP, Bamford K, Brannigan ET, et al. Forecasting carbapenem resistance from antimicrobial consumption surveillance: lessons learnt from an OXA-48-producing *Klebsiella pneumoniae* outbreak in a West London renal unit. Int J Antimicrob Agents. 2015;46:150–6.

75. Plüss-Suard C, Pannatier A, Kronenberg A, Mühlemann K, Zanetti G. Impact of antibiotic use on carbapenem resistance in *Pseudomonas aeruginosa*: is there a role for antibiotic diversity? Antimicrob Agents Chemother. 2013;57:1709–13.

76. Wexler HM, Finegold SM. Impact of imipenem/cilastatin therapy on normal fecal flora. Am J Med. 1985;78:41–6.

77. DiNubile MJ, Chow JW, Satishchandran V, Polis A, Motyl MR, Abramson MA, et al. Acquisition of resistant bowel flora during a double-blind randomized clinical trial of ertapenem versus piperacillin–tazobactam therapy for intraabdominal infections. Antimicrob Agents Chemother. 2005;49:3217–21.

78. Pultz NJ, Donskey CJ. Effects of imipenem-cilastatin, ertapenem, piperacillin–tazobactam, and ceftriaxone treatments on persistence of intestinal colonization by extended-spectrum-beta-lactamase-producing *Klebsiella pneumoniae* strains in mice. Antimicrob Agents Chemother. 2007;51:3044–5.

79. Gagliotti C, Giordani S, Ciccarese V, Barozzi A, Giovinazzi A, Pietrantonio AM, et al. Risk factors for colonization with carbapenemase-producing *Klebsiella pneumoniae* in hospital: a matched case-control study. Am J Infect Control. 2014;42:1006–8.

80. Mittal G, Gaind R, Kumar D, Kaushik G, Gupta KB, Verma PK, et al. Risk factors for fecal carriage of carbapenemase producing enterobacteriaceae among intensive care unit patients from a tertiary care center in India. BMC Microbiol. 2016;16:138.

81. Ling ML, Tee YM, Tan SG, Amin IM, How KB, Tan KY, et al. Risk factors for acquisition of carbapenem resistant enterobacteriaceae in an acute tertiary care hospital in Singapore. Antimicrob Resist Infect Control. 2015;4:26.

82. Jiao Y, Qin Y, Liu J, Li Q, Dong Y, Shang Y, et al. Risk factors for carbapenem-resistant *Klebsiella pneumoniae* infection/colonization and predictors of mortality: a retrospective study. Pathog Glob Health. 2015;109:68–74.

83. Candevir Ulu A, Kurtaran B, Inal AS, Kömür S, Kibar F, Yapıcı Çiçekdemir H, et al. Risk factors of carbapenem-resistant *Klebsiella pneumoniae* infection: a serious threat in ICUs. Med Sci Monit Int Med J Exp Clin Res. 2015;21:219–24.

84. Gómez Rueda V, Zuleta Tobón JJ. Risk factors for infection with carbapenem-resistant *Klebsiella pneumoniae*: a case-case-control study. Colomb Méd Cali Colomb. 2014;45:54–60.

85. Ahn JY, Song JE, Kim MH, Choi H, Kim JK, Ann HW, et al. Risk factors for the acquisition of carbapenem-resistant *Escherichia coli* at a tertiary care center in South Korea: a matched case-control study. Am J Infect Control. 2014;42:621–5.

86. Mantzarlis K, Makris D, Manoulakas E, Karvouniaris M, Zakynthinos E.

Risk factors for the first episode of *Klebsiella pneumoniae* resistant to carbapenems infection in critically ill patients: a prospective study. Biomed Res Int. 2013;2013:850547.

87. Dizbay M, Guzel Tunccan O, Karasahin O, Aktas F. Emergence of carbapenem-resistant *Klebsiella* spp infections in a Turkish university hospital: epidemiology and risk factors. J Infect Dev Ctries. 2014;8:44–9.

88. Orsi GB, Bencardino A, Vena A, Carattoli A, Venditti C, Falcone M, et al. Patient risk factors for outer membrane permeability and KPC-producing carbapenem-resistant *Klebsiella pneumoniae* isolation: results of a double case-control study. Infection. 2013;41:61–7.

89. Chang H-J, Hsu P-C, Yang C-C, Kuo A-J, Chia J-H, Wu T-L, et al. Risk factors and outcomes of carbapenem-nonsusceptible *Escherichia coli* bacteremia: a matched case-control study. J Microbiol Immunol Infect Wei Mian Yu Gan Ran Za Zhi. 2011;44:125–30.

90. Tuon FF, Rocha JL, Toledo P, Arend LN, Dias CH, Leite TM, et al. Risk factors for KPC-producing *Klebsiella pneumoniae* bacteremia. Braz J Infect Dis Off Publ Braz SocInfect Dis. 2012;16:416–9.

91. Papadimitriou-Olivgeris M, Marangos M, Christofidou M, Fligou F, Bartzavali C, Panteli ES, et al. Risk factors for infection and predictors of mortality among patients with KPC-producing *Klebsiella pneumoniae* bloodstream infections in the intensive care unit. Scand J Infect Dis. 2014;46:642–8.

92. Maseda E, Salgado P, Anillo V, Ruiz-Carrascoso G, Gómez-Gil R, Martín-Funke C, et al. Risk factors for colonization by carbapenemase-producing enterobacteria at admission to a Surgical ICU: a retrospective study. Clin: Enferm Infecc Microbiol; 2016.

93. Popejoy MW, Paterson DL, Cloutier D, Huntington JA, Miller B, Bliss CA, et al. Efficacy of ceftolozane/tazobactam against urinary tract and intra-abdominal infections caused by ESBL-producing *Escherichia coli* and *Klebsiella pneumoniae*: a pooled analysis of Phase 3 clinical trials. J Antimicrob Chemother. 2017;72:268–72.

94. Balakrishnan I, Awad-El-Kariem FM, Aali A, Kumari P, Mulla R, Tan B, et al. Temocillin use in England: clinical and microbiological efficacies in infections caused by extended-spectrum and/or derepressed AmpC β-lactamase-producing Enterobacteriaceae. J Antimicrob Chemother. 2011;66:2628–31.

95. Bin C, Hui W, Renyuan Z, Yongzhong N, Xiuli X, Yingchun X, et al. Outcome of cephalosporin treatment of bacteremia due to CTX-M-type extended-spectrum beta-lactamase-producing *Escherichia coli*. Diagn Microbiol Infect Dis. 2006;56:351–7.

96. Chaubey VP, Pitout JD, Dalton B, Ross T, Church DL, Gregson DB, et al. Clinical outcome of empiric antimicrobial therapy of bacteremia due to extended-spectrum beta-lactamase producing *Escherichia coli* and *Klebsiella pneumoniae*. BMC Res Notes. 2010;3:116.

97. Chung H-C, Lai C-H, Lin J-N, Huang C-K, Liang S-H, Chen W-F, et al. Bacteremia caused by extended-spectrum-β-lactamase-producing *Escherichia coli* sequence type ST131 and non-ST131 clones: comparison of demographic data, clinical features, and mortality. Antimicrob Agents Chemother. 2012;56:618–22.

98. De Rosa FG, Pagani N, Fossati L, Raviolo S, Cometto C, Cavallerio P, et al. The effect of inappropriate therapy on bacteremia by ESBL-producing bacteria. Infection. 2011;39:555–61.

99. Endimiani A, Luzzaro F, Brigante G, Perilli M, Lombardi G, Amicosante G, et al. Proteus mirabilis bloodstream infections: risk factors and treatment outcome related to the expression of extended-spectrum beta-lactamases. Antimicrob Agents Chemother. 2005;49:2598–605.

100. Ferrández O, Grau S, Saballs P, Luque S, Terradas R, Salas E. Mortality risk factors for bloodstream infections caused by extended-spectrum beta-lactamase-producing microorganisms. Rev Clín Esp. 2011;211:119–26.

101. Gudiol C, Calatayud L, Garcia-Vidal C, Lora-Tamayo J, Cisnal M, Duarte R, et al. Bacteraemia due to extended-spectrum beta-lactamase-producing *Escherichia coli* (ESBL-EC) in cancer patients: clinical features, risk factors, molecular epidemiology and outcome. J Antimicrob Chemother. 2010;65:333–41.

102. Harris PNA, Yin M, Jureen R, Chew J, Ali J, Paynter S, et al. Comparable outcomes for β-lactam/β-lactamase inhibitor combinations and carbapenems in definitive treatment of bloodstream infections caused by cefotaxime-resistant *Escherichia coli* or *Klebsiella pneumoniae*. Antimicrob Resist Infect Control. 2015;4:14.

103. Lee C-H, Lee Y-T, Kung C-H, Ku W-W, Kuo S-C, Chen T-L, et al. Risk factors of community-onset urinary tract infections caused by plasmid-mediated AmpC β-lactamase-producing Enterobacteriaceae. J Microbiol Immunol Infect. 2015;48:269–75.

104. Matsumura Y, Yamamoto M, Nagao M, Komori T, Fujita N, Hayashi A, et al. Multicenter retrospective study of cefmetazole and flomoxef for treatment of extended-spectrum-β-lactamase-producing *Escherichia coli* bacteremia. Antimicrob Agents Chemother. 2015;59:5107–13.

105. Qureshi ZA, Paterson DL, Pakstis DL, Adams-Haduch JM, Sandkovsky G, Sordillo E, et al. Risk factors and outcome of extended-spectrum β-lactamase-producing *Enterobacter cloacae* bloodstream infections. Int J Antimicrob Agents. 2011;37:26–32.

106. Pilmis B, Parize P, Zahar JR, Lortholary O. Alternatives to carbapenems for infections caused by ESBL-producing enterobacteriaceae. Microbiol: Eur J Clin Microbiol Infect Dis Off Publ Eur Soc Clin; 2014.

107. Retamar P, López-Cerero L, Muniain MA, Pascual Á, Rodríguez-Baño J, ESBL-REIPI/GEIH Group. Impact of the MIC of piperacillin–tazobactam on the outcome of patients with bacteremia due to extended-spectrum-β-lactamase-producing *Escherichia coli*. Antimicrob Agents Chemother. 2013;57:3402–4.

108. Tsai H-Y, Chen Y-H, Tang H-J, Huang C-C, Liao C-H, Chu F-Y, et al. Carbapenems and piperacillin/tazobactam for the treatment of bacteremia caused by extended-spectrum β-lactamase-producing Proteus mirabilis. Diagn Microbiol Infect Dis. 2014;80:222–6.

109. Tumbarello M, Sanguinetti M, Montuori E, Trecarichi EM, Posteraro B, Fiori B, et al. Predictors of mortality in patients with bloodstream infections caused by extended-spectrum-beta-lactamase-producing Enterobacteriaceae: importance of inadequate initial antimicrobial treatment. Antimicrob Agents Chemother. 2007;51:1987–94.

110. Tuon FF, Bianchet LC, Penteado-Filho SR. Epidemiology of extended spectrum beta-lactamase producing enterobacter bacteremia in a brazilian hospital. Rev Soc Bras Med Trop. 2010;43:452–4.

111. van Duin D, Bonomo RA. Ceftazidime/avibactam and ceftolozane/tazobactam: second-generation β-lactam/β-lactamase inhibitor combinations. Clin Infect Dis Off Publ Infect Dis Soc Am. 2016;63:234–41.

17

De-escalation of antifungal treatment in critically ill patients with suspected invasive *Candida* infection: incidence, associated factors, and safety

Karim Jaffal[1], Julien Poissy[1,2,3], Anahita Rouze[1,2,3], Sébastien Preau[1,2,3], Boualem Sendid[2,3,4], Marjorie Cornu[2,3,4] and Saad Nseir[1,2,3]* 🆔

Abstract

Background: Antifungal treatment is common in critically ill patients, but only a small proportion of patients receiving antifungals have a proven fungal infection. However, antifungal treatment has side effects such as toxicity, emergence of resistance, and high cost. Moreover, empirical antifungal treatment is still a matter for debate in these patients. Our study aimed to determine the incidence, associated factors, and safety of de-escalation of antifungals in critically ill patients.

Methods: This retrospective study was conducted in a 30-bed mixed ICU, from January 2012 through January 2013. Patients hospitalized for > 5 days and treated with antifungals for first suspected or proven invasive *Candida* infection were included. Exclusion criteria were prophylactic antifungals, suspected invasive aspergillosis, and neutropenia. De-escalation was defined as switch from initial systemic antifungals (except fluconazole) to triazoles, or stopping initial drugs within the 5 days following their initiation.

Results: One hundred and ninety patients were included. Antifungal treatment was empirical, preemptive, and targeted in 55, 27, and 24% of study patients, respectively. Caspofungin (53%), fluconazole (43%), voriconazole (4%), and liposomal amphotericin B (0.5%) were the more frequently used antifungals. De-escalation was performed in 38 (20%) patients. Invasive mechanical ventilation was independently associated with lower rates of de-escalation (OR 0.25 [95% CI 0.08–0.85], $p = 0.013$). Total duration of antifungal treatment was significantly shorter in patients with de-escalation, compared with those with no de-escalation (med [IQR] 6 (5, 18) vs. 13 days (7, 25), $p = 0.023$). No significant difference was found in duration of mechanical ventilation (22 [5–31] vs. 20 days [10–35], $p = 0.43$), length of ICU stay (25 [14–40] vs. 25 days [11–40], $p = 0.99$), ICU mortality (45 vs. 59%, $p = 0.13$), or 1-year mortality (55 vs. 64%, $p = 0.33$) between patients with de-escalation and those with no de-escalation, respectively.

Conclusions: De-escalation was performed in 20% of patients receiving systemic antifungals for suspected or proven invasive *Candida* infection. Mechanical ventilation was independently associated with lower rates of de-escalation. De-escalation of antifungal treatment seems to be safe in critically ill patients.

Background

Invasive fungal infections are common in critically ill patients [1–3]. Candidiasis is the most frequent fungal infection in hospitalized patients worldwide [4]. Despite a frequency twice less important than the frequency of bacteremia, mortality linked to candidemia is twice higher than that linked to bacteremia [5]. In case of septic shock, this mortality can reach 60% [6]. Despite the introduction of several extended-spectrum triazoles and echinocandin antifungal agents with superior safety,

*Correspondence: s-nseir@chru-lille.fr
[1] Critical Care Center, CHU Lille, 59000 Lille, France

spectrum, and potency, the incidence of invasive *Candida* infection and the associated mortality have not decreased over the past two decades [2]. The high mortality rate is related to comorbidities and also to the difficulty in diagnosis coupled with challenges in prompt adequate antifungal therapy [7].

Clinical signs of invasive *Candida* infection are non-specific, risk factors are common, the predictive positive value of all scores set to help clinicians remains insufficient [8, 9], and blood cultures have insufficient diagnostic accuracy [10, 11]. Because prompt antifungal treatment has a major impact on mortality [6, 12], guidelines recommend initiating systemic antifungal therapy, for critically ill patients with risk factors for invasive *Candida* infection and no other known cause for fever [13]. Criteria for initiating such therapy in clinical practice remain poorly defined. Consequently, the lack of rapid, sensitive, and specific diagnostic tests can lead to possible overuse of antifungal agents without further confirmation of invasive *Candida* infection [14]. Moreover, the overuse of antifungal agents is associated with increased prevalence of *Candida* non-albicans species and antifungal resistance [15–18]. Other potential consequences of inappropriate use of antifungals are increased cost, drug toxicity, and adverse drug interactions [19, 20].

A cross-sectional multicenter study showed that antifungal treatment was administered to 7.5% of ICU patients, although two-thirds of them had no documented invasive candidiasis [14]. In addition, recent studies suggested no benefit of empirical antifungal treatment in these patients [21, 22]. Reducing antifungal use in the ICU with an antifungal stewardship is feasible and would allow avoiding drawbacks. The European Society for Clinical Microbiology and Infectious Diseases (ESCMID) and the Infectious Diseases Society of America (IDSA) guidelines recommend a de-escalation strategy (5 days in stabilized patients for the IDSA and 10 days overall for the ESCMID) [13, 23], but the level of recommendations is low. The safety of de-escalation in the case of proven invasive *Candida* infection has been suggested by prospective recent studies [24–26]. However, some limitations, such as non-comparative or post hoc design, preclude definite conclusions. Therefore, we hypothesized that de-escalation of antifungal treatment might be safe in patients with suspected invasive *Candida* infection and conducted this retrospective study to identify the incidence and associated factors, and to assess safety of antifungal treatment de-escalation in ICU patients.

Methods
Study design
This retrospective observational study was performed in a 30-bed mixed ICU, located in the University Hospital of Lille, France. All data were retrospectively collected during a one-year period (from January 2012 through January 2013). The study was approved by the local Institutional Review Board (Comité de Protection des Personnes Nord-ouest IV). Because of the retrospective observational design of the study, and in accordance with the French law, written informed consent was not required by the local IRB.

Definitions and studied population
De-escalation of antifungal treatment was defined as either a switch from initial antifungals, except fluconazole, to triazoles, or discontinuation of initial antifungal treatment within the 5 days following their initiation [26]. Proven and suspected fungal infections were defined according to the revised criteria of the European Organization for Research and Treatment of invasive fungal infections Cooperative Group (EORTC) [27]. All patients hospitalized for more than 5 days and requiring systemic antifungal treatment for the first documented or suspected invasive *Candida* infection during their ICU stay were eligible. Patients receiving prophylactic antifungal treatment were excluded, as well as those with suspected mold infection, or neutropenia.

Study objectives
The primary objective was to evaluate the factors independently associated with antifungal de-escalation. Secondary objectives were to evaluate the incidence of de-escalation of antifungal treatment, and its impact on ICU length of stay, duration of mechanical ventilation, and mortality.

Data collection
All data were retrospectively recorded from archived medical records of University Hospital of Lille and its mycology laboratory. Patients were identified using the electronic pharmacy database setup to guide and monitor antifungal prescriptions. Only first episodes of proven or suspected invasive *Candida* infection were considered. Initial antifungal treatment was based on local guidelines, driven from international guidelines [28].

The following characteristics were recorded at ICU admission: age, gender, severity of acute illness based on simplified acute physiology score (SAPS) II, comorbidities (diabetes, chronic obstructive pulmonary disease (COPD), chronic heart failure, cirrhosis, chronic renal failure requiring dialysis, or immunosuppression), location before ICU admission, admission category (medical or surgical), reason for ICU admission (acute exacerbation of COPD, acute respiratory distress syndrome, pneumonia, congestive heart failure, neurologic failure, poisoning, shock, and infection), and prior antibiotic or antifungal treatment used in the last 3 months. During ICU stay, data were collected on type of antifungal treatment (empirical, preemptive, or curative), suspected (probable and possible categories of the EORTC definitions) or proven invasive *Candida* infection, successive antifungal treatments prescribed, duration of each antifungal treatment, total duration of antifungal therapy, and appropriateness of the initial antifungal treatment. The following data were collected regarding de-escalation: date of onset and reasons for de-escalation. We also collected the results of mycological cultures from sterile sites (blood, cerebrospinal, pleural, peritoneal and pericardial fluid, surgical site) and the sites usually checked for the multifocal colonization status (skin, urine, trachea, catheter, anus), and data on antibiotic treatment, severe sepsis, total parenteral nutrition, surgery, renal replacement therapy, length of mechanical ventilation, duration of treatment with vasoactive drugs, length of ICU stay, occurrence of apyrexia, ICU, and 30-day and 1-year mortality.

Statistical analysis

SPSS software (SPSS, Chicago, IL, USA) was used for data analysis. Categorical variables were described as frequency (%). Kolmogorov–Smirnov test was used to evaluate the distribution of continuous variables. Normally distributed and skewed continuous variables were described as mean ± standard deviation (SD), or as median and interquartile range (IQR), respectively.

To determine factors associated with de-escalation, patients with de-escalation were compared with those with no de-escalation using univariate and multivariate analyses. Student's *t* test or the Mann–Whitney *U* test was used to compare normally distributed and skewed continuous variables, respectively. The Chi-square (χ^2) test or Fischer's exact test was used to compare qualitative variables, as appropriate. The odds ratio (OR) and 95% confidence interval (CI) were calculated for all qualitative variables significant in univariate analysis and for all variables significant in multivariate analysis. Differences were considered significant if *p* values were < 0.05, with two-tailed tests. Exposure to potential factors associated with antifungal de-escalation was considered until the occurrence of de-escalation, or until ICU discharge in patients with no de-escalation. All variables with *p* values < 0.2 by univariate analysis were included in a backward multivariate logistic regression model. Potential interactions were tested, and the Hosmer–Lemeshow goodness of fit and *c*-statistics were calculated. Cox proportional hazards models were performed to determine factors associated with ICU mortality.

Results

Among the 582 patients hospitalized for > 5 days during the study period, 244 (42%) patients received antifungal treatment. Fifty-four (22%) patients were excluded, because they received prophylactic antifungal treatment ($n = 18$, 8%), had suspected filamentous fungal infection ($n = 20$, 8%), or were neutropenic ($n = 16$, 7%). The remaining 190 patients were all included in the study (Fig. 1). One hundred and five (55%), 52 (27%), and 46 (24%) patients received empirical, preemptive, and targeted treatment, respectively. Caspofungin ($n = 101$, 53%), fluconazole ($n = 81$, 43%), voriconazole ($n = 7$, 4%), and liposomal amphotericin B ($n = 1$, 0.5%) were the most frequently used antifungals.

Patient characteristics and incidence of de-escalation

De-escalation was performed in 38 (20%) of the 190 included patients. Initial antifungal treatment was stopped in 19 (50%) patients within 5 days and switched to an azole in 19 (50%) patients. Reasons for de-escalation were susceptible strain based on antifungal

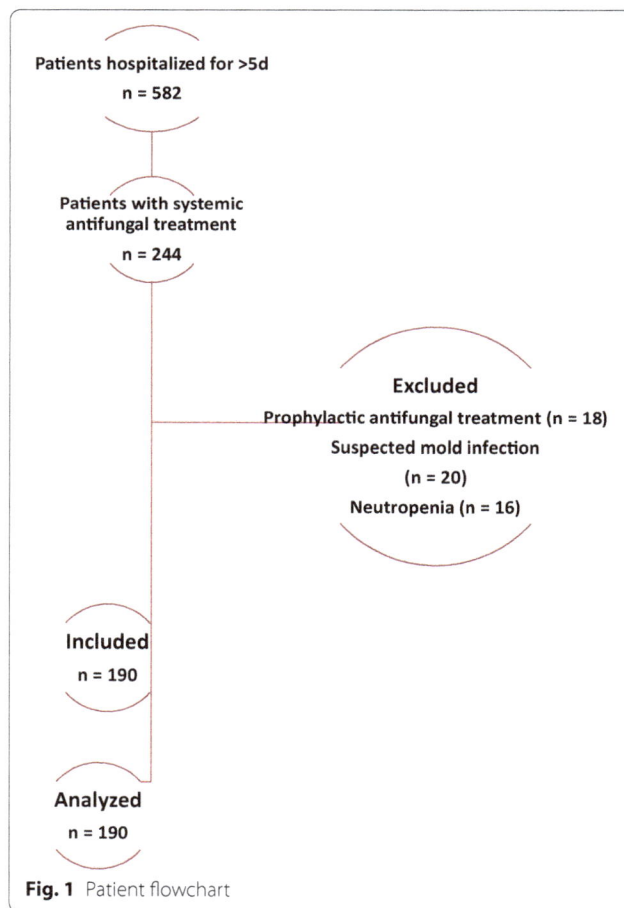

Patients hospitalized for >5d
n = 582

Patients with systemic antifungal treatment
n = 244

Excluded
Prophylactic antifungal treatment (n = 18)
Suspected mold infection
(n = 20)
Neutropenia (n = 16)

Included
n = 190

Analyzed
n = 190

Fig. 1 Patient flowchart

susceptibility testing in 16 (42%) patients, proven bacterial infection with no evidence for fungal infection in 10 (26%) patients, and negative mycological investigations in 12 (32%) patients.

Patient characteristics are presented in Table 1.

Mycological results

Thirty-four (18%) of the 187 samples taken from sterile sites were positive, of which 26 (76%) were positive to *Candida albicans*, 2 (6%) to *Candida glabrata*, and 6 (18%) to other *Candida* species. Of 192 samples taken from non-sterile sites, 170 (89%) samples were positive, including 99 (58%) to *C. albicans*, 27 (16%) to *C. parapsilosis*, 20 (12%) to *C. glabrata*, 17 (10%) to *C. tropicalis*, and 7 (4%) to other *Candida* species.

Factors associated with antifungal de-escalation

By univariate analysis, factors associated with higher rate of de-escalation were chronic dialysis, negative mycological samples, proven bacterial infection, apyrexia for >72 h, and vasoactive drug discontinuation at 72 h after initiation of antifungal treatment. Multifocal *Candida* colonization, preemptive treatment, and mechanical ventilation were associated with significantly lower rate of de-escalation (Tables 1 and 2). By multivariate analysis, only mechanical ventilation was independently associated with de-escalation (OR 0.25 (95% CI 0.08–0.74), $p = 0.023$; Hosmer–Lemeshow goodness-of-fit test, $p = 0.95$, c-statistics 0.85).

Impact of de-escalation on outcomes

There was no significant impact of de-escalation on ICU length of stay, duration of mechanical ventilation, ICU mortality, 30-day mortality, or 1-year mortality rate (Table 3). In multivariable Cox proportional hazards model, only SAPS II and catecholamines withdrawal at day 3 were independently associated with ICU mortality, even when de-escalation was forced in the model (Table 4).

Discussion

Our results suggest that de-escalation is performed in 20% of critically ill patients receiving empirical, preemptive, or targeted antifungal treatment for suspected or proven invasive *Candida* infection. Mechanical ventilation was the only factor independently associated with lower rates of de-escalation of antifungal treatment. No negative impact of de-escalation was found on duration of mechanical ventilation, ICU length of stay, ICU mortality, 28-day mortality, or 1-year mortality rates.

The incidence of de-escalation of antifungal treatment in our study is in line with that reported recently by Bailly et al. (22%) [26]. In another recent retrospective study performed in 262 critically ill patients receiving empirical or targeted antifungal treatment, the incidence of de-escalation was lower at 10% [29]. Azoulay et al. performed a large multicenter cross-sectional one-day study to determine the incidence of ICU patients without documented antifungal infection who receive antifungals. Antifungal treatment was used in 154 (7.5%) of study patients, including 100 (65%) patients without documented fungal infection. These results suggest that de-escalation of antifungal treatment could probably be performed in a larger proportion of critically ill patients.

Table 1 Characteristics of study patients at ICU admission

Characteristics	De-escalation		p
	Yes (n = 38)	No (n = 152)	
Age, years	63 [56–68]	63 [55–72]	0.57
Female gender n (%)	8 (21)	55 (36)	0.067
SAPS II	49 [30–68]	54 [36–71]	0.38
Comorbidities n (%)			
Diabetes	8 (21)	30 (20)	0.87
COPD	9 (24)	33 (22)	0.79
Chronic heart failure	8 (21)	30 (20)	0.87
Cirrhosis	4 (11)	10 (6)	0.49
Chronic dialysis	9 (24)	14 (9)	0.014*
Immunosuppression n (%)			
Chemotherapy	7 (18)	13 (9)	0.076
Corticosteroid therapy	9 (24)	29 (19)	0.53
Transfer from			0.66
Home	4 (11)	21 (14)	
Other wards	25 (66)	104 (68)	
Other ICUs	9 (24)	27 (18)	
Admission category			0.75
Medical	22 (58)	98 (64)	
Surgical	15 (39)	51 (34)	
Other (trauma, burn)	1 (3)	3 (2)	
Cause for ICU admission			
Acute exacerbation of COPD	3 (8)	26 (17)	0.16
Acute respiratory distress syndrome	12 (32)	41 (27)	0.57
Community-acquired pneumonia	11 (29)	32 (21)	0.30
Hospital-acquired pneumonia	6 (16)	38 (25)	0.23
Congestive heart failure	0 (0)	7 (5)	0.18
Neurologic failure	0 (0)	7 (5)	0.18
Poisoning	1 (3)	15 (10)	0.15
Septic shock	22 (58)	89 (59)	0.94
Infection at ICU admission	37 (97)	135 (89)	0.17
Prior antibiotic treatment	16 (42)	69 (45)	0.72
Prior antifungal treatment	5 (13)	15 (10)	0.56

Data are N (%), or median (interquartile range)

COPD chronic obstructive pulmonary disease, *ICU* intensive care unit, *SAPS* simplified acute physiology score

* Odds ratio (95% confidence interval) 3.1 (1.21–7.74)

Table 2 Patient characteristics during ICU stay

Characteristics	De-escalation		p	OR [95% CI]
	Yes (n = 38)	No (n = 152)		
Multifocal colonization	19 (50)	115 (76)	0.002	0.32 [0.15–0.67]
Negative yeast samples	16 (42)	30 (20)	0.004	2.95 [1.4–6.3]
Empirical antifungal treatment	12 (32)	68 (45)	0.14	
Preemptive antifungal treatment	4 (11)	48 (32)	0.008	0.26 [0.09–0.78]
Targeted antifungal treatment	10 (26)	36 (24)	0.73	
Proven bacterial infection	10 (26)	0 (0)	<0.001	NA
Apyrexia >72 h	37 (97)	123 (81)	0.013	8.7 [1.2–66]
Catecholamine withdrawal at 72 h	29 (76)	89 (59)	0.026	2.57 [1.1–5.98]
Mechanical ventilation	30 (79)	142 (93)	0.006	0.26 [0.09–0.73]
Antibiotic treatment	38 (100)	150 (99)	0.96	
Total parenteral nutrition	18 (47)	81 (53)	0.51	
Surgery	21 (55)	76 (50)	0.56	
Renal replacement therapy	21 (55)	76 (50)	0.56	
Shock	31 (82)	121 (80)	0.79	

Data are N (%)

CI confidence interval, *OR* odds ratio

Table 3 Impact of de-escalation on outcome

Characteristics	De-escalation		p
	Yes (n = 38)	No (n = 152)	
Length of ICU stay	25 [14–40]	25 [14–40]	0.99
Duration of mechanical ventilation	22 [5–31]	20 [10–35]	0.43
Total duration of antifungal treatment	6 [5–18]	13 [7–25]	0.023
ICU mortality	17 (45)	89 (59)	0.13
30-day mortality	9 (24)	56 (37)	0.13
1-year mortality	21 (55)	97 (64)	0.33

Data are *N* (%), or median (interquartile range)

Invasive mechanical ventilation was the only factor independently associated with lower rates of de-escalation of antifungal treatment. This result could be related to the higher severity of patients receiving invasive mechanical ventilation, which might have prevented attending physicians from de-escalating antifungal treatment. The superiority of echinocandins over fluconazole has been demonstrated in a single head-to-head clinical trial of anidulafungin that showed significantly better overall response rates (76 vs. 60%; $p = 0.01$) [30]. A further post hoc analysis showed better global responses (70.8 vs. 54.1%) and reduced 14-day all-cause mortality (10.1 vs. 20.3%, $p = 0.08$) in critically ill patients [31]. However, a recent large multicenter observational study,

Table 4 Factors associated with ICU mortality by Cox proportional hazards models

Factors	Univariate analysis		Multivariate analysis	
	HR (95% CI)	p	HR (95% CI)	p
At ICU admission				
SAPS II	1.01* (1.004–1.02)	0.005	1.01* (1–1.02)	0.040
Surgical patients	0.46 (0.3–0.69)	<0.001	–	–
ARDS	1.81 (1.22–2.68)	0.003	–	–
During ICU stay				
Renal replacement therapy	1.64 (1.1–2.47)	0.018	–	–
Preemptive antifungal treatment	0.50 (0.32–0.80)	0.004	–	–
Apyrexia >72 h	0.36 (0.23–0.57)	<0.001	–	–
Catecholamine withdrawal at 72 h	0.35 (0.27–0.52)	<0.001	0.47 (0.29–0.76)	0.002
De-escalation of antifungal treatment**	0.75 (0.44–1.26)	0.28	–	–

ICU intensive care medicine, *SAPS* simplified acute physiology score, *ARDS* acute respiratory distress syndrome

* Per point of SAPS II; *HR* hazard ratio, *CI* confidence interval

** De-escalation of antifungal treatment was forced in the final Cox model using a propensity-score derived analysis, did not report increased mortality using fluconazole as empirical or targeted treatment, as compared with echinocandins, in adult patients with candidemia [32]. Similar results were also reported in the subgroup of patients with sepsis or septic shock.

Recent observational and randomized controlled studies have questioned the beneficial effects of empirical antifungal treatment on mortality, even in patients in septic shock with high colonization index [33, 34]. However, the randomized controlled EMPIRICUS trial found significantly reduced rate of invasive candidiasis in patients who received micafungin, as compared with those who received placebo [34]. Our results suggest that de-escalation of antifungal treatment is safe. Overall, our results confirm previous studies, suggesting that early de-escalation to azole is possible and safe. For proven invasive *Candida* infection, three studies reported that de-escalation is safe in *Candida spp.* fluconazole-sensitive infections [24, 25, 35]. Bailly et al. [26] also reported that de-escalation could be safely performed in critically ill patients, as no negative impact was found on ICU mortality, duration of mechanical ventilation, or length of ICU stay. In addition, antifungal de-escalation was associated with significant decrease in the antifungal consumption, which might be helpful in reducing toxicity, drug interaction, fungal resistance, and cost [36]. A recent randomized controlled trial aimed to determine the usefulness of fungal biomarkers in early discontinuation of empirical antifungal treatment [37]. Patients were randomized to receive routine care (control group) or biomarker-based strategy (intervention group), in which a recommendation was given based on $(1,3)$-β-D-glucan, mannan, and anti-mannan serum assays performed on day 0 and day 4. The percentage of patients with early discontinuation of empirical antifungal treatment was significantly higher in intervention, compared with control group (54 vs. 2%, $p < 0.0001$), with no negative impact on mortality or morbidity. However, this open-label study was performed in a single center, and patients with immunosuppression were excluded. Therefore, further randomized controlled trials are needed to confirm these results.

Our study has some limitations. First, it was a retrospective study performed in a single center. Therefore, our results could not be generalized and further prospective multicenter studies are needed to confirm these findings. Second, the number of patients with de-escalation was relatively low. Therefore, analysis of subgroups with early stop, or reduction in antifungal spectrum was not possible. Third, potential benefit of de-escalation of antifungal treatment on cost was not evaluated. However, given the significant reduction in duration of antifungal treatment of 6 days in patients with de-escalation, compared with those with no de-escalation, a lower cost could be expected in these patients. Finally, no data were collected on dose or duration of corticosteroids. Corticosteroids use is a risk factor for invasive Candida infection and could impact on prognosis of patients with these infections. However, it is unlikely that corticosteroids have influenced de-escalation of antifungal treatment.

Conclusions

De-escalation was performed in 20% of patients receiving systemic antifungals for suspected invasive *Candida* infection. Invasive mechanical ventilation was independently associated with reduced de-escalation of antifungal treatment. De-escalation was associated with decreased antifungal treatment duration. De-escalation of antifungal treatment seems to be feasible and safe in critically ill patients. However, further large prospective studies are required to confirm these findings.

Authors' contributions
KJ and SN designed the study. KJ and MC collected the data. SN performed the statistical analysis. KF and SN wrote the manuscript. All authors participated in the final revision of the manuscript. All authors read and approved the final manuscript.

Author details
[1] Critical Care Center, CHU Lille, 59000 Lille, France. [2] U995-LIRIC-Lille Inflammation Research International Center, Univ. Lille, 59000 Lille, France. [3] Inserm, U995, 59000 Lille, France. [4] Laboratory of Mycology and Parasitology, CHU Lille, 59000 Lille, France.

Acknowledgments
None.

Competing interests
SN, Medtronic, and MSD (lecture); CielMedical and Bayer (advisory board); other authors: none.

Funding
None.

References
1. León C, Ostrosky-Zeichner L, Schuster M. What's new in the clinical and diagnostic management of invasive candidiasis in critically ill patients. Intensive Care Med. 2014;40:808–19.
2. Lortholary O, Renaudat C, Sitbon K, Madec Y, Denoeud-Ndam L, Wolff M, et al. Worrisome trends in incidence and mortality of candidemia in intensive care units (Paris area, 2002–2010). Intensive Care Med. 2014;40:1303–12.
3. Leroy O, Bailly S, Gangneux J-P, Mira J-P, Devos P, Dupont H, et al. Systemic antifungal therapy for proven or suspected invasive candidiasis: the AmarCAND 2 study. Ann Intensive Care. 2016;6:2.
4. Vincent J-L, Rello J, Marshall J, Silva E, Anzueto A, Martin CD, et al. International study of the prevalence and outcomes of infection in intensive care units. JAMA. 2009;302:2323–9.

5. Kett DH, Azoulay E, Echeverria PM, Vincent J-L. Candida bloodstream infections in intensive care units: analysis of the extended prevalence of infection in intensive care unit study. Crit Care Med. 2011;39:665–70.

6. Bassetti M, Righi E, Ansaldi F, Merelli M, Trucchi C, Cecilia T, et al. A multicenter study of septic shock due to candidemia: outcomes and predictors of mortality. Intensive Care Med. 2014;40:839–45.

7. Ostrosky-Zeichner L, Kullberg BJ, Bow EJ, Hadley S, León C, Nucci M, et al. Early treatment of candidemia in adults: a review. Med Mycol. 2011;49:113–20.

8. Ostrosky-Zeichner L. Invasive mycoses: diagnostic challenges. Am J Med. 2012;125:S14–24.

9. León C, Álvarez-Lerma F, Ruiz-Santana S, León MÁ, Nolla J, Jordá R, et al. Fungal colonization and/or infection in non-neutropenic critically ill patients: results of the EPCAN observational study. Eur J Clin Microbiol Infect Dis. 2009;28:233–42.

10. Arvanitis M, Anagnostou T, Fuchs BB, Caliendo AM, Mylonakis E. Molecular and nonmolecular diagnostic methods for invasive fungal infections. Clin Microbiol Rev. 2014;27:490–526.

11. Clancy CJ, Nguyen MH. Finding the "missing 50%" of invasive candidiasis: how nonculture diagnostics will improve understanding of disease spectrum and transform patient care. Clin Infect Dis. 2013;56:1284–92.

12. Kollef M, Micek S, Hampton N, Doherty JA, Kumar A. Septic shock attributed to Candida infection: importance of empiric therapy and source control. Clin Infect Dis. 2012;54:1739–46.

13. Pappas PG, Kauffman CA, Andes DR, Clancy CJ, Marr KA, Ostrosky-Zeichner L, et al. Clinical practice guideline for the management of candidiasis: 2016 update by the infectious diseases society of America. Clin Infect Dis. 2016;62:e1–50.

14. Azoulay E, Dupont H, Tabah A, Lortholary O, Stahl J-P, Francais A, et al. Systemic antifungal therapy in critically ill patients without invasive fungal infection. Crit Care Med. 2012;40:813–22.

15. Arendrup MC, Dzajic E, Jensen RH, Johansen HK, Kjaeldgaard P, Knudsen JD, et al. Epidemiological changes with potential implication for antifungal prescription recommendations for fungaemia: data from a nationwide fungaemia surveillance programme. Clin Microbiol Infect. 2013;19:E343–53.

16. Ostrosky-Zeichner L. Candida glabrata and FKS mutations: witnessing the emergence of the true multidrug-resistant Candida. Clin Infect Dis. 2013;56:1733–4.

17. Lortholary O, Desnos-Ollivier M, Sitbon K, Fontanet A, Bretagne S, Dromer F, et al. Recent exposure to caspofungin or fluconazole influences the epidemiology of candidemia: a prospective multicenter study involving 2,441 patients. Antimicrob Agents Chemother. 2011;55:532–8.

18. Dannaoui E, Desnos-Ollivier M, Garcia-Hermoso D, Grenouillet F, Cassaing S, Baixench M-T, et al. Candida spp. with acquired echinocandin resistance, France, 2004–2010. Emerg Infect Dis. 2012;18:86–90.

19. Drgona L, Khachatryan A, Stephens J, Charbonneau C, Kantecki M, Haider S, et al. Clinical and economic burden of invasive fungal diseases in Europe: focus on pre-emptive and empirical treatment of Aspergillus and Candida species. Eur J Clin Microbiol Infect Dis. 2014;33:7–21. https://doi.org/10.1007/s10096-013-1944-3.

20. Valerio M, Rodriguez-Gonzalez CG, Munoz P, Caliz B, Sanjurjo M, Bouza E, et al. Evaluation of antifungal use in a tertiary care institution: antifungal stewardship urgently needed. J Antimicrob Chemother. 2014;69:1993–9.

21. Playford EG, Webster AC, Sorrell TC, Craig JC. Antifungal agents for preventing fungal infections in non-neutropenic critically ill and surgical patients: systematic review and meta-analysis of randomized clinical trials. J Antimicrob Chemother. 2006;57:628–38.

22. Schuster MG, Edwards JE, Sobel JD, Darouiche RO, Karchmer AW, Hadley S, et al. Empirical fluconazole versus placebo for intensive care unit patients: a randomized trial. Ann Intern Med. 2008;149:83–90.

23. Cornely OA, Bassetti M, Calandra T, Garbino J, Kullberg BJ, Lortholary O, et al. ESCMID guideline for the diagnosis and management of Candida diseases 2012: non-neutropenic adult patients. Clin Microbiol Infect. 2012;18:19–37.

24. Takesue Y, Ueda T, Mikamo H, Oda S, Takakura S, Kitagawa Y, et al. Management bundles for candidaemia: the impact of compliance on clinical outcomes. J Antimicrob Chemother [Internet]. 2015;70:587–93.

25. Vazquez J, Reboli AC, Pappas PG, Patterson TF, Reinhardt J, Chin-Hong P, et al. Evaluation of an early step-down strategy from intravenous anidulafungin to oral azole therapy for the treatment of candidemia and other forms of invasive candidiasis: results from an open-label trial. BMC Infect Dis. 2014;14:97.

26. Bailly S, Leroy O, Montravers P, Constantin J-M, Dupont H, Guillemot D, et al. Antifungal de-escalation was not associated with adverse outcome in critically ill patients treated for invasive candidiasis: post hoc analyses of the AmarCAND2 study data. Intensive Care Med. 2015;41:1931–40. https://doi.org/10.1007/s00134-015-4053-1.

27. De Pauw B, Walsh TJ, Donnelly JP, Stevens DA, Edwards JE, Calandra T, et al. Revised definitions of invasive fungal disease from the European Organization for Research and Treatment of Cancer/Invasive Fungal Infections Cooperative Group and the National Institute of Allergy and Infectious Diseases Mycoses Study Group (EORTC/MSG) Consensus Group. Clin Infect Dis. 2008;46:1813–21. https://doi.org/10.1086/588660.

28. Pappas PG, Kauffman CA, Andes D, Benjamin DK Jr, Calandra TF, Edwards JE Jr, et al. Clinical practice guidelines for the management of candidiasis: 2009 update by the infectious diseases society of America. Clin Infect Dis. 2009;48:503–35.

29. Zein M, Parmentier-Decrucq E, Kalaoun A, Bouton O, Wallyn F, Baranzelli A, et al. Factors predicting prolonged empirical antifungal treatment in critically ill patients. Ann Clin Microbiol Antimicrob. 2014;13:11.

30. Reboli AC, Rotstein C, Pappas PG, Chapman SW, Kett DH, Kumar D, et al. Anidulafungin versus fluconazole for invasive candidiasis. N Engl J Med. 2007;356:2472–82. https://doi.org/10.1056/NEJMoa066906.

31. Kett DH, Shorr AF, Reboli AC, Reisman AL, Biswas P, Schlamm HT. Anidulafungin compared with fluconazole in severely ill patients with candidemia and other forms of invasive candidiasis: support for the 2009 IDSA treatment guidelines for candidiasis. Crit Care. 2011;15:R253. https://doi.org/10.1186/cc10514.

32. López-Cortés LE, Almirante B, Cuenca-Estrella M, Garnacho-Montero J, Padilla B, Puig-Asensio M, et al. Empirical and targeted therapy of candidemia with fluconazole versus echinocandins: a propensity score-derived analysis of a population-based, multicentre prospective cohort. Clin Microbiol Infect. 2016;22(733):e1–8.

33. Bailly S, Bouadma L, Azoulay E, Orgeas MG, Adrie C, Souweine B, et al. Failure of empirical systemic antifungal therapy in mechanically ventilated critically ill patients. Am J Respir Crit Care Med. 2015;191:1139–46. https://doi.org/10.1164/rccm.201409-1701OC.

34. Timsit J-F, Azoulay E, Schwebel C, Charles PE, Cornet M, Souweine B, et al. Empirical micafungin treatment and survival without invasive fungal infection in adults with ICU-acquired sepsis, Candida colonization, and multiple organ failure. JAMA. 2016;316:1555.

35. Bal AM, Shankland GS, Scott G, Imtiaz T, Macaulay R, McGill M. Antifungal step-down therapy based on hospital intravenous to oral switch policy and susceptibility testing in adult patients with candidaemia: a single centre experience. Int J Clin Pract. 2014;68:20–7.

36. Rouzé A, Jaffal K, Nseir S. How could we reduce antifungal treatment in the intensive care unit. World J Clin Infect Dis. 2015;5:55–8.

37. Rouzé A, Loridant S, Poissy J, Dervaux B, Sendid B, Cornu M, et al. Biomarker-based strategy for early discontinuation of empirical antifungal treatment in critically ill patients: a randomized controlled trial. Intensive Care Med. 2017;43(11):1668–77.

Pleural effusion during weaning from mechanical ventilation

Keyvan Razazi[1,2,3]* iD, Florence Boissier[4,5], Mathilde Neuville[6], Sébastien Jochmans[2,7], Martial Tchir[8], Faten May[1,2], Nicolas de Prost[1,2], Christian Brun-Buisson[1,2], Guillaume Carteaux[1,2] and Armand Mekontso Dessap[1,2,3]

Abstract

Background: Pleural effusion is common during invasive mechanical ventilation, but its role during weaning is unclear. We aimed at assessing the prevalence and risk factors for pleural effusion at initiation of weaning. We also assessed its impact on weaning outcomes and its evolution in patients with difficult weaning.

Methods: We performed a prospective multicenter study in five intensive care units in France. Two hundred and forty-nine patients were explored using ultrasonography. Presence of moderate-to-large pleural effusion (defined as a maximal interpleural distance ≥ 15 mm) was assessed at weaning start and during difficult weaning.

Results: Seventy-three (29%) patients failed weaning, including 46 (18%) who failed the first spontaneous breathing trial (SBT) and 39 (16%) who failed extubation. Moderate-to-large pleural effusion was detected in 81 (33%) patients at weaning start. Moderate-to-large pleural effusion was associated with more failures of the first SBT [27 (33%) vs. 19 (11%), $p < 0.001$], more weaning failures [37 (47%) vs. 36 (22%), $p < 0.001$], less ventilator-free days at day 28 [21 (5–24) vs. 23 (16–26), $p = 0.01$], and a higher mortality at day 28 [14 (17%) vs. 14 (8%), $p = 0.04$]. The association of pleural effusion with weaning failure persisted in multivariable analysis and sensitivity analyses. Short-term (48 h) fluid balance change was not associated with the evolution of interpleural distance in patients with difficult weaning.

Conclusions: In this multicenter observational study, pleural effusion was frequent during the weaning process and was associated with worse weaning outcomes.

Keywords: Mechanical ventilation, Pleural effusion, Weaning, Ultrasonography

Introduction

Several factors may contribute to the occurrence of pleural effusions in critically ill patients, including heart failure, pneumonia, hypoalbuminemia, and fluid overload [1]. Its incidence in mechanically ventilated patients varies depending on the screening method, from approximately 8% with physical examination to more than 60% with routine ultrasonography [1, 2]. Pleural effusion was found in 83% of patients with acute respiratory distress syndrome (ARDS) explored with computed tomography scans [3].

The presence of pleural effusion is associated with a longer duration of mechanical ventilation and intensive care unit (ICU) stay [2]. Although a causal relationship cannot be established, this prolongation may result from altered respiratory mechanics [4] and impeded diaphragmatic contraction [5]. Indeed, pleural effusion increases the total thoracic volume, leading inspiratory muscles to operate in a less advantageous portion of their length-tension curve. Thus, the capacity of the diaphragm to generate pressure decreases when pleural effusion increases [5, 6]. Drainage of large pleural effusions improves oxygenation and respiratory mechanics in mechanically ventilated patients [4, 7].

*Correspondence: keyvan.razazi@aphp.fr
[1] AP-HP, DHU A-TVB, Service de Réanimation Médicale, Hôpitaux Universitaires Henri Mondor, 94010 Créteil, France

Weaning accounts for approximately 40% of the total duration of mechanical ventilation [8], but data on pleural effusion during the weaning process are scarce [9]. The main objective of the present observational multicenter study was to assess the prevalence and risk factors of pleural effusion at initiation of weaning. The second objective was to explore the association of pleural effusion with weaning outcomes, and its evolution during difficult weaning.

Materials and methods

This prospective multicenter observational study recruited patients admitted in five ICUs in France. Inclusion criteria were endotracheal mechanical ventilation for at least 24 h, and the fulfillment of weaning criteria [10] allowing a first spontaneous breathing trial (SBT). Noninclusion criteria were pregnancy or lactation, age less than 18 years, pleural effusion drainage before the first SBT, and a do-not-reintubate decision at time of inclusion.

Weaning protocol and definitions

Weaning initiation was defined as the day of first SBT. The first SBT used a T-piece trial in three centers and a low-level pressure support (7–10 cm H_2O) with zero end-expiratory pressure in two centers, as per usual care. Failure of the SBT was based on predefined criteria (see the online supplement, Additional file 1). Extubation failure was defined as death or reintubation within the 7 days following extubation; this delay was used instead of 48–72 h because prophylactic noninvasive ventilation may postpone reintubation [11]. Indications for prophylactic noninvasive ventilation included patients older than 65 years and those with underlying cardiac or respiratory disease [12]. According to the International Consensus Conference [10], weaning success was defined as a first successful SBT followed by successful extubation. Failure of the weaning process was defined [10] as failure of the first SBT or extubation failure. Because some patients could not be classified with this definition, weaning was also categorized according to the WIND definition [13] as follows: short when the first SBT resulted in a successful termination of the weaning process or death within 1 day after the first SBT; difficult in case of successful weaning or death after more than 1 day but in less than 1 week after the first SBT; prolonged if weaning was still not terminated 7 days after the first SBT. Ventilator-free days at day 28 were computed as days without invasive mechanical ventilation during the 28 days following first SBT; patients who died before day 28 or were dependent on mechanical ventilation for more

than 28 days after the first SBT had zero ventilator-free days [14]. Other definitions (e.g., Mac Cabe classification, ARDS, ventilator-associated pneumonia, failure of SBT) and data collection process are reported in the online supplement (Additional file 1).

Lung ultrasonography

Lung ultrasonography was performed on the day of first SBT and repeated on the 2 days following a SBT failure and on the day of extubation, if applicable. Maximal end-expiratory interpleural distance, sonographic patterns of effusion (homogeneously anechoic, complex nonseptated, complex septated, or homogeneously echogenic) [15], and of lung parenchyma (condensation or atelectasis) [16] were assessed on each side with the patient in the semirecumbent position. A moderate-to-large pleural effusion was defined as a maximal interpleural distance $\geq$ 15 mm (predicting an effusion volume of 300 mL or more) [17]; a large pleural effusion was defined by a maximal interpleural distance $\geq$ 25 mm [4, 17]. A pleural effusion was deemed drainable if the maximal interpleural distance was $\geq$ 15 mm, and the effusion was visible over at least three intercostal spaces [18]. When possible, a transthoracic echocardiography was also performed to assess left ventricle ejection fraction (see the online supplement, Additional file 1). In patients with SBT failure, attempts at depletion (by diuretics or ultrafiltration) and fluid balance were collected during the 2 days following the SBT. There was no mandatory depletive strategy for the management of pleural effusion.

Statistical analysis

The primary endpoint was the prevalence of pleural effusion at weaning start. The sample size was calculated by hypothesizing a prevalence of pleural effusion of 40% [1–3], and considering a precision of 8%. The study required a minimum of 170 patients (for an alpha risk of 5%, i.e., a confidence interval of 95%) and a maximum of 260 patients (for an alpha risk of 1%, i.e., a confidence interval of 99%). Continuous data were expressed as medians [25th–75th centiles] unless otherwise specified, and were compared using the Mann–Whitney test. Categorical variables, expressed as percentages, were compared using the Chi-square test or Fisher exact test. To evaluate independent factors associated with the presence of moderate-to-large pleural effusion at weaning start or with failure of the weaning process, significant or marginally significant ($p < 0.10$) bivariate risk factors (using the above mentioned tests) were examined using univariate and multivariable backward stepwise logistic regression analysis. Among related univariate factors, only the most statistically robust (yet clinically relevant) was entered into the regression model in order to minimize the effect of colinearity. The selection process was guided by consistency (less than 5% missing values) and maximal imbalances between groups (as estimated by absolute standardized differences, which are independent of the sample size and variable unit) [19]. Coefficients were computed by the method of maximum likelihood. The calibration of models was assessed by the Hosmer–Lemeshow goodness-of-fit statistic (good fit was defined as p value > 0.05), and discrimination was assessed by the area under the receiver operating characteristics curve (with a value of 1 indicating perfect discrimination, and a value of 0.5 indicating the effects of chance alone). Correlations were tested using the Spearman's method. Two-tailed p values < 0.05 were considered significant. Data were analyzed using the IBM SPSS Statistics for Windows (Version 19.0, IBM Corp Armonk, NY, USA).

Results

Study population

The inclusion period lasted from 2 to 12 months depending on centers, between June 2015 and May 2016. Four hundred seventy-seven patients mechanically ventilated for more than 24 h were screened (Fig. 1). Sixty-seven patients died before weaning start, and 161 patients were excluded because of either a do-not-reintubate decision at time of inclusion ($n = 72$), unavailability of pleural ultrasound ($n = 63$), or drainage of pleural effusion before inclusion ($n = 26$). Thus, the present study comprises 249 patients assessed with lung ultrasonography at weaning initiation. Median duration of mechanical ventilation before weaning was 4 [2–7] days. The weaning trajectories are summarized in Fig. 1. Two hundred and three patients succeeded the first SBT, and 200 of them were extubated (the remainder three patients were not extubated despite the success of the first SBT because of borderline cough, and experienced a novel complication leading to death before any extubation attempt).

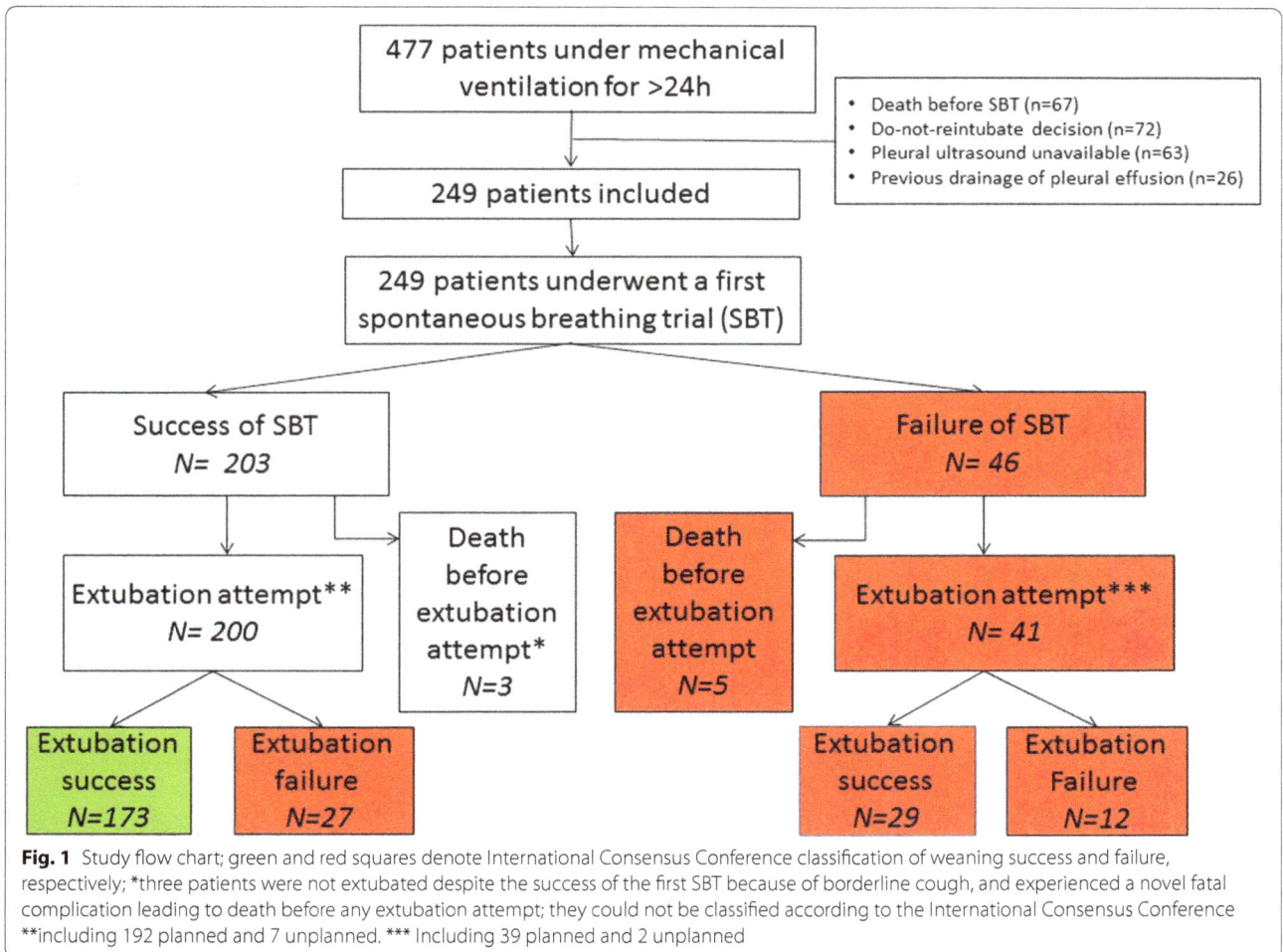

Fig. 1 Study flow chart; green and red squares denote International Consensus Conference classification of weaning success and failure, respectively; *three patients were not extubated despite the success of the first SBT because of borderline cough, and experienced a novel fatal complication leading to death before any extubation attempt; they could not be classified according to the International Consensus Conference **including 192 planned and 7 unplanned. *** Including 39 planned and 2 unplanned

Forty-six patients (18%) failed the first SBT; 41 of them succeeded a subsequent SBT and were extubated latter in the course of weaning, while the remainder five patients died before any extubation attempt. Reasons for SBT failure were respiratory rate > 35 breaths/min with increased accessory muscle activity ($n = 17$), $SpO_2 < 90\%$, while on $FiO_2 \geq 0.5$ ($n = 6$), systolic blood pressure < 90 mmHg or > 180 mmHg ($n = 2$), or a combination of those reasons ($n = 22$).

Overall, 241 patients were extubated during the weaning process, while eight patients died before any extubation attempt. Among the 241 patients extubated, 232 were planned and nine unplanned (including one accidental and eight self-extubations). After extubation, 95 (40%) patients received noninvasive ventilation prophylactically, while twelve (5%) received it for post-extubation acute respiratory failure. A total of 39 (16%) patients failed extubation. The main reason for reintubation was acute respiratory failure ($n = 23$, 73%).

Prevalence and risk factors for pleural effusion

A moderate-to-large pleural effusion was detected in 81 of 249 patients assessed at weaning initiation, for a prevalence of 33%, 95% confidence interval: 27–39%. Most of pleural effusions were homogeneously anechoic ($n = 74$, 93%) and associated with pulmonary condensation or atelectasis ($n = 68$, 85%) (see the online supplement, Table e1, Additional file 1). Seventy-six (31%) patients had a bilateral pleural effusion. The maximal interpleural distance was equally located either on the left ($n = 41$, 51%) or right side ($n = 40$, 49%). Patients with moderate-to-large pleural effusions at weaning initiation were older, had more baseline comorbidities and more organ failures before weaning as compared to their counterparts (see the online supplement, Table e4). In multivariable analysis, older age, McCabe class 2, cardiac disease, acute respiratory failure as cause of intubation, and need for dialysis before the first SBT were the five independent factors associated with a moderate-to-large pleural effusion at initiation of weaning (Table 1).

Outcome of weaning

According to the International Consensus Conference, the 249 patients were classified as follows: 173 (69%) weaning successes (a first successful SBT followed by successful extubation); 76 (31%) weaning failures (including 46 who failed the first SBT and 27 who succeeded the first SBT but failed extubation); three unclassifiable patients (despite the success of the first SBT, they were not extubated because of borderline

Table 1 Univariate and multivariable analysis of factors associated with moderate-to-large pleural effusion

Variables	Missing values, n (%)	Absolute standardized differences	Odd ratio (95% confidence interval), p value by logistic regression	
			Univariate	Multivariable
Age (per year)	0	60.5	1.04 (1.02–1.06), $p < 0.001$	1.03 (1.01–1.05), $p = 0.017$
SAPS II (per point)	0	26.9	1.02 (1.0–1.03), $p = 0.048$	I/NR
Mc Cabe class II (yes vs. no)	0	51.8	4.7 (2.1–10.3), $p < 0.001$	4.2 (1.8–9.9), $p = 0.001$
Cancer or hematological malignancy (yes vs. no)	0	47	3.5 (1.7–7.2), $p = 0.001$	NI
Cardiac disease (yes vs. no)	0	55.1	3.3 (1.1–3.3), $p < 0.001$	2.2 (1.1–4.4), $p = 0.02$
Left ventricle ejection fraction at cardiac ultrasound (%),	44 (18%)	52.9	0.96 (0.93–0.98), $p < 0.001$	NI
Supra-ventricular arrhythmias (yes vs. no)	0	35.8	2.3 (1.3–4.2), $p = 0.007$	NI
Acute respiratory failure as cause of intubation (yes vs. no)	0	31.9	1.9 (1.3–3.9), $p = 0.02$	1.8 (0.98–3.2), $p = 0.059$
Dialysis (yes vs. no)	0	31.5	2.5 (1.2–5.4), $p = 0.02$	2.0 (0.9–4.6), $p = 0.088$
Serum Creatinine (per µmol/L)	0	25.8	1.0 (0.99–1.00), $p = 0.20$	NI
Septic shock (yes vs. no)	0	25.4	1.7 (0.98–2.9), $p = 0.06$	I/NR
ARDS (yes vs. no)	0	22.2	1.7 (0.91–3.1), $p = 0.098$	I/NR
Duration of MV before first SBT (per day)	0	19	1.04 (0.99–1.1), $p = 0.15$	NI

SAPS II simplified acute physiology score, *COPD* chronic obstructive pulmonary disease, *ARDS* acute respiratory distress syndrome, *SBT* spontaneous breathing trial, *NI* not included, *I/NR* included, but not retained by the final model

Among related univariate factors, only the most statistically robust (yet clinically relevant) was entered into the regression model in order to minimize the effect of colinearity. The selection process was guided by consistency (less than 5% missing values) and maximal imbalances between groups (as estimated by absolute standardized differences) as follows: Mc Cabe class II was selected among Mc Cabe class II, cancer and hematological malignancy; dialysis was selected among creatininemia and dialysis; cardiac disease was selected among supra-ventricular arrhythmias, left ventricle ejection fraction and cardiac disease; ARDS was selected among duration of mechanical ventilation before the first spontaneous breathing trial and ARDS before inclusion. The multivariable model showed a good calibration as assessed by the Hosmer and Lemeshow goodness-of-fit test [χ^2 (8 df) = 6.42, $p = 0.60$] and a fair discrimination as assessed by the receiver operating characteristics curve [area under the curve of 0.74 (0.67–0.80), $p < 0.001$]

cough, and experienced a novel complication leading to death before any extubation attempt) (Fig. 1). According to the WIND classification, 161 (65%) patients had a short weaning, 60 (24%) had a difficult weaning, and 28 (11%) had a prolonged weaning. The presence of a moderate-to-large pleural effusion at weaning initiation was associated with more failures of the first SBT [27 (33%) vs. 19 (11%), $p < 0.001$], more weaning failures [37 (47%) vs. 36 (22%), $p < 0.001$], less ventilator-free days at day 28 (21 [5–24] vs. 23 [16–26], $p = 0.01$), and a higher mortality at day 28 [14 (17%) vs. 14 (8%), $p = 0.04$] (Table 2, Fig. 2). All variables associated with weaning failure are shown in Table 3 and Table e5. In multivariable analysis, PaO_2/FiO_2 ratio, chronic obstructive pulmonary disease, a longer duration of mechanical ventilation prior to weaning, and the presence of moderate-to-large pleural effusion at weaning initiation were the four independent factors associated with weaning failure (Table 4). In sensitivity analyses, the association of pleural effusion with weaning failure also persisted after adjustment on SAPS II, in selected centers using the T-piece trial, or in those using a low-level pressure support, and when considering pleural effusions deemed drainable (as defined by a maximal interpleural distance ≥ 15 mm with the effusion visible over three intercostal spaces) or those considered large (as defined by a maximal interpleural distance ≥ 25 mm) [4, 17] (Table e3). A moderate-to-large pleural effusion was detected in 60 (28%) of 218 patients assessed on the day of first extubation attempt. The extubation failure rate was higher in patients with a moderate-to-large pleural effusion on the day of extubation as compared to their counterparts [14 (23%) vs. 19 (12%), $p = 0.04$]; of note, this extubation failure rate was similar in patients with or without pleural effusion assessed earlier, at weaning initiation [24 (15%) vs 15 (20%), $p = 0.31$]. As compared to patients without effusion ($n = 168$), those with a unilateral ($n = 21$) or bilateral ($n = 60$) moderate-to-large pleural effusion had similarly altered weaning outcomes, including SBT failure [19 (11.3%) vs. 8 (38.1%) vs. 19 (31.7%), $p < 0.001$] and weaning failure [37 (22.0%) vs. 11 (52.4%) vs. 28 (46.7%), $p < 0.001$].

Evolution of pleural effusion during difficult weaning

Among the 46 patients who failed the first SBT, lung ultrasonography was repeated 24 and 48 h later in 41 and 31 patients, respectively. Patients in whom diuretics and/or ultrafiltration were used had a lower fluid balance as compared with their counterparts (-484 [$-1210–330$] vs. 858 [205–1806] mL after 24 h, $p < 0.001$), but this depletive strategy did not alter the interpleural distance

(see the online supplement, Table e2, Additional file 1). Fluid balance was not significantly correlated with changes in interpleural distance (ρ 0.13, $p = 0$, 17, see Figure e1 of the online supplement, Additional file 2). Pleural effusion was drained in only four patients during weaning.

Discussion

We herein report the largest study assessing pleural effusion during weaning from mechanical ventilation. A moderate-to-large pleural effusion was detected by ultrasound examination in one-third of 249 patients at initiation of weaning and was associated with weaning failure by multivariable analysis. Depletive strategies did not alter pleural effusion volume on the short term in patients with difficult weaning.

Prevalence and risk factors for pleural effusion

In our study, one-third of patients had a moderate-to-large pleural effusion at the initiation of the weaning process. This prevalence is higher than that of 13% reported by Dres et al. [9]. This discrepancy may be explained by differences in definitions used. Volume of pleural fluid was estimated in our report according to interpleural distance, which may be more sensitive than the classification of the British Thoracic Society [20] used in the latter study; indeed, patients with moderate-to-large pleural effusion in our study had a median interpleural distance inferior to the value found in the Dres' study (27 [20–41] vs. 45 [30–60] mm). Other differences between these two studies include patient's comorbidities (with more patients included with cardiac diseases in our report) and/or timing of inclusion (with less patients excluded because of prior pleural drainage before SBT in our study).

Risk factors for pleural effusion found in our study are in accordance with previous reports [1, 2]. Congestive heart failure is one of the leading factors associated with the occurrence of pleural effusion in ICU [1]. All patients intubated for acute respiratory failure had acute cardiac failure or pneumonia, two common risk factors for pleural effusion [1]. Our study suggests that diastolic dysfunction may be of importance in the association of cardiac failure with pleural effusion. Acute renal failure has also been previously reported as a risk factor for nonmalignant pleural effusions, an association possibly mediated by fluid overload [21]. The association of Mc Cabe class (i.e., a rapidly fatal underlying disease) with pleural effusion may be driven by other comorbidities like liver cirrhosis, cancer, and hypoalbuminemia [22, 23].

Table 2 Characteristics and outcome of 249 mechanically ventilated patients with or without moderate-to-large pleural effusion at first spontaneous breathing trial

Variables	Moderate-to-large pleural effusion		p value
	Absent (n = 168)	Present (n = 81)	
Male gender	98 (58%)	52 (64%)	0.38
Age (years)	61 [50–72]	69 [60–80]	< 0.001
SAPS II score at ICU admission	49 [37–62]	52 [41–67]	0.07
Comorbidities			
Neurological disease	22 (13%)	6 (7%)	0.18
Cardiac disease	93 (55%)	65 (80%)	< 0.001
Cirrhosis	12 (7%)	9 (11%)	0.29
Chronic renal failure	22 (13%)	16 (20%)	0.17
Cancer or hematological malignancy	16 (10%)	22 (27%)	< 0.001
Main reason for intubation			
Coma	54 (32%)	9 (11%)	< 0.001
Acute respiratory failure	51 (30%)	37 (46%)	0.02
Septic shock	22 (13%)	12 (15%)	0.71
Others	41 (24%)	23 (28%)	0.5
From ICU admission to first SBT			
ARDS	32 (19%)	23 (28%)	0.096
Duration of MV before the first SBT	4 [2–7]	4 [3–9]	0.09
Dialysis	15 (9%)	16 (20%)	0.015
Biological and ultrasound data at first SBT			
Serum creatinine (μmol/L)	74 [55–119]	90 [60–164]	0.07
Serum protide (mg/L)	59 [54–66]	59 [51–63]	0.19
Bilateral pleural effusion	16 (10%)	60 (74%)	< 0.001
Maximal interpleural distance (mm)	0 [0–5]	27 [20–41]	< 0.001
Condensation or atelectasis of lung adjacent to the pleural effusion at ultrasound	–	68 (84%)	
Left ventricle ejection fraction (%)	60 [50–60]	50 [39–60]	< 0.001
Outcome			
Pleural effusion drainage during weaning	0	4 (5%)	0.005
Prophylactic NIV post-extubation	62 (38%)	33 (43%)	0.39
Failure of the first SBT	19 (11%)	27 (33%)	< 0.001
Extubation failure	24 (15%)	15 (20%)	0.31
Weaning failure[a]	36 (22%)	37 (47%)	< 0.001
Weaning group[b]			0.03
Short weaning	118 (70%)	43 (53%)	
Difficult weaning	38 (20%)	26 (32%)	
Prolonged weaning	16 (10%)	12 (15%)	
Tracheotomy	4 (2%)	2 (3%)	0.97
VFD from first SBT to day 28 (days)	23 [16–26]	21 [5–24]	0.01
Death in ICU	14 (8%)	13 (16%)	0.07
Death at day 28	14 (8%)	14 (17%)	0.04

Values are indicating number (%) or median [1st–3rd quartile]

[a] According to the international conference consensus (three patients could not be classified)

[b] According to the WIND study classification

SAPS II simplified acute physiology score, *ARDS* acute respiratory distress syndrome, *SBT* spontaneous breathing trial, *NIV* noninvasive ventilation, *ICU* intensive care unit, *VFD* ventilator-free days

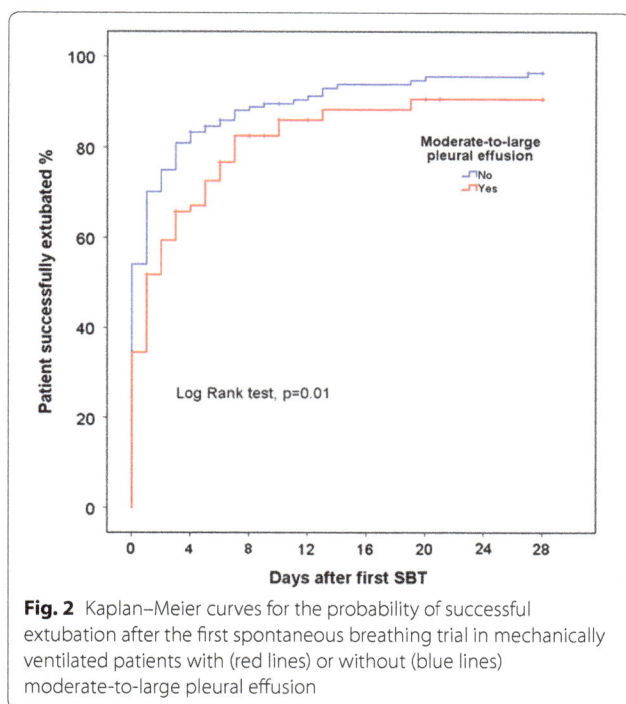

Fig. 2 Kaplan–Meier curves for the probability of successful extubation after the first spontaneous breathing trial in mechanically ventilated patients with (red lines) or without (blue lines) moderate-to-large pleural effusion

Pleural effusion and weaning outcomes

Our study is the first to show an association between moderate-to-large pleural effusion on the one hand and worse weaning outcomes and survival on the other hand. Dres et al. found similar weaning outcomes in patients with or without pleural effusion, but the limited number of patients with pleural effusions in their report ($n = 18$) weakened their conclusions [9]. Our findings are consistent with a previous report by Mattison et al., suggesting an association between pleural effusion and a longer duration of mechanical ventilation [2]. Although pleural effusion in patients with early ARDS do not seem to significantly influence lung physiology and gas exchange [3], its role in the latter stages of mechanical ventilation seems more relevant [4]. Physiological alterations associated with pleural effusion may worsen the respiratory load during the weaning process. Indeed, physiological studies showed that pleural effusion increases chest wall volume and decreases the length of inspiratory muscles and thus their efficiency and power [5, 6]. Umbrello et al. recently showed that during weaning, drainage of a unilateral pleural effusion

improves diaphragmatic contractile activity [24]. This improvement could decrease dyspnea and mitigate weaning failure. Pleural fluid accumulation may also result in relaxation atelectasis of the adjacent lung. In our study, most pleural effusions (85%) were associated with condensation or atelectasis.

Clinical implications

There was no significant association between fluid balance and the evolution of pleural effusion during the 48 h following SBT failure. However, the negative fluid balance achieved was modest in the depletive group and this limitation precludes any definite conclusion. Pleural drainage with ultrasonography guidance has a low risk of complication under mechanical ventilator support [7] and may improve oxygenation, respiratory mechanics [4], and diaphragm performance [6, 24]. Removal of pleural fluid may therefore decrease the work of breathing and increase the ability of patients to succeed weaning. Further studies are needed to test whether a strategy of aggressive diuretic management or drainage of pleural effusions, in mechanically ventilated patients entering the weaning process, with others risk factors of weaning failure or a SBT failure, has the potential to decrease its duration [25].

Strengths and limitations

Strengths of our study include the large sample size, the prospective and multicentric design, and the use of ultrasound, which is currently considered the most sensitive method to detect pleural effusion at bedside. Our study has several limitations. First, only 249 of the 477 screened patients were included, a fact that may alter the external validity of our prevalence estimation. Second, the inter- or intra-observer agreement for pleural ultrasonography was not evaluated, but several reports previously demonstrated an excellent agreement for the measurement of left or right maximal interpleural distance [26]. Third, the physicians in charge of the patient were not fully blinded to the ultrasound examination results, and this may have theoretically influenced extubation decision and outcomes. However, criteria for SBT result were defined a priori and independent from ultrasound findings. Fourth, no estimation of respiratory drive (e.g., with airway occlusion pressure) nor respiratory muscle strength (e.g., with maximal inspiratory

Table 3 Variables associated with weaning failure in 246 mechanically ventilated patients (three patients could not be classified according to the international conference consensus definition)

Variables	Weaning success (n = 173)	Weaning failure (n = 73)	p value
Male gender	98 (57%)	49 (67%)	0.13
Age (years)	61 [52–73]	69 [60–79]	0.006
Body mass index (kg/m^2)	26 [22–29]	27 [22–32]	0.07
SAPS II at ICU admission	49 [38–62]	49 [39–65]	0.73
Comorbidities			
COPD	23 (13%)	23 (32%)	0.001
Cardiac disease	101 (58%)	55 (75%)	0.01
Main reason for intubation			
Coma	54 (31%)	9 (12%)	0.002
Acute respiratory failure	48 (27%)	39 (53%)	< 0.001
Septic shock	24 (14%)	8 (11%)	0.54
Others	47 (27%)	17 (23%)	0.53
From ICU admission to first SBT			
ARDS	28 (16%)	27 (37%)	< 0.001
Neuromuscular blockade	26 (15%)	28 (38%)	< 0.001
Septic shock	61 (35%)	39 (53%)	0.01
VAP	17 (10%)	16 (22%)	0.01
Supra-ventricular arrhythmias	32 (19%)	22 (30%)	0.04
Duration of MV before first SBT	3 [2–6]	6 [3–12]	< 0.001
Dialysis	22 (13%)	8 (11%)	0.70
Fluid balance between ICU admission and first SBT (L)	2.8 [0.9–6.4]	5.7 [0.7–11.4]	0.01
Biological and ultrasound data at first SBT			
PaO$_2$/FiO$_2$ ratio (mmHg)	307 [242–385]	247 [200–299]	< 0.001
Moderate-to-large pleural effusion	42 (24%)	37 (51%)	< 0.001
Drainable pleural effusion	36 (21%)	29 (40%)	0.002
Large pleural effusion	21 (12%)	25 (34%)	< 0.001
Left ventricle ejection fraction (%, n = 205)	60 [50–60]	55 [40–60]	0.06
Outcome			
Pleural effusion drainage during weaning	0	4 (6%)	0.01
Prophylactic NIV post-extubation	65 (38%)	30 (44%)	0.35
Tracheotomy	1 (1%)	5 (7%)	0.01
VFD from first SBT to day 28 (days)	23 [20–26]	11 [0–21]	< 0.001
Death in ICU	5 (3%)	19 (26%)	< 0.001
Death at day 28	8 (5%)	17 (23%)	< 0.001

Values are indicating number (%), or median [1st–3rd quartile]

SAPS II simplified acute physiology score, *COPD* chronic obstructive pulmonary disease, *ARDS* acute respiratory distress syndrome, *VAP* ventilator-associated pneumonia, *SBT* spontaneous breathing trial, *NIV* noninvasive ventilation, *ICU* intensive care unit, *VFD* ventilator-free days

pressures) was performed. Last, a significant decrease in pleural effusion during difficult weaning may have required more time, and/or more intense depletive fluid management [27].

Conclusion

Moderate-to-large pleural effusion was found in one-third of patients at initiation of weaning and associated with worse outcomes. Depletive strategies did not rapidly alter its evolution. Further studies should test the clinical

Table 4 Univariate and multivariable logistic regression of factors associated with weaning failure (n = 246)

Variables	Missing values, n (%)	Absolute standardized differences	Odd ratio (95% confidence interval), p value by logistic regression	
			Univariate	Multivariable
Age (per year)	0	47	1.03 (1.01–1.05), $p = 0.01$	1.02 (0.997–1.05), $p = 0.08$
Body mass index (per kg/m^2)	6 (2%)	32	1.06 (1.01–1.11), $p = 0.02$	I/NR
COPD (yes vs. no)	0	48	3.0 (1.6–5.8), $p = 0.001$	2.2 (1.02–4.7), $p = 0.045$
Cardiac disease (yes vs. no)	0	37	2.2 (1.2–4.0), $p = 0.01$	I/NR
Left ventricle ejection fraction at cardiac ultrasound (%)	44 (18%)	27	0.98 (0.96–1.0), $p = 0.09$	NI
Supra–ventricular arrhythmias (yes vs. no)	0	26	1.9 (1.01–3.6), $p = 0.046$	NI
Septic shock (yes vs. no)	0	37	2.1 (1.2–3.7), $p = 0.01$	I/NR
Fluid balance between ICU admission and first SBT (per L)	15 (6%)	44	1.07 (1.03–1.12), $p = 0.002$	NI
Acute respiratory failure as cause of intubation (yes vs. no)	0	55	3.0 (1.7–5.2), $p < 0.001$	NI
PaO$_2$/FiO$_2$ ratio (per mmHg)	3 (1%)	58	0.994 (0.991–0.997), $p < 0.001$	0.996 (0.993–1.0), $p = 0.03$
Duration of MV before the first SBT (per day)	0	57	1.11 (1.06–1.17), $p < 0.001$	1.11 (1.05–1.17), $p < 0.001$
ARDS before the first SBT (yes vs. no)	0	49	3.0 (1.6–5.7), $p < 0.001$	NI
Neuromuscular blockade before the first SBT (yes vs. no)	0	54	3.5 (1.9–6.6), $p < 0.001$	NI
VAP before the first SBT (yes vs. no)	0	33	2.6 (1.2–5.4), $p = 0.01$	NI
Moderate-to-large pleural effusion (yes vs. no)	0	58	3.2 (1.8–5.7), $p < 0.001$	3.0 (1.5–5.8), $p = 0.001$

SAPS II simplified acute physiology score, *COPD* chronic obstructive pulmonary disease, *ARDS* acute respiratory distress syndrome, *VAP* ventilator-associated pneumonia, *SBT* spontaneous breathing trial, *NI* not included, *I/NR* included, but not retained by the final model

Among related univariate factors, only the most statistically robust (yet clinically relevant) was entered into the regression model in order to minimize the effect of colinearity. The selection process was guided by consistency (less than 5% missing values) and maximal imbalances between groups (as estimated by absolute standardized differences), as follows: cardiac disease was selected among supra-ventricular arrhythmias, left ventricle ejection fraction and cardiac disease; septic shock was selected among fluid balance between ICU admission and first SBT and septic shock; PaO$_2$/FiO$_2$ ratio was selected among acute respiratory failure as cause of intubation and PaO$_2$/FiO$_2$ ratio; duration of MV before the first SBT was selected among neuromuscular blockade, duration of MV before the first SBT, VAP, and ARDS. The multivariable model showed a good calibration as assessed by the Hosmer and Lemeshow goodness-of-fit test [χ^2 (8 df) = 6.8, $p = 0.56$] and a fair discrimination as assessed by the receiver operating characteristics curve [area under the curve of 0.76 (0.69–0.82), $p < 0.001$]

usefulness and safety of reducing moderate-to-large pleural effusion at initiation of ventilator weaning, either by aggressive depletion or drainage.

Abbreviations
SBT: spontaneous breathing trial; ARDS: acute respiratory distress syndrome; ICU: intensive care unit.

Authors' contributions
Dr Razazi had full access to all of the data in the study and takes responsibility for the integrity of the data and the accuracy of the data analysis. Dr Razazi, Dr Mekontso Dessap contributed to initial study design, analysis, interpretation of data, drafting of the submitted article, critical revisions for intellectual content. Dr Florence Boissier, Dr Mathilde Neuville, Dr Sébastien Jochmans, Dr Martial Tchir, Dr Faten May, Dr Nicolas de Prost, Dr Christian Brun-Buisson, MD, Dr Guillaume Carteaux contributed to study design and analysis, interpretation of data, drafting of the submitted article, critical revisions for intellectual content. All authors read and approved the final manuscript.

Author details
[1] AP-HP, DHU A-TVB, Service de Réanimation Médicale, Hôpitaux Universitaires Henri Mondor, 94010 Créteil, France. [2] Faculté de Médecine de Créteil, IMRB, GRC CARMAS, Université Paris Est Créteil, 94010 Créteil, France. [3] Unité U955 (Institut Mondor de Recherche Biomédicale), INSERM, Créteil, France. [4] Service de Réanimation Médicale, Centre Hospitalier Universitaire de Poitiers, Poitiers 86021, France. [5] AP-HP, Service de Réanimation Médicale, Hôpital Européen Georges Pompidou, 75015 Paris, France. [6] AP-HP, Réanimation Médicale et des Maladies Infectieuses, Hôpital Bichat Claude Bernard, Paris, France. [7] Département de Médecine Intensive, Groupe Hospitalier Sud Ile-de-France, Hôpital de Melun, 77011 Melun, France. [8] Service de Réanimation, Centre Hospitalier de Villeneuve-Saint-Georges, 94190 Villeneuve-Saint-Georges, France.

Acknowledgements
This study was carried out as part of our routine clinical work.

Competing interests
The authors declare that they have no competing interests.

Funding
None.

References
1. Fartoukh M, Azoulay E, Galliot R, Le Gall J-R, Baud F, Chevret S, et al. Clinically documented pleural effusions in medical ICU patients: how useful is routine thoracentesis? Chest. 2002;121:178–84.
2. Mattison LE, Coppage L, Alderman DF, Herlong JO, Sahn SA. Pleural effusions in the medical ICU: prevalence, causes, and clinical implications. Chest. 1997;111:1018–23.

3. Chiumello D, Marino A, Cressoni M, Mietto C, Berto V, Gallazzi E, et al. Pleural effusion in patients with acute lung injury: a CT scan study. Crit Care Med. 2013;41:935–44.

4. Razazi K, Thille AW, Carteaux G, Beji O, Brun-Buisson C, Brochard L, et al. Effects of pleural effusion drainage on oxygenation, respiratory mechanics, and hemodynamics in mechanically ventilated patients. Ann Am Thorac Soc. 2014;11:1018–24.

5. De Troyer A, Leduc D, Cappello M, Gevenois PA. Mechanics of the canine diaphragm in pleural effusion. J Appl Physiol Bethesda Md. 1985;2012(113):785–90.

6. Estenne M, Yernault JC, De Troyer A. Mechanism of relief of dyspnea after thoracocentesis in patients with large pleural effusions. Am J Med. 1983;74:813–9.

7. Goligher EC, Leis JA, Fowler RA, Pinto R, Adhikari NKJ, Ferguson ND. Utility and safety of draining pleural effusions in mechanically ventilated patients: a systematic review and meta-analysis. Crit Care Lond Engl. 2011;15:R46.

8. Esteban A, Alía I, Ibañez J, Benito S, Tobin MJ. Modes of mechanical ventilation and weaning. A national survey of Spanish hospitals. The Spanish lung failure collaborative group. Chest. 1994;106:1188–93.

9. Dres M, Roux D, Pham T, Beurton A, Ricard J-D, Fartoukh M, et al. Prevalence and impact on weaning of pleural effusion at the time of liberation from mechanical ventilation: a multicenter prospective observational study. Anesthesiology. 2017;126:1107–15.

10. Boles J-M, Bion J, Connors A, Herridge M, Marsh B, Melot C, et al. Weaning from mechanical ventilation. Eur Respir J. 2007;29:1033–56.

11. Girault C, Bubenheim M, Abroug F, Diehl JL, Elatrous S, Beuret P, et al. Noninvasive ventilation and weaning in patients with chronic hypercapnic respiratory failure: a randomized multicenter trial. Am J Respir Crit Care Med. 2011;184:672–9.

12. Thille AW, Boissier F, Ben-Ghezala H, Razazi K, Mekontso-Dessap A, Brun-Buisson C, et al. Easily identified at-risk patients for extubation failure may benefit from noninvasive ventilation: a prospective before-after study. Crit Care Lond Engl. 2016;20:48.

13. Béduneau G, Pham T, Schortgen F, Piquilloud L, Zogheib E, Jonas M, et al. Epidemiology of Weaning Outcome according to a New Definition. The WIND Study. Am J Respir Crit Care Med. 2017;195:772–83.

14. Mekontso Dessap A, Roche-Campo F, Kouatchet A, Tomicic V, Beduneau G, Sonneville R, et al. Natriuretic peptide-driven fluid management during ventilator weaning: a randomized controlled trial. Am J Respir Crit Care Med. 2012;186:1256–63.

15. Yang PC, Luh KT, Chang DB, Wu HD, Yu CJ, Kuo SH. Value of sonography in determining the nature of pleural effusion: analysis of 320 cases. AJR Am J Roentgenol. 1992;159:29–33.

16. Volpicelli G, Elbarbary M, Blaivas M, Lichtenstein DA, Mathis G, Kirkpatrick AW, et al. International evidence-based recommendations for point-of-care lung ultrasound. Intensive Care Med. 2012;38:577–91.

17. Balik M, Plasil P, Waldauf P, Pazout J, Fric M, Otahal M, et al. Ultrasound estimation of volume of pleural fluid in mechanically ventilated patients. Intensive Care Med. 2006;32:318–21.

18. Lichtenstein D, Hulot JS, Rabiller A, Tostivint I, Mezière G. Feasibility and safety of ultrasound-aided thoracentesis in mechanically ventilated patients. Intensive Care Med. 1999;25:955–8.

19. Austin PC. Balance diagnostics for comparing the distribution of baseline covariates between treatment groups in propensity-score matched samples. Stat Med. 2009;28:3083–107.

20. Havelock T, Teoh R, Laws D, Gleeson F, BTS Pleural Disease Guideline Group. Pleural procedures and thoracic ultrasound: British Thoracic Society Pleural Disease Guideline 2010. Thorax. 2010;65(Suppl 2):ii61–76.

21. Walker SP, Morley AJ, Stadon L, De Fonseka D, Arnold DA, Medford AR, et al. Non-malignant pleural effusions (NMPE): a prospective study of 356 consecutive unselected patients. Chest. 2017;151(5):1099–105.

22. Mccabe WR, Jackson G. Gram-negative bacteremia: I. etiology and ecology. Arch Intern Med. 1962;110:847–55.

23. Light RW. Clinical practice. Pleural effusion. N Engl J Med. 2002;346:1971–7.

24. Umbrello M, Mistraletti G, Galimberti A, Piva IR, Cozzi O, Formenti P. Drainage of pleural effusion improves diaphragmatic function in mechanically ventilated patients. Crit Care Resusc J Australas Acad Crit Care Med. 2017;19:64–70.

25. Mayo P, Volpicelli G, Lerolle N, Schreiber A, Doelken P, Vieillard-Baron A. Ultrasonography evaluation during the weaning process: the heart, the diaphragm, the pleura and the lung. Intensive Care Med. 2016;42:1107–17.

26. Begot E, Grumann A, Duvoid T, Dalmay F, Pichon N, François B, et al. Ultrasonographic identification and semiquantitative assessment of unloculated pleural effusions in critically ill patients by residents after a focused training. Intensive Care Med. 2014;40:1475–80.

27. Giglioli C, Spini V, Landi D, Chiostri M, Romano SM, Calabretta R, et al. Congestive heart failure and decongestion ability of two different treatments: continuous renal replacement and diuretic therapy: experience of a cardiac step down unit. Acta Cardiol. 2013;68:355–64.

19

MicroDAIMON study: Microcirculatory DAIly MONitoring in critically ill patients

Claudia Scorcella[1], Elisa Damiani[1], Roberta Domizi[1], Silvia Pierantozzi[1], Stefania Tondi[1], Andrea Carsetti[1], Silvia Ciucani[1], Valentina Monaldi[1], Mara Rogani[1], Benedetto Marini[1], Erica Adrario[1], Rocco Romano[1], Can Ince[2], E. Christiaan Boerma[3] and Abele Donati[1]*

Abstract

Background: Until now, the prognostic value of microcirculatory alterations in critically ill patients has been mainly evaluated in highly selected subgroups. Aim of this study is to monitor the microcirculation daily in mixed group of Intensive Care Unit (ICU)-patients and to establish the association between (the evolution of) microcirculatory alterations and outcome.

Methods: This is a prospective longitudinal observational single-centre study in adult patients admitted to a 12-bed ICU in an Italian teaching hospital. Sublingual microcirculation was evaluated daily, from admission to discharge/death, using Sidestream Dark Field imaging. Videos were analysed offline to assess flow and density variables. Laboratory and clinical data were recorded simultaneously. A priori, a Microvascular Flow Index (MFI) < 2.6 was defined as abnormal. A binary logistic regression analysis was performed to evaluate the association between microcirculatory variables and outcomes; a Kaplan–Meier survival curve was built. Outcomes were ICU and 90-day mortality.

Results: A total of 97 patients were included. An abnormal MFI was present on day 1 in 20.6%, and in 55.7% of cases during ICU admission. Patients with a baseline MFI < 2.6 had higher ICU, in-hospital and 90-day mortality (45 vs. 15.6%, $p = 0.012$; 55 vs. 28.6%, $p = 0.035$; 55 vs. 26%, $p = 0.017$, respectively). An independent association between baseline MFI < 2.6 and outcome was confirmed in a binary logistic analysis (odds ratio 4.594 [1.340–15.754], $p = 0.015$). A heart rate (HR) ≥ 90 bpm was an adjunctive predictor of mortality. However, a model with stepwise inclusion of mean arterial pressure < 65 mmHg, HR ≥ 90 bpm, lactate > 2 mmol/L and MFI < 2.6 did not detect significant differences in ICU mortality. In case an abnormal MFI was present on day 1, ICU mortality was significantly higher in comparison with patients with an abnormal MFI after day 1 (38 vs. 6%, $p = 0.001$), indicating a time-dependent significant difference in prognostic value.

Conclusions: In a general ICU population, an abnormal microcirculation at baseline is an independent predictor for mortality. In this setting, additional routine daily microcirculatory monitoring did not reveal extra prognostic information. Further research is needed to integrate microcirculatory monitoring in a set of commonly available hemodynamic variables.

Keywords: Microcirculation, Physiologic monitoring, Critical illness, Tachycardia, Video microscopy, Capillaries

*Correspondence: a.donati@univpm.it
[1] Anaesthesia and Intensive Care, Department of Biomedical Sciences and Public Health, Università Politecnica delle Marche, via Tronto 10/a, 60126 Ancona, Italy

Background

The microcirculation is a vast network of small vessels (terminal arterioles, capillaries and venules < 100 μm diameter) in which the exchange of oxygen and nutrients with tissues takes place [1]. Its derangement, defined as "microcirculatory shock" [2], is recognised as an important cause of organ dysfunction in critically ill patients, affected by various disease states, such as sepsis, severe trauma, haemorrhagic shock and post-cardiac arrest [2–5]. Furthermore, microcirculatory abnormalities and its persistence despite adequate macro-hemodynamic resuscitation were independently associated with morbidity and mortality in many critical conditions [6–12].

Today, the development of new technologies of in vivo video microscopy and its integration in easy-to-handle microscopes as in Sidestream Dark Field (SDF) imaging allow us to assess the (sublingual) microcirculation at the bedside, in a non-invasive way [13]. However, until 2015, data on microcirculatory alterations in the Intensive Care Unit (ICU) were restricted to small sample-sized studies in high-risk patients [7, 8, 14].

The MicroSOAP study by Vellinga and colleagues [15] gave a first insight in the *prevalence* of microcirculatory alterations in a large number of ICU patients. However, due to its design with a single time-point observation, the *incidence* in a time-dependent manner remains to be elucidated. Primary aim of the study was to detect a difference in the incidence of microvascular flow abnormalities between ICU survivors and non-survivors. Secondary outcomes were long-term mortality (in-hospital mortality and 90-day mortality) and development of organ dysfunction (described by sequential organ failure assessment, SOFA).

Methods
Patients enrolment and data collection

The MicroDAIMON (Microcirculation DAIly MONitoring in critically ill patients) is a single-centre prospective observational study (clinicaltrials.gov, NCT 02649088 registered on 23 December; retrospectively registered). The recruiting phase was performed in a 9-month period in 2013 (from 1 April to 31 December) in a 12-bed mixed ICU of an Italian teaching hospital with a mean number of yearly-admitted patients of 400. The ICU was structured in three subunits of four beds each, caring for respiratory, traumatology and medical critically ill patients, respectively. For the study purpose, each subunit was subsequently included and monitored during a 3-month period for patients' screening and the recruitment: from 1 April to 30 June 2013, the medical subunit, from 1 July to 30 September 2013, the traumatology subunit and from 1st October to 31st December 2013, the respiratory subunit.

Patients were screened and included in the study within the first 12 h from ICU admission. Exclusion criteria were age < 18 years, lack of informed consent and pathophysiological conditions that may interfere with the sublingual microcirculation videos acquisition (maxillofacial traumas/surgery, oral bleeding, mucositis, etc.). In context to the microcirculatory assessments, demographic, laboratory, microbiologic, hemodynamic and other clinical data were recorded. All patients were followed up for 90 days after the ICU admission.

The study protocol was approved by the Local Ethics Committee and conducted in respect of the principles of Helsinki declaration (last revision, Edinburgh 2000). A written informed consent was obtained from all the included subjects or their next of kin in compliance with national applicable laws.

Microcirculation assessment

The sublingual microcirculation was evaluated at the moment of the inclusion and every 24 h until discharge/death with SDF imaging (Microscan®, Microvision Medical, Amsterdam, The Netherlands) [13].

The video acquisition technique is extensively described in previous papers [16]. For every session, videos from at least five different sites were registered trying to obtain a good video quality and to avoid artefacts that may affect flow or vessels density variables [16].

The three best videos were chosen from each session, in compliance with recommendations from Massey et al. [17] and blindly analysed offline with a dedicated software (Automated Vascular Analysis, AVA Software 3.0, MicroVision Medical, Amsterdam, The Netherlands) by a restricted group of four experienced investigators. Interobserver variability was calculated, based on the simultaneous analysis of ten randomly selected SDF videos by all the investigators. Variables of flow (Microvascular Flow Index, MFI and proportion of perfused vessels, PPV), as well as capillary density (total vessel density, TVD, perfused vessel density, PVD) and flow distribution (Heterogeneity Index, HI) were calculated according to international criteria [18, 19]. Flow was scored per quadrant as 0 (no flow), 1 (intermittent flow), 2 (sluggish flow) and 3 (continuous flow). The MFI is the average over 4 quadrants × 3 areas of interest. Total vessel density (TVD, mm/mm^2) was calculated as the total length of vessels divided by the total area of the image. The percentage of perfused vessels (PPV) was estimated as follows: $100 \times$ [(total number of grid crossings − [no flow + intermittent flow])/total number of grid crossings] and expressed as percentage. The perfused vessel density (PVD, mm/mm^2) was estimated by multiplying TVD by PPV as estimated with the De Backer method. The Flow Heterogeneity Index (FHI, arbitrary units) was calculated as the highest MFI minus the lowest MFI, divided by the mean MFI of all sublingual sites [18].

Analogous to previous data, a threshold for the MFI < 2.6 was a priori established to define an abnormal microcirculation [3, 8, 15, 20].

Statistical analysis

Data analysis was conducted with SPSS Software 17.0 (IBM, New York, NY) and GraphPad Prism 6 (Graph-Pad Software, La Jolla, CA). All data are presented as mean ± standard deviation (SD) or median [interquartile range, IQR].

Descriptive statistics were performed to obtain patients' baseline characteristics. Quantitative variables distribution was tested with Kolmogorov–Smirnov normality test. Parametric (Student's t test with Welch's correction) and nonparametric tests (Mann–Whitney U test) were applied to describe the differences between groups for the variables of interest as appropriate. Fisher's exact test was performed for comparisons between categorical variables, and the results are presented as percentage, odds ratio (OR) and 95% confidence interval (CI). Kaplan–Meier 90-day survival curves with Tarone–Ware test for the comparison of the hazard ratio between groups were built for the survival analysis.

Binary logistic regression analysis was performed with a forward stepwise entry method. A p value of less than 0.05 was considered statistically significant.

Results

Population characteristics

During the study period, 40, 37 and 38 patients were admitted, respectively, in the medical, traumatology and respiratory ICU subunits, for a total amount of 115 patients. Hundred patients met the inclusion criteria. All the patients were included in the study within 12 h from ICU admission, with no exceptions due to timing or organizational issues. Three patients were a posteriori excluded because no SDF videos were available for the baseline assessment. Therefore, 97 patients were included in the final analysis. The flow chart for the patients' inclusion process is illustrated in Additional file 1.

Baseline characteristics of the patients are illustrated in Table 1. Patients were predominantly male (66%) with a median age of 67 years [46–75], a mean acute physiology and chronic health evaluation (APACHE) II score of 16 ± 7 and a median SOFA score of 7 [4–10]; the most frequent cause of ICU admission was trauma (38.1%). Patients admitted for sepsis represented the 9.3% of the sample. During the ICU stay, ten more patients developed sepsis: two trauma patients (5.4%), one neurologic patient (4.8%), two respiratory patients (18.2%) and five other patients (26.3%).

Median ICU length of stay was 7 [4–15] days; ICU mortality was 21.6%, in-hospital mortality 34%, 90-day mortality 31.9% (two patients died in the hospital after 90 days from ICU admission).

Microcirculatory abnormalities at baseline and outcome

2455 videos were collected and analysed offline to obtain microcirculatory variables. The coefficient of variation (inter-observer variability) for MFI was 1.4 ± 3% for small vessels. Baseline microcirculatory variables are described in Table 1. The incidence of MFI abnormality at the day of ICU admission was 20.6%.

ICU non-survivors showed a higher baseline APACHE II score and SOFA score, higher age, heart rate (HR), Cumulative Vasopressor Index [21], arterial lactate level, serum creatinine and lower platelets count (Table 1).

Subsequently, patients were divided into two groups based on normal (≥ 2.6) or abnormal (< 2.6) baseline MFI. In comparison with patients with a normal MFI at baseline, patients with an abnormal MFI showed a higher ICU mortality (45 vs. 15.6%, $p = 0.012$) (Table 1), in-hospital mortality (55 vs. 28.6%, $p = 0.035$) and 90-day mortality (55 vs. 26%, $p = 0.017$). (Additional files 2, 3)

Survival analysis, by Kaplan–Meier method, confirmed a significant difference between the two groups for 90-day mortality (Tarone–Ware $\chi^2 = 6.15$, $p = 0.003$) (Fig. 1a). In the binary logistic regression analysis, the presence of an abnormal MFI at baseline was associated with ICU mortality (OR 4.594 [95% CI 1.340–15.754], $p = 0.015$) independently of the APACHE II score (Table 2).

The role of tachycardia in combination with an abnormal microcirculation was additionally tested. Patients were divided into four groups based on the presence of tachycardia (defined as the presence of an HR ≥ 90 beats per minute, bpm) [22–25] and/or MFI abnormality at the baseline. ICU mortality was significantly different between the four groups (overall $\chi^2 = 12.76$, $p = 0.002$). Survival analysis confirmed a significant difference between the groups in terms of 90-day mortality (Tarone–Ware $\chi^2 = 24.98$, $p < 0.0001$) with a survival rate as low as 12.5% among patients with tachycardia plus abnormal MFI (Fig. 1b). The combination of tachycardia and an abnormal MFI on day 1 was associated with an increased risk for ICU mortality (OR 10.732 [95% CI 1.685–68.354], $p = 0.012$) independently of the APACHE II score (Table 2).

Integration of an abnormal microcirculation in a set of common hemodynamic variables

In order to clarify the additional prognostic value of an abnormal microcirculation (MFI < 2.6) at baseline in a set of commonly available hemodynamic variables, i.e. mean arterial blood pressure (MAP), HR and lactate,

Table 1 Baseline characteristics and comparison between ICU survivors versus non-survivors

Patients characteristics	n	All (97)	ICU survivors (76)	ICU non-survivors (21)	p
Male gender (n, %)	97	64 (66)	50 (65.8)	14 (66.7)	1
Age (years, n)	97	67 [46–75]	64 [44–73]	71 [56–81]	0.034
APACHE II (pts)	97	16 ± 7	14 ± 7	22 ± 6	< 0.001
SOFA (pts)	97	7 [4–10]	6 [4–9]	12 [8–15]	< 0.001
ICU admission diagnosis, n (%)	97				0.046
		Trauma 37 (38.1)	34	3 (8.1)	
		Neurologic 21 (21.6)	17	4 (19)	
		Respiratory 11 (11.3)	8	3 (27.3)	
		Sepsis 9 (9.3)	6	3 (33.3)	
		Other 19 (19.7)	11	8 (42.1)	
Heart rate (bpm)	97	79 [61–102]	77 [61–95]	96 [69–107]	0.045
Mean arterial pressure (mmHg)	97	84 ± 19	86 ± 17	79 ± 27	0.255
Vasoactive drugs (treated)	54		38 (50)	16 (76.2)	0.046
Noradrenaline (mcg/kg/min)	52	0.28 [0.14–0.61]			
Dopamine (mcg/kg/min)	5	6.1 [4.8–7.4]			
Dobutamine (mcg/kg/min)	8	2.54 [2–4.5]			
Cumulative Vasopressor Index	54	4 [4]	1 [0–4]	4 [2–4]	0.008
Glasgow Coma Scale (pts)	97	10 [3–15]	10 [4–15]	4 [3–14]	0.074
Mechanical ventilation (n, %)	97	91 (93.8)	71 (93.4)	21 (100)	0.581
Peep (cmH₂O)	91	7 [6–9]	7 [6–9]	8 [7–10]	0.095
Haemoglobin (g/dL)	97	11 ± 1.78	11.1 ± 1.7	10.8 ± 2.2	0.58
White blood cells ($n \times 10^3$/mmc)	97	12.1 [8.83–14.81]	11.3 [8.8–15.7]	12.7 [9.5–14.6]	0.518
Platelets ($n \times 10^3$/mmc)	97	150 [102–199]	165 [110–201]	115 [56–173]	0.02
Creatinine (mg/dL)	97	1.0 [0.8–1.45]	1 [0.8–1.2]	1.4 [1.1–1.8]	< 0.001
Bilirubine (mg/dL)	97	0.8 [0.5–1.2]	0.75 [0.5–1.1]	0.9 [0.4–1.8]	0.264
PaO₂ (mmHg)	97	146 [104–175]	147 [106–176]	140 [93–172]	0.63
Arterial lactates (mmol/L)	97	1.4 [1.0–2.15]	1.3 [0.9–1.67]	3.1 [1.4–5.6]	< 0.001
ScvO₂ (%)	60	77.2 [71–82.3]	77.7 [72.3–82.5]	75.6 [62.7–80.8]	0.24
Microcirculatory variables					
TVD (small) (mm/mm²)	97	20.4 ± 3.7	20.5 [17.2–22.7]	20.9 [17.8–22.7]	0.817
PVD (small) (mm/mm²)	97	19.3 ± 4.4	19.3 ± 4	19.3 ± 6	0.951
De Backer score (small) (n/mm)	97	11.9 ± 2	11.8 ± 2	12.2 ± 2	0.489
PPV (small) (%)	97	98.3 [95.4–100]	98.2 [94.8–100]	98.3 [97–100]	0.688
MFI (small) (AU)	97	3 [2.7–3.0]	3 [2.75–3]	2.93 [2.3–3]	0.155
HI (small)	97	0 [0.0–0.2]	0 [0–0.2]	0 [0–0.3]	0.417
Abnormal MFI (n, %)	97	20 (20.6)	11 (14.5)	9 (42.9)	0.012

Data are presented as mean ± or as median [IQR] unless stated otherwise

APACHE acute physiologic and chronic health evaluation II, calculated over the first 24 h from ICU admission; *SOFA* sequential organ failure assessment, calculated over the first 24 h from ICU admission; *CVI* cumulative vasopressor index; *ICU* Intensive Care Unit; *COPD*, chronic obstructive pulmonary disease. *TVD* total vessel density; *PVD* perfused vessel density; *PPV* proportion of perfused vessel; *HI* Heterogeneity Index; *MFI* Microvascular Flow Index. Abnormal MFI is defined as MFI < 2.6. Cut-off value for small vessels diameter < 20 μm

we divided these variables into normal and abnormal: MAP ≥ 65 mmHg = normal, < 65 mmHg = abnormal; HR < 90 bpm = normal, ≥ 90 bpm = abnormal; and arterial lactate ≤ 2 mmol/L = normal, > 2 mmol/L = abnormal. In the first model, all variables were normal. A stepwise addition of each variable was associated with a non-significant reduction in ICU mortality (Fig. 2). In the second model, all variables were abnormal. A stepwise addition of each variable was associated with a non-significant increment in ICU mortality (Fig. 2). The comparison between the two models revealed in each step a significantly higher ICU mortality in the 'abnormal' model (Fig. 2).

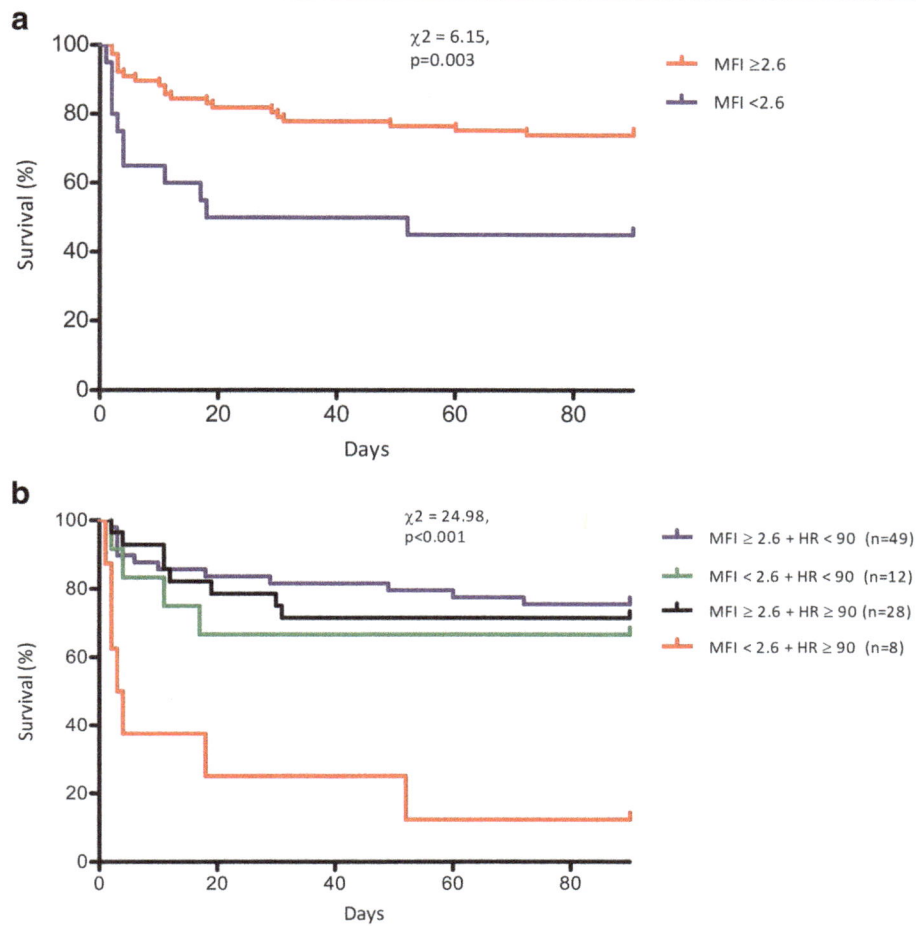

Fig. 1 Kaplan–Meier survival analysis. **a** Represents two subgroups, separated by microvascular blood flow (MFI) < 2.6 versus MFI ≥ 2.6. **b** Represents four subgroups, separated by MFI with identical cut-off value and heart rate (HR) ≥ 90 versus < 90 bpm

Table 2 Binary logistic regression analysis for ICU mortality

Variables	Odds ratio (95% CI)	p value
ICU MORTALITY (abnormal MFI)		
APACHE II score	1.204 (1.089–1.331)	< 0.001
MFI < 2.6	4.594 (1.340–15.754)	0.015
ICU MORTALITY (abnormal MFI + tachycardia)		
APACHE II score	1.191 (1.077–1.316)	0.001
MFI < 2.6 + tachycardia	10.732 (1.685–68.354)	0.012

In the upper model baseline, MFI abnormality was the independent variable. Model AUC 0.836 [0.747–0.904], Nagelkerke R^2 0.359, Hosmer and Lemeshow χ^2 4.733, $p = 0.822$. In the lower model, the presence of abnormal MFI plus tachycardia was the independent variable. Model AUC 0.836 [0.747–0.903], Nagelkerke R^2 0.374, Hosmer and Lemeshow χ^2 2.670, $p = 0.914$

APACHE acute physiologic and chronic health evaluation II, calculated in the first 24 h from ICU admission; *ICU* Intensive Care Unit; *MFI* Microvascular Flow Index. Abnormal MFI is defined as MFI < 2.6 for small vessels (diameter < 20 μm). Tachycardia is defined as a heart rate ≥ 90 bpm

Microcirculatory longitudinal monitoring and outcome

The median duration of follow-up for each patient category was: 6 [3–12] days for trauma, 8 [3–14] days for neurologic, 5 [1–6] days for respiratory, 8 [3–11] days for septic and 4 [2–8] days for other patients.

The total *incidence* of an abnormal microcirculation during the entire ICU stay was 55.7% (20.6% on day 1, 35.1% after day 1). Microcirculatory imaging was restricted to day 1 in ten patients (six died, four were discharged); missing data (SOFA and/or MFI) prevented further analysis in 19 patients. MFI and SOFA score over time are depicted in Fig. 3. Twenty-two patients showed an increment in MFI between days 1 and 2 (ΔMFI (+)), 21 patients showed a reduction in MFI between days 1 and 2 (ΔMFI (−)) and 25 remained indifferent. ΔMFI (+) was not associated with a significant reduction in SOFA score between days 2 and 3 (corresponding with the same time frame of MFI days 1 and 2) or mortality,

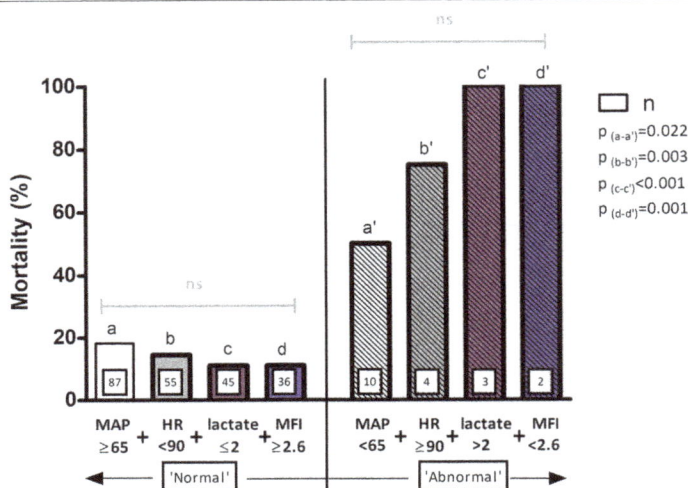

Fig. 2 Prognostic model with stepwise inclusion of consecutive hemodynamic variables: mean arterial pressure (MAP) in mmHg, heart rate (HR) in bpm, (arterial) lactate in mmol/L and Microvascular Flow Index (MFI) in AU

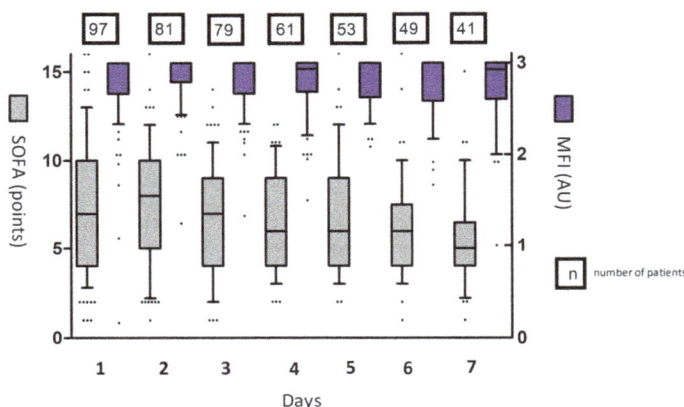

Fig. 3 Evolvement over time of sequential organ failure assessment (SOFA) score and Microvascular Flow Index (MFI) in the first 7 days of ICU admission. Box and 10–90th percentile whisker plots with individual outliers

as compared to patients with a ΔMFI $(-)$. Any increase/decrease in MFI was considered relevant for this analysis.

Post hoc, patients were divided into four groups according to the timing of the presence of an abnormal MFI. Group 1: patients with a normal MFI on day 1 and later on ($n=36$). Group 2: patients with a normal MFI on day 1 but with one or more episodes of an abnormal MFI later on ($n=34$). Group 3: patients with an abnormal MFI on day 1 and a normal MFI later on ($n=6$). Group 4: patients with an abnormal MFI on day 1 and one or more episodes of an abnormal MFI later on ($n=10$). Mortality was significantly different across groups ($p<0.001$). If an abnormal MFI was present on day one (groups 3 and 4), mortality was 6/16 (38%), whereas in patients with an abnormal MFI only after day 1 (group 2), ICU mortality

was 2/34 (6%, $p=0.001$), indicating a significant difference in prognostic value of an abnormal MFI on day 1 in comparison with an abnormal MFI after day 1.

Discussion

This MicroDAIMON study is currently the largest prospective longitudinal observational study to describe the incidence of microcirculatory derangements among a mixed group of critically ill patients, offering a day-by-day follow-up. The incidence of baseline microcirculatory flow abnormalities was 20.6%, and more than half (55.7%) of the patients displayed an abnormal MFI in at least one observation during ICU stay. The main finding of this study is that in this mixed ICU population, an abnormal baseline MFI is independently associated with unfavourable outcome in terms of ICU, in-hospital and 90-day mortality. In addition, the contemporary presence of tachycardia showed an additive predictive power towards mortality in the survival analysis. However, the change of MFI over time was not associated with outcome, in terms of both organ failure (SOFA) and mortality. In contrast to an abnormal MFI on day 1, we could not associate an abnormal MFI after day 1 with unfavourable outcome. No associations were found between the other microvascular variables and outcome.

In 2015, the MicroSOAP study provided the first and largest database on the prevalence and the significance of the microcirculatory alterations in a heterogeneous ICU population, with a time-point observation across 36 ICUs worldwide [15]. The authors reported a prevalence of MFI abnormalities of 17%, using the same predefined cut-off value [15, 26]. This difference in reported percentage of MFI abnormalities can be explained by the difference in study design (longitudinal vs. point prevalence). Our data confirm previous observations, showing an important prognostic role of the microcirculation in various subsets of critically ill patients [4–9, 14]. In contrast to the existing literature, these findings extend the predictive value of early microcirculatory alterations towards 90-day mortality. Patients with an abnormal MFI at baseline showed an absolute risk of non-survival almost three times higher in comparison with patients with a normal MFI.

However, in the present study, routine day-by-day microcirculatory monitoring does not confirm previous observations. In 2004, Sakr et al. [11] introduced for the first time the concept of serial observations of microcirculation in a cohort of 49 patients with septic shock. In this highly selected group of patients, the persistence of microcirculatory alterations was associated with persistence of shock, development of multiple organ failure and mortality.

Conversely, ICU survivors showed early improvement of microcirculation. These data were confirmed by others [21]. Duranteau and colleagues observed in another selected cohort of 18 patients with traumatic haemorrhagic shock, early derangements of microcirculatory flow and vessel density, as well as its persistence, were able to predict a worse SOFA score after 96 h from ICU admission [5]. A possible explanation for this discrepancy may lie in the heterogeneous composition of our study population and in considerable differences in microcirculatory baseline abnormalities. Alternatively, microvascular alterations represent differences in underlying pathology between study populations. Careful selection of patients at risk may contribute to the prognostic power of microcirculatory observation. As of now, our data indicate that routine daily monitoring of the microcirculation

in an unselected group of ICU patients is of limited prognostic value.

This study has several limitations. Although this study contains the largest reported database on day-by-day monitoring of the microcirculation in critically ill, it appears to have insufficient sample size to correlate differences in the evolution of microcirculatory conditions over time with clinically relevant endpoints (SOFA, mortality) also due to the considerable number of patients lost to follow-up, due to death/discharge. And although the independent predictive value of an abnormal MFI on day 1 was established, the integration of such variable in a model with more commonly used hemodynamic variables was clearly limited by the sample size as well. Further research is needed to establish the additive value of microcirculatory imaging on top of the existing hemodynamic variables. In addition, it is conceivable that other microvascular variables and different cut-off yield different results. We did not found any significant association between the other microcirculatory variables (TVD, PVD, PPV) and the outcome either on day 1 or in the following days. This could be explained by the fact that the MFI, especially if used as a dichotomous variable based on an a priori cut-off of 2,6, could have been the most sensitive variable to detect an association with the outcome in a such heterogeneous population which is expected to cause a "dilution effect" on the microcirculatory alterations. It is also possible that a vessel-by-vessel MFI calculation could have been more precise and provide different results depending on a more accurate evaluation of the capillary blood flow, especially in the presence of marked heterogeneity. In this respect, the burden of time-consuming offline analysis remains a major practical limitation for the study population sample size until the time of the development and full validation of automated analysis software. Real-time "eyeballing" the microcirculation by bedside assessment of MFI is a major advantage in the development of a bedside tool and showed good agreement with the gold standard offline analysis [27]. Post hoc analysis of our data confirmed 2.6 as the optimal cut-off for the discrimination between survivors and non-survivors. Finally, this was a pure observational study: patients were treated following the international guidelines and principles of good clinical practice, and clinicians had no information about the microcirculation during the study. Therefore, our study design is insufficient to draw conclusions on the applicability of microcirculatory monitoring as a tool to guide resuscitation. Even in the setting where there is an absence of additional prognostic information, derived from microcirculatory monitoring, the observation itself may contain valuable information about the underlying pathophysiologic mechanisms. For example, an increased lactate may adequately predict outcome, but does not reveal its underlying mechanism. Under these conditions, additional assessment of microvascular blood flow may not be useful to predict outcome, but may be helpful for the clinician to select the appropriate resuscitation strategy. Further research is needed to address this topic. Careful selection of subgroups and adequate timing remain of the essence in this process.

Conclusions

This MicroDAIMON study provides data about incidence of microcirculatory alterations in a heterogeneous group of critically ill patients. Microcirculatory flow abnormalities at the baseline were independently associated with an increased risk of unfavourable outcome. Simultaneous presence of tachycardia enhanced this predictive value. However, neither the evolution of MFI over time nor the development or new abnormalities after day 1 was associated with organ function or mortality in our population with a sample size limitation. Further studies are needed to incorporate microcirculatory monitoring into a set of currently available hemodynamic variables and to establish its value as a tool to guide specific resuscitation strategies.

Abbreviations

SDF: Sidestream Dark Field; ICU: Intensive Care Unit; SOFA: sequential organ failure assessment; MFI: Microvascular Flow Index; PPV: proportion of perfused vessels; TVD: total vessel density; PVD: perfused vessel density; SD: standard deviation; IQR: interquartile range; OR: odds ratio; CI: confidence interval; APACHE II: acute physiology and chronic evaluation score; HR: heart rate; MAP: mean arterial pressure.

Authors' contributions

CS, AD, ED, RR, EA designed the study, contributed to the interpretation of the results and critically revised the manuscript. CS and ED performed the statistical analysis, drafted the manuscript and interpreted the data. ED, CS, RD, AC, SP, ST, VM, SC, MR, BM made a substantial contributions to the acquisition of the data and the analysis of SDF videos and revised the manuscript for important intellectual content. CB made a substantial contribution in drafting the manuscript and interpreting the results. CI made a substantial contribution in the study design and critically revised the manuscript for important intellectual content. All authors had full access to the data, take responsibility for the integrity of the data and the accuracy of the analysis. All authors read and approved the final manuscript.

Author details

[1] Anaesthesia and Intensive Care, Department of Biomedical Sciences and Public Health, Università Politecnica delle Marche, via Tronto 10/a, 60126 Ancona, Italy. [2] Department of Translational Physiology, Academic Medical Centre, University of Amsterdam, Meibergdreef 9, 1105 AZ Amsterdam, The Netherlands. [3] Department of Intensive Care, Medical Centre Leeuwarden, Henri Dunantweg 2, 8934 AD Leeuwarden, The Netherlands.

Acknowledgements

We would like to thank Luca Giovannelli, MD, and Marco Zacchilli, MD, Università Politecnica delle Marche, Department of Biomedical Science and Public Health, for the precious help in the SDF video analysis all the medical doctors, residents and nurses of the Clinic of General, Respiratory and Trauma Intensive Care of Ospedali Riuniti of Ancona for the kind support.

Competing interests

CI is the inventor of Sidestream Dark Field imaging technology. He has been a consultant for MicroVision Medical in the past but he has actually no contact with this company for more than 5 years, except that he still holds shares. He has no other competing interests in this field other than his commitment to promoting the importance of the microcirculation during patient care; and there are no other relationships or activities that could appear to have influenced the submitted work. The other authors have no competing interests to declare.

Funding

Local departmental funding.

References

1. Ince C. The microcirculation is the motor of sepsis. Crit Care. 2005;9(Suppl 4):S13–9.
2. Kanoore Edul VS, Ince C, Dubin A. What is microcirculatory shock? Curr Opin Crit Care. 2015;21(3):245–52.
3. Spanos A, Jhanji S, Vivian-Smith A, et al. Early microvascular changes in sepsis and severe sepsis. Shock. 2010;33(4):387–91.
4. Bateman RM, Sharpe MD, Ellis CG. Bench-to-bedside review: microvascular dysfunction in sepsis—hemodynamics, oxygen transport, and nitric oxide. Crit Care. 2003;7(5):359–73.
5. Tachon G, Harrois A, Tanaka S, et al. Microcirculatory alterations in traumatic hemorrhagic shock. Crit Care Med. 2014;42(6):1433–41.
6. van Genderen ME, Lima A, Akkerhuis M, et al. Persistent peripheral and microcirculatory perfusion alterations after out-of-hospital cardiac arrest are associated with poor survival. Crit Care Med. 2012;40(8):2287–94.
7. De Backer D, Donadello K, Sakr Y, et al. Microcirculatory alterations in patients with severe sepsis: impact of time of assessment and relationship with outcome. Crit Care Med. 2013;41(3):791–9.
8. Trzeciak S, Dellinger RP, Parrillo JE, et al. Early microcirculatory perfusion derangements in patients with severe sepsis and septic shock: relationship to hemodynamics, oxygen transport, and survival. Ann Emerg Med. 2007;49(1):88–98.
9. Jhanji S, Lee C, Watson D, et al. Microvascular flow and tissue oxygenation after major abdominal surgery: association with post-operative complications. Intensive Care Med. 2009;35(4):671–7.
10. den Uil CA, Lagrand WK, van der Ent M, et al. Impaired microcirculation predicts poor outcome of patients with acute myocardial infarction complicated by cardiogenic shock. Eur Heart J. 2010;31(24):3032–9.
11. Sakr Y, Dubois MJ, De Backer D, et al. Persistent microcirculatory alterations are associated with organ failure and death in patients with septic shock. Crit Care Med. 2004;32(9):1825–31.
12. Top APC, Ince C, de Meij N, et al. Persistent low microcirculatory vessel density in nonsurvivors of sepsis in pediatric intensive care. Crit Care Med. 2011;39(1):8–13.
13. Goedhart PT, Khalilzada M, Bezemer R, et al. Sidestream Dark Field (SDF) imaging: a novel stroboscopic LED ring-based imaging modality for clinical assessment of the microcirculation. Opt Express. 2007;15(23):15101–14.
14. De Backer D, Creteur J, Dubois MJ, et al. Microvascular alterations in patients with acute severe heart failure and cardiogenic shock. Am Heart J. 2004;147(1):91–9.
15. Vellinga NAR, Boerma EC, Koopmans M, et al. International study on microcirculatory shock occurrence in acutely ill patients. Crit Care Med. 2015;43(1):48–56.
16. Damiani E, Ince C, Scorcella C, et al. Impact of microcirculatory video quality on the evaluation of sublingual microcirculation in critically ill patients. J Clin Monit Comput. 2017;31(5):981–8.
17. Massey MJ, Shapiro NI. A guide to human in vivo microcirculatory flow image analysis. Crit Care. 2016;20:35.

18. De Backer D, Hollenberg S, Boerma C, et al. How to evaluate the microcirculation: report of a round table conference. Crit Care. 2007;11(5):R101.

19. Boerma EC, Mathura KR, van der Voort PHJ, et al. Quantifying bedside-derived imaging of microcirculatory abnormalities in septic patients: a prospective validation study. Crit Care. 2005;9(6):R601–6.

20. Pranskunas A, Koopmans M, Koetsier PM, et al. Microcirculatory blood flow as a tool to select ICU patients eligible for fluid therapy. Intensive Care Med. 2013;39(4):612–9.

21. Trzeciak S, McCoy JV, Phillip Dellinger R, et al. Early increases in microcirculatory perfusion during protocol-directed resuscitation are associated with reduced multi-organ failure at 24 h in patients with sepsis. Intensive Care Med. 2008;34(12):2210–7.

22. Hoke RS, Müller-Werdan U, Lautenschläger C, et al. Heart rate as an independent risk factor in patients with multiple organ dysfunction: a prospective, observational study. Clin Res Cardiol. 2012;101(2):139–47.

23. Schmittinger CA, Torgersen C, Luckner G, et al. Adverse cardiac events during catecholamine vasopressor therapy: a prospective observational study. Intensive Care Med. 2012;38(6):950–8.

24. Disegni E, Goldbourt U, Reicher-Reiss H, et al. The predictive value of admission heart rate on mortality in patients with acute myocardial infarction. SPRINT Study Group. Secondary Prevention Reinfarction Israeli Nifedipine Trial. J Clin Epidemiol. 1995;48(10):1197–205.

25. Bone RC, Balk RA, Cerra FB, et al. Definitions for sepsis and organ failure and guidelines for the use of innovative therapies in sepsis. The ACCP/SCCM Consensus Conference Committee. American College of Chest Physicians/Society of Critical Care Medicine. Chest. 1992;101(6):1644–55.

26. Edul VSK, Enrico C, Laviolle B, et al. Quantitative assessment of the microcirculation in healthy volunteers and in patients with septic shock. Crit Care Med. 2012;40(5):1443–8.

27. Arnold RC, Parrillo JE, Phillip Dellinger R, et al. Point-of-care assessment of microvascular blood flow in critically ill patients. Intensive Care Med. 2009;35(10):1761–6.

20

Clinical impact of upper gastrointestinal endoscopy in critically ill patients with suspected bleeding

Sylvain Jean-Baptiste[1], Jonathan Messika[1,2,3†] (ID), David Hajage[4,5,6,7†], Stéphane Gaudry[1,6,7], Julie Barbieri[8], Henri Duboc[9], Didier Dreyfuss[1,2,3], Benoit Coffin[8,9] and Jean-Damien Ricard[1,2,3*]

Abstract

Background and Aims: Upper gastrointestinal endoscopies' (UGE) profitability is undisputable in patients admitted for an overt upper digestive tract bleeding. In critically ill subjects admitted for other causes, its performances have scarcely been investigated despite its broad use. We sought to question the performance of bedside UGE in intensive care unit (ICU) patients, admitted for another reason than overt bleeding.

Methods: This was a six-year (January 2007–December 2012) retrospective observational study of all UGE performed in a medico-surgical ICU. Exclusion of those performed: in patients admitted for a patent upper digestive bleeding; for a second-look gastroscopy of a known lesion; as a planned interventional procedure. Main demographic and clinical data were recorded; UGE indication and profitability were rated according to its findings and therapeutic impact. Operative values of the indications of UGE were calculated. This study received approval from the Ethics Committee of the French Society of Intensive Care (n° 12-363).

Results: Eighty-four patients (74% male, mean age 61 ± 14 years) underwent a diagnostic UGE, all for a suspected upper digestive tract bleeding. The main symptoms justifying the procedure were anemia (52%), digestive bleeding (27%), vomiting (15%), hemodynamic instability (3%) and hyperuremia (3%). The profitability of UGE was rated as major ($n = 5$; 5.8%); minor ($n = 34$; 40.5%); or null ($n = 45$; 53.6%).

Conclusions: When ICU admission is not warranted by a digestive bleeding, UGE has limited diagnostic and therapeutic interest, despite being often performed.

Keywords: Upper gastrointestinal endoscopy, Intensive care unit, Profitability

Background

Bedside upper gastrointestinal endoscopy (UGE) is a procedure frequently performed in critically ill patients admitted to the intensive care unit (ICU). It has both a diagnostic (macroscopic examination of the lesions and biopsy sampling) and a therapeutic role (hemostatic vasoconstrictor injection, clipping, ligation of esophageal varices, etc.).

Its performance is well demonstrated for the management of patients admitted for upper digestive tract bleeding [1–9]. Nevertheless, apart from this specific context, a bedside UGE is also frequently performed in patients admitted for another reason, in which an upper digestive bleeding suspicion is raised during the course of ICU stay. The reasons for such suspicion might be the occurrence of exteriorized bleeding, an acute anemia, an hemodynamic instability or an hyperuremia without renal failure [10–12].

The performance and added value of UGE in this indication are much more debated [10, 13–16]. Indeed, critically ill patients often present with complex medical situations, many reasons to account for these signs (such

*Correspondence: jean-damien.ricard@aphp.fr
†Jonathan Messika and David Hajage have contributed equally to this work
[1] Medico-Surgical Intensive Care Unit, AP-HP, Hôpital Louis Mourier, 178 rue des Renouillers, 92700 Colombes, France

as bleeding from another site, inflammatory anemia, sepsis and acute kidney injury). Furthermore, the discovery of a mucosal lesion might not require any endoscopic nor pharmacological treatment (gastritis, esophagitis, nasogastric tube-associated ulcerations) [17, 18] and hypothetic benefits of this procedure must be weighed against its inherent costs and risks [19]. We therefore questioned the performance of a bedside UGE in critically ill patients, admitted for another reason than upper digestive bleeding in the ICU. Our hypothesis was that a majority of procedures, performed in a general ICU population to confirm or exclude a GI bleeding, would only find nonspecific, ICU-associated lesions that would not significantly influence the patients' management.

Patients and methods

We conducted a retrospective, monocenter study, in a single teaching-based, 12-bed medico-surgical ICU, of all UGE performed between January 2007 and December 2012. The Ethics Committee of the French Society of Intensive Care (SRLF) approved the study (n° 12-363). An informed consent was waived due to the retrospective design of the study.

All the patients who underwent a gastroscopy were identified through the endoscopy unit's database, in which all UGEs performed in our institution are registered. All the patients who had an UGE performed during their ICU stay were included, and their whole medical records were analyzed. Excluded patients were those admitted for a patent upper digestive bleeding or those who underwent a second-look gastroscopy of a known lesion or for a planned interventional procedure (such as a gastric tube or esophageal prosthesis placement). When a patient underwent several procedures, only the first one was taken into account.

Data collected were age, gender, the reason for ICU admission, the Sequential Organ Failure Assessment (SOFA) score [20] at ICU admission and the number of organ failures according to the individual organ score of the SOFA score [20]. We also recorded the symptoms and conditions that motivated the UGE, its findings and the subsequent procedures performed if any. Vital status at ICU discharge was also recorded.

UGE was performed by a gastroenterologist (in most cases by a senior physician and in rare instances, by a trainee under a senior's supervision) with standard Fuji video gastroscope. It was performed under general anesthesia with orotracheal intubation or under sedation in patients with no previous intubation. If gastric hemorrhage was suspected, a 2.5 mg/kg IV infusion of erythromycin was performed 30–60 min before endoscopy.

For each UGE, its profitability was rated. It was considered as "major" if it allowed a hemostatic procedure or

the diagnosis of a cancer; "minor" if it allowed a diagnosis of a peptic disorder, which could be pharmacologically treated; or "null" if it was normal or if the findings had no therapeutic consequence.

Continuous data are presented as mean and standard deviation unless otherwise indicated. Dichotomous data are presented as number and percentage. For each reason motivating the UGE, we calculated the operative values (sensibility, specificity, positive and negative predictive value) associated with a major or minor profitability of the UGE. The analyses were performed with R version 3.2.0.

Results
Patient demographics and characteristics
Patients' flowchart is shown in Fig. 1, and patients' characteristics are summarized in Table 1. Among 3352 ICU admissions, 84 patients (74% male, mean age 61 ± 14 years) had not been admitted for upper digestive bleeding and underwent a diagnostic UGE during their ICU stay, after a mean of 13 ± 16 days of ICU admission. Main reason for ICU admission was sepsis (81%), 38% were surgical patients, and 7% were admitted in ICU following a gastroesophageal surgery. A multiorgan failure was present in most of them, as 92% received invasive mechanical ventilation and 62% had vasopressors. The mean SOFA score at admission was 7.7 ± 3.7. In our cohort, ICU mortality was 29%.

UGE indication
The reasons for performing the UGE are shown in Table 2. In every case, an upper bleeding was suspected.

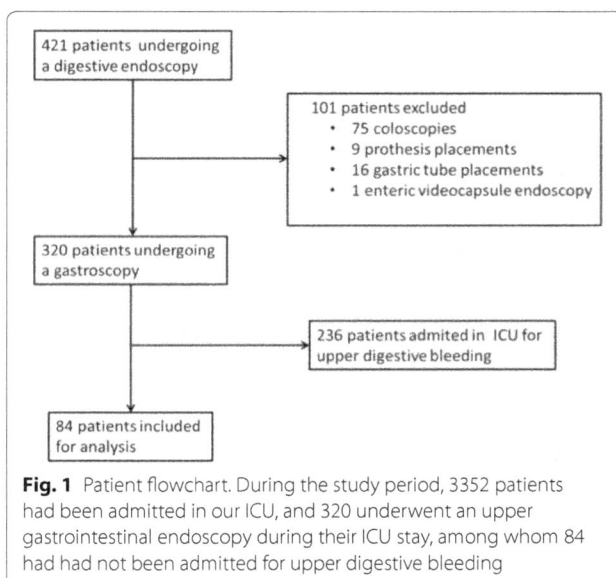

Fig. 1 Patient flowchart. During the study period, 3352 patients had been admitted in our ICU, and 320 underwent an upper gastrointestinal endoscopy during their ICU stay, among whom 84 had had not been admitted for upper digestive bleeding

Table 1 Characteristics of the 84 critically ill patients undergoing a bedside upper gastrointestinal endoscopy

Patients' characteristics. $n = 84$	
Age (years)	61.7 ± 14
Male sex	62 (74%)
Medical patients	52 (62%)
Surgical patients	32 (38%)
Esogastric surgery	6 (7%)
SOFA score	7.7 ± 3.7
Mechanical ventilation	77 (92%)
Vasopressor	52 (62%)
Acute kidney injury	50 (60%)
Sepsis	68 (81%)

Data are expressed as mean $\pm$ SD, or n (%); SOFA: Sequential Organ Failure Assessment SOFA scores can range from 0 (no organ failure) to 24 (most severe level of multiorgan failure)

Table 2 Reasons for performing the upper gastrointestinal endoscopy in the 84 critically ill patients

Acute anemia	50 (60%)
Digestive bleeding	26 (31%)
Vomiting	14 (17%)
Hemodynamic instability	3 (4%)
Hyperuremia	3 (4%)

One patient could have various reasons for performing the upper gastrointestinal endoscopy. Data are presented in n (%)

Table 3 Findings of the 84 upper gastrointestinal endoscopy performed

Normal	25 (30%)
Esophagitis or gastritis	14 (17%)
Nasogastric tube erosion	18 (21%)
Peptic ulcer	13 (15%)
Esophagogastric varices	4 (5%)
Amyloidosis	1 (1%)
Esophageal candidosis	7 (8%)
Cancer	2 (2%)

Data are presented as n (%)

The main symptoms justifying the procedure according to the attending physician were acute anemia (52%), digestive bleeding (27%), vomiting (15%), hemodynamic instability (3%) and hyperuremia (3%).

UGE findings

The findings of the UGE are shown in Table 3. It was considered normal in 30% of those ($n = 25$). Among abnormal findings, the most frequent were nasogastric tube erosions ($n = 18$), peptic gastritis or esophagitis ($n = 14$),

peptic gastric ulcer ($n = 13$), esophageal candidiasis ($n = 7$), esogastric varices ($n = 4$). According to our pre-specified classification, we considered that 5 UGE had a major profitability (5.8%) and 34 (40.5%) had a minor profitability, and for 45 (53.6%), this profitability was null.

Diagnostic and predictive value

Sensibility, specificity, positive and negative predictive value (PPV and NPV) of the symptoms and conditions that motivated the procedures are shown in Table 4. Hemodynamic instability had a PPV of 100% but was present in only 3 patients and always associated with at least another sign (drop in hemoglobin in 3 and overt digestive bleeding in 2). The second best PPV was 66.7% for hyperuremia. It has to be noted that that acute anemia and digestive bleeding have not a high PPV (61.5 and 48%, respectively).

Discussion

In our 6-year retrospective review of all UGE performed in a single medico-surgical ICU, we showed that although regularly performed, UGE for critically ill patients initially hospitalized for another reason than upper digestive bleeding but for whom the question of upper digestive bleeding is raised during their ICU stay has limited diagnostic and therapeutic interest during ICU stay.

This is, to our knowledge, the largest study assessing the profitability of this procedure in this specific patient population.

In this population of non-selected ICU patients, with the suspicion of ICU-acquired upper digestive bleeding, we found that UGE was strictly normal in one third of procedures. When performed in patients in whom gastrointestinal bleeding was not suspected, Ovenden et al. reported that UGE was normal in two-thirds of procedures [18]. The vast majority of abnormal findings we observed ($n = 45$; 76%) were either peptic lesions (*i.e.,* ulcer or esophagitis/gastritis) or nasogastric tube-associated erosions. Similar lesions were reported by Ovenden et al. In this series of 74 patients who underwent an UGE, a pathological finding was found in 34% of the subjects, either gastritis/erosions in 14%, nasogastric tube trauma in 8 (11%), esophagitis in 4 (5%) and non-bleeding duodenal ulceration in 3 (4%) [18].

In our series, an active bleeding was only retrieved in three of the 13 peptic ulcers at the time of the UGE, therefore requiring an instrumental hemostasis procedure (submucosal adrenaline injection and clip application). Nasogastric tube erosions were always considered incidental findings that could not be held responsible for the symptoms and that did not change the patients' management. The other lesions found were mostly incidental that did not account for any significant digestive

Table 4 Diagnostic and predictive values of upper gastrointestinal endoscopy in critically ill subjects

	Sensibility	Specificity	PPV	NPV
Esogastric surgery	7.7	93.3	50.0	53.8
Acute kidney injury	46.2	28.9	36.0	38.2
Coagulopathy	20.5	80.0	47.1	53.7
Sepsis	79.5	17.8	45.6	50
Shock	61.5	37.8	46.2	53.1
Mechanical ventilation	87.2	4.4	44.2	28.6
Cirrhosis	10.3	86.7	40.0	52.7
History of ulcer	7.7	93.3	50.0	53.8
Acute anemia	61.5	42.2	48.0	55.9
Hyperuremia	5.1	97.8	66.7	54.3
Hemodynamic instability	7.7	100	100	55.6
Digestive bleeding	25.6	64.4	38.5	50.0
Vomiting	15.4	82.2	42.9	52.9

Data are presented as %

PPV positive predictive value, *NPV* negative predictive value

bleeding. We can infer that not only the suspicion of active bleeding is very infrequent, but also, when suspected its occurrence, is very rare.

These results are of importance since UGE is a costly and time-consuming procedure, for both ICU and endoscopy teams, that can cause significant morbidity if performed unduly [21]. Its poor performance can probably be explained by the large prescription of prophylactic proton pump inhibitors in our unit for the patients that present several risk factors for the so-called stress related mucosal disease. Although prevention with prophylactic proton pump inhibitor has been showed to be safe [4, 5, 22], its use is still being challenged [23–25]. Our study population was composed of patients presenting multiple organ failure so the results cannot be explained by a lack of severity of the patients, as attested by the high SOFA score.

Whereas previous reports focused on UGE performed in the ICU for overt gastrointestinal bleeding [7, 16], Plaisier et al. [15] described the indications and results of 411 gastroscopies performed in 4 ICUs of a single Dutch hospital. Unlike our series, most patients were admitted for a gastrointestinal hemorrhage. Nevertheless, in patients undergoing the UGE for another reason, esophagitis, gastritis and gastric ulcer were the most frequent coincidental findings, as in our series. Of interest, in this setting, UGE was also widely used (in 35% of cases) for the placement of feeding tubes, which was a very uncommon indication in our series.

The operative values of the symptoms and conditions that justified performing the UGE are disappointingly poor. None of them was found to be discriminating enough to be useful, alone, in clinical practice.

It is interesting to note that we observed an unexpectedly high number of esophageal candidiasis. None of these patients had an HIV infection or hematologic malignancy, and this diagnosis was never evoked before the UGE was performed. Although this was considered an incidental finding and an unlikely cause of digestive bleeding, all of them were treated by fluconazole [26, 27]. Risk factors and incidence of esophageal candidiasis in ICU patients are poorly studied [27], and our work raises the concern that this condition might be underdiagnosed and undertreated.

Our study holds several limitations. First, the retrospective design does not allow to drawing any definitive conclusion concerning the efficacy of upper digestive endoscopy in ICU patients suspected of ICU-acquired upper digestive bleeding. Nevertheless, the review of the whole charts and the gastroscopy report of the patients included enables to retrace the exact motives of the endoscopy.

Second, although we do acknowledge the number of patients is small ($n = 84$) with regard to the number of subjects admitted in our ICU during the study period ($n = 3352$), we can explain it with our policy of proton pump inhibitor prescription in subjects with a risk factor for digestive bleeding, and of active enteral nutrition of all patients for whom the digestive tract can be used. Third, our data reflect the experience of a single center, and the decision to perform the endoscopies or the hemostatic procedures were left to the attending intensivist and endoscopist and we cannot rule out that the results might have been different in another patient population treated by another medical team and our findings may not be generalized. Nevertheless, the decision to perform a gastroscopy is generally taken within the whole ICU medical team, with habits that did not change during the study period, and hemostatic procedures were performed according to the standard guidelines.

These limitations taken into account, we propose that UGE is of very limited use in ICU patients suspected of ICU-acquired upper digestive bleeding. The low yield of UGE in our center suggests that these patients can be managed with a watchful waiting when hemodynamically stable.

Conclusions

Bedside UGE has very poor diagnostic and therapeutic performances when performed in a population of intensive care patient suspected of ICU-acquired upper digestive bleeding. These results should be confirmed by a prospective multicenter observational cohort.

Abbreviations
ICU: Intensive care unit; SOFA: Sequential Organ Failure Assessment; UGE: upper gastrointestinal endoscopy.

Authors' contributions
SJ-B, JM and J-DR contributed to study concept and design; SJ-B, SG, JB and HD contributed to acquisition of data; SJ-B, JM, DH and J-DR contributed to analysis and interpretation of data; SJ-B, JM, DH and J-DR contributed to drafting of the manuscript; SG, HD, DD, BC and J-DR contributed to critical revision of the manuscript for important intellectual content; DH contributed to statistical analysis; SG, JB, HD and BC contributed to administrative, technical or material support; and J-DR contributed to study supervision. All authors read and approved the final manuscript.

Author details
[1] Medico-Surgical Intensive Care Unit, AP-HP, Hôpital Louis Mourier, 178 rue des Renouillers, 92700 Colombes, France. [2] IAME, UMR 1137, INSERM, 75018 Paris, France. [3] IAME, UMR 1137, Univ Paris Diderot, Sorbonne Paris Cité, 75018 Paris, France. [4] Département de Biostatistiques, Santé Publique et Information Médicale, AP-HP, Hôpital Pitié-Salpêtrière, 75013 Paris, France. [5] Univ Pierre et Marie Curie, Sorbonne Universités, 75013 Paris, France. [6] ECEVE, U1123, CIC-EC 1425, INSERM, 75010 Paris, France. [7] ECEVE, UMRS 1123, Univ Paris Diderot, Sorbonne Paris Cité, 75010 Paris, France. [8] Gastroenterology Unit, AP-HP, Hôpital Louis Mourier, 178 rue des Renouillers, 92700 Colombes, France. [9] Univ Paris Diderot, Sorbonne Paris Cité, 75018 Paris, France.

Competing interests
The authors declare that they have no competing interests.

Funding
None.

References
1. Lau JYW, Barkun A, Fan D, Kuipers EJ, Yang Y, Chan FKL. Challenges in the management of acute peptic ulcer bleeding. Lancet Lond Engl. 2013;381:2033–43.
2. Gralnek IM, Barkun AN, Bardou M. Management of acute bleeding from a peptic ulcer. N Engl J Med. 2008;359:928–37. http://www.nejm.org/doi/abs/10.1056/NEJMra0706113. Cited 29 March 2017.
3. Cook DJ, Fuller HD, Guyatt GH, Marshall JC, Leasa D, Hall R, et al. Risk factors for gastrointestinal bleeding in critically ill patients. N Engl J Med. 1994;330:377–81. http://www.nejm.org/doi/abs/10.1056/NEJM199402103300601. Cited 29 March 2017.
4. Barkun AN, Bardou M, Pham CQD, Martel M. Proton pump inhibitors vs. histamine 2 receptor antagonists for stress-related mucosal bleeding prophylaxis in critically ill patients: a meta-analysis. Am J Gastroenterol. 2012;107:507–20 (quiz 521).
5. Alhazzani W, Alenezi F, Jaeschke RZ, Moayyedi P, Cook DJ. Proton pump inhibitors versus histamine 2 receptor antagonists for stress ulcer prophylaxis in critically ill patients: a systematic review and meta-analysis. Crit Care Med. 2013;41:693–705.
6. Spiegel BM, Vakil NB, Ofman JJ. Endoscopy for acute nonvariceal upper gastrointestinal tract hemorrhage: is sooner better? A systematic review. Arch Intern Med. 2001;161:1393–404.
7. Lin HJ, Wang K, Perng CL, Chua RT, Lee FY, Lee CH, et al. Early or delayed endoscopy for patients with peptic ulcer bleeding. A prospective randomized study. J Clin Gastroenterol. 1996;22:267–71.
8. Lu Y, Loffroy R, Lau JYW, Barkun A. Multidisciplinary management strategies for acute non-variceal upper gastrointestinal bleeding. Br J Surg. 2014;101:e34–50.
9. Barkun AN, Bardou M, Kuipers EJ, Sung J, Hunt RH, Martel M, et al. International consensus recommendations on the management of patients with nonvariceal upper gastrointestinal bleeding. Ann Intern Med. 2010;152:101–13.
10. Richards RJ, Donica MB, Grayer D. Can the blood urea nitrogen/creatinine ratio distinguish upper from lower gastrointestinal bleeding? J Clin Gastroenterol. 1990;12:500–4.
11. Mortensen PB, Nøhr M, Møller-Petersen JF, Balslev I. The diagnostic value of serum urea/creatinine ratio in distinguishing between upper and lower gastrointestinal bleeding. A prospective study. Dan Med Bull. 1994;41:237–40.
12. Witting MD, Magder L, Heins AE, Mattu A, Granja CA, Baumgarten M. ED predictors of upper gastrointestinal tract bleeding in patients without hematemesis. Am J Emerg Med. 2006;24:280–5. http://linkinghub.elsevier.com/retrieve/pii/S0735675705004274. Cited 29 March 2017.
13. Lee Y-C, Wang H-P, Wu M-S, Yang C-S, Chang Y-T, Lin J-T. Urgent bedside endoscopy for clinically significant upper gastrointestinal hemorrhage after admission to the intensive care unit. Intensive Care Med. 2003;29:1723–8.
14. Zaltman C, Souza HSP de, Castro MEC, Sobral M de FS, Dias PCP, Lemos V. Upper gastrointestinal bleeding in a Brazilian hospital: a retrospective study of endoscopic records. Arq Gastroenterol. 2002;39:74–80.
15. Plaisier PW, van Buuren HR, Bruining HA. Upper gastrointestinal endoscopy at four intensive care units in one hospital: frequency and indication. Eur J Gastroenterol Hepatol. 1998;10:997–1000.
16. Lewis JD, Shin EJ, Metz DC. Characterization of gastrointestinal bleeding in severely ill hospitalized patients. Crit Care Med. 2000;28:46–50.
17. Hayden SJ, Albert TJ, Watkins TR, Swenson ER. Anemia in critical illness: insights into etiology, consequences, and management. Am J Respir Crit Care Med. 2012;185:1049–57.
18. Ovenden C, Plummer MP, Selvanderan S, Donaldson TA, Nguyen NQ, Weinel LM, et al. Occult upper gastrointestinal mucosal abnormalities in critically ill patients. Acta Anaesthesiol Scand. 2017;61:216–23. http://doi.wiley.com/10.1111/aas.12844. Cited 9 June 2018.
19. Tam WY, Bertholini D. Tension pneumoperitoneum, pneumomediastinum, subcutaneous emphysema and cardiorespiratory collapse following gastroscopy. Anaesth Intensive Care. 2007;35:307–9.
20. Vincent JL, Moreno R, Takala J, Willatts S, De Mendonca A, Bruining H, et al. The SOFA (Sepsis-related Organ Failure Assessment) score to describe organ dysfunction/failure. On behalf of the Working Group on Sepsis-Related Problems of the European Society of Intensive Care Medicine. Intensive Care Med. 1996;22:707–10. http://www.ncbi.nlm.nih.gov/entrez/query.fcgi?cmd=Retrieve&db=PubMed&dopt=Citation&list_uids=8844239.
21. Rehman A, Iscimen R, Yilmaz M, Khan H, Belsher J, Gomez JF, et al. Prophylactic endotracheal intubation in critically ill patients undergoing endoscopy for upper GI hemorrhage. Gastrointest Endosc. 2009;69:e55–9.
22. Selvanderan SP, Summers MJ, Finnis ME, Plummer MP, Ali Abdelhamid Y, Anderson MB, et al. Pantoprazole or placebo for stress ulcer prophylaxis (POP-UP): randomized double-blind exploratory study*. Crit Care Med. 2016;44:1842–50. http://Insights.ovid.com/crossref?an=00003246-20161 0000-00006. Cited 1 June 2018.
23. Krag M, Perner A, Wetterslev J, Wise MP, Borthwick M, Bendel S, et al. Stress ulcer prophylaxis with a proton pump inhibitor versus placebo in critically ill patients (SUP-ICU trial): study protocol for a randomised controlled trial. Trials. 2016;17:205.
24. Alhazzani W, Guyatt G, Alshahrani M, Deane AM, Marshall JC, Hall R, et al. Withholding pantoprazole for stress ulcer prophylaxis in critically ill patients: a pilot randomized clinical trial and meta-analysis*. Crit Care Med. 2017;45:1121–9. http://Insights.ovid.com/crossref?an=00003246-20170 7000-00003. Cited 1 June 2018.
25. El-Kersh K, Jalil B, McClave SA, Cavallazzi R, Guardiola J, Guilkey K, et al. Enteral nutrition as stress ulcer prophylaxis in critically ill patients: a randomized controlled exploratory study. J Crit Care. 2018;43:108–13. http://linkinghub.elsevier.com/retrieve/pii/S0883944117305294. Cited 1 June 2018.
26. Cuenca-Estrella M, Verweij PE, Arendrup MC, Arikan-Akdagli S, Bille J, Donnelly JP, et al. ESCMID* guideline for the diagnosis and management of Candida diseases 2012: diagnostic procedures. Clin Microbiol Infect Off Publ Eur Soc Clin Microbiol Infect Dis. 2012;18(Suppl 7):9–18.
27. Weerasuriya N, Snape J. Oesophageal candidiasis in elderly patients: risk factors, prevention and management. Drugs Aging. 2008;25:119–30.

21

Renal failure in critically ill patients, beware of applying (central venous) pressure on the kidney

Xiukai Chen[1*], Xiaoting Wang[2], Patrick M. Honore[3], Herbert D. Spapen[4] and Dawei Liu[2*]

Abstract

The central venous pressure (CVP) is traditionally used as a surrogate of intravascular volume. CVP measurements therefore are often applied at the bedside to guide fluid administration in postoperative and critically ill patients. Pursuing high CVP levels has recently been challenged. A high CVP might impede venous return to the heart and disturb microcirculatory blood flow which may cause tissue congestion and organ failure. By imposing an increased "afterload" on the kidney, an elevated CVP will particularly harm kidney hemodynamics and promote acute kidney injury (AKI) even in the absence of volume overload. Maintaining the lowest possible CVP should become routine to prevent and treat AKI, especially when associated with septic shock, cardiac surgery, mechanical ventilation, and intra-abdominal hypertension.

Keywords: Acute kidney injury, Central venous pressure, Afterload

Background

Acute kidney injury (AKI) is a common complication in critically ill patients with high attributable morbidity and mortality [1, 2]. Systemic and renal perfusion considerably determines the development and course of AKI. Yet, optimal hemodynamic targets to minimize the risk of AKI are not precisely defined [3, 4]. In critical care, hypotension and shock are the "rogue enemies." Resuscitation primarily focuses on optimizing mean arterial pressure (MAP) to improve renal perfusion [5]. However, there is little evidence that MAP correctly reflects organ perfusion. Moreover, aggressive fluid loading may contribute to an increased central venous pressure (CVP). By accepting high CVP levels [6–10], clinicians neglect that volume treatment and AKI are closely intertwined.

CVP is traditionally used for assessing volume status and volume responsiveness at the bedside [11]. However,

CVP measurements to direct volume management in critically ill patients have repeatedly been found unreliable [12]. Whether and how CVP monitoring should be adapted to a particular patient (e.g., postsurgical, cardiac, septic) population is topic of controversy and debate [13, 14]. Monitoring CVP also does not guarantee preservation of renal function. A recent study reported a higher incidence of AKI in patients undergoing CVP monitoring as compared with unmonitored subjects. A 1 cm H_2O higher CVP was associated with a 1.02 (95% CI 1.00–1.03, $p = 0.02$) risk of AKI. No association was found between pulmonary edema and AKI [13]. Till recently, the innate pressure character of CVP and its pathophysiological impact have been largely underestimated. What follows is a thorough discussion about the role of CVP, beyond its value as volume indicator, in various diseases.

Main text

CVP is a pressure used to estimate volume

The CVP is the pressure recorded from the superior vena cava or right atrium which, in the absence of tricuspid stenosis, equals right ventricular end-diastolic pressure. CVP is determined by the interaction between cardiac function and venous return which both depend

---

*Correspondence: xic91@pitt.edu; dwliu98@163.com
[1] Pittsburgh Heart, Lung, Blood and Vascular Medicine Institute, University of Pittsburgh, 200 Lothrop Street, BST E1240, Pittsburgh, PA 15261, USA
[2] Department of Critical Care Medicine, Peking Union Medical College Hospital, Peking Union Medical College, Chinese Academy of Medical Sciences, 1 Shuaifuyuan, Dongcheng District, Beijing 100073, China

on changes in total blood volume, vascular tone, cardiac output (CO), right ventricular compliance, intrathoracic and pericardial pressure [15]. CVP measurements are especially useful when followed over time and combined with a CO recording. A properly measured CVP can successfully guide right ventricular filling [16]. Within a certain range, CVP increases with expanding blood volume. However, excessive fluid administration may augment CVP and end-diastolic pressure without increasing end-diastolic or stroke volume. On the other hand, an increased CVP is often associated with decreased right ventricular compliance. Additionally, CVP is the downstream pressure for venous return and close to the minimum pressure in the global circulation [17].

CVP and kidney "afterload"
CVP must be lower than renal venous pressure (RVP) in order to allow an adequate venous renal blood flow (RBF) to the heart. Accordingly, the presence of a high CVP requires a much higher RVP to ensure this flow. Renal perfusion pressure (RPP) approximates the difference between renal arterial pressure and RVP. As such, a higher RVP lowers RPP. In analogy with cardiac physiology, this forms the basis for the renal "afterload" concept [18]. Recent studies focusing on kidney "afterload" have revived interest in older studies which suggested that kidney dysfunction resulted from venous congestion transmitted to the renal venous compartment. Almost a century ago, it was indeed demonstrated that an hypervolemia-induced increase in RVP caused AKI independently of CO or RBF [19].

Effect of CVP on pressure and flow in the kidney
Kidney perfusion is pressure and flow dependent. If intravascular volume augments without excessive CVP elevation, the unstressed volume (i.e., the fluid volume to fill the vascular bed to the point where it exerts force on the vessel walls) may incrementally follow a CO increase and RBF will rise. When CVP is already high, however, any additional volume load may increase CVP without a subsequent increase in CO and RBF. Right ventricular function then may deteriorate and evolve into acute cor pulmonale [17]. The difference between mean system filling pressure (MSFP) and CVP is the driving force behind venous return. Thus, with increasing CVP, a venous return will drop [20, 21]. With the heart functioning on the steep portion of the Starling curve, volume expansion will increase MSFP more than CVP. In contrast, changes in MSFP are approximately similar to CVP changes on the flat part of the Starling curve with no or minimal effects on CO [22, 23]. If fluid administration fails to obtain a higher MSFP, CVP must be kept low to enhance venous return, cardiac preload and CO.

In isolated kidneys of healthy dogs, renal venous and tissue pressures were unaffected over a large range of increased venous pressures. However, RBF fell when RVP approached or exceeded renal venous and tissue pressure [24]. Critically ill patients even have a more narrow pressure autoregulation range [25]. In the cardiorenal syndrome, an elevated CVP causes lowering of RPP below the kidney autoregulation threshold, resulting in pressure-dependent renal perfusion [26]. The rise in CVP is transmitted to the renal veins, sustains the cardiorenal syndrome, and induces a detrimental feedback loop via the renin–angiotensin–aldosterone and neuroendocrine pathways that leads to refractory heart failure. Worsening congestion also enhances sodium retention which exacerbates heart failure.

CVP can be more than a volume "indicator"
Many studies report a weak relationship between CVP and blood volume. CVP itself or changes in CVP evolution over time also failed to predict the hemodynamic response to a fluid challenge or to correctly estimate cardiac filling. As a result, it was suggested to abandon CVP to guide fluid resuscitation in critically ill patients [11, 27]. However, a more thorough understanding of various parameters and variables (i.e., preload, measurements in fluid-filled systems, impact of respiration, physiological determinants of CVP, and the point on the tracing that best estimates cardiac preload) may revalue CVP as a reproducible indicator of cardiac preload [16]. This is best illustrated by looking at the relationship between CVP and AKI in cardiac disease and sepsis.

Heart failure and cardiorenal syndrome
Since pressure/volume relationships are largely determined by heart compliance, a high CVP indicates volume overload, cardiac dysfunction, or both [28, 29]. Traditionally, AKI in congestive heart failure or cardiorenal syndrome is attributed to a reduction in CO and MAP which elicits a series of neurohumoral events resulting in increased renal vascular resistance and decreased renal function [30]. The degree of AKI is closely associated with congestive venous "backward failure." In 2557 patients who underwent right heart catheterization, Damman et al. found that an increased CVP was not only associated with impaired renal function but also independently related to all-cause mortality [31]. A study in patients with advanced decompensated heart failure showed that those with worsening renal function had a higher CVP on admission and after intensive medical therapy [32]. Worsening renal function occurred less frequently in patients in whom CVP was kept below 8 mmHg. An apparent potential of CVP for AKI risk stratification was noted across the spectrum of systemic

blood pressure, pulmonary capillary wedge pressure, cardiac index, and estimated glomerular filtration rate [32]. In adults with chronic heart disease after biventricular repair, Ohuchi et al. found that a high CVP predicted kidney enlargement and abnormal intrarenal flow dynamics that were closely associated with severity of heart failure and with cardiovascular events [33]. Right ventricular dysfunction and increased CVP are frequently observed in cardiac surgery patients and may lead to congestive renal dysfunction [34]. Studies in patients with acute right ventricular failure suggest that a high CVP is associated with a marked reduction in RBF by increasing renal backward pressure [35, 36]. A strong relationship was observed between CVP and RBF in both acute and chronic heart failure. Reducing CVP markedly improved renal function [35]. Cardiovascular surgery patients with progressive AKI had greater diastolic perfusion pressure deficits as compared to patients without AKI progression. Almost 25% of the diastolic perfusion pressure deficit was due to an increase in CVP [36]. This underscores the strong relationship between back (renal venous) pressure and CVP in the development of AKI.

Taken together, more attention must be paid to the pressure effect of CVP in heart failure/cardiorenal syndrome, regardless of whether fluid overload is present or not.

Sepsis and septic shock

Based on the landmark article of Rivers et al. which highlighted a striking mortality benefit of early goal-directed therapy (EGDT) in severe sepsis and septic shock [37], the Surviving Sepsis Campaign guidelines endorsed a CVP of 8–12 mmHg (12–15 mmHg in mechanically ventilated patients) as a key resuscitation target [38]. However, fluid load after 72 h in the Rivers study was equally high (approximately 13.5 L) in the EGDT and control arm. A major drawback of the study was the lack of data on occurrence and incidence of AKI. Recently, EGDT was assessed in the multicenter ProCESS [39, 40], ARISE [41], and ProMISE [42] trials which all used a CVP target ≥ 8 mmHg for guiding fluid resuscitation. The results of these trials, while reporting an all-time low sepsis mortality, question the need to use all elements of EGDT or the need for protocolized care in general. Limited data suggest that EGDT does not improve incidence of AKI and outcome of patients with AKI [43]. A CVP > 8 mmHg decreased microcirculatory and renal blood flow and increased AKI and mortality risk [44]. After adjustment for fluid balance and positive end-expiratory pressure ventilation, a lower diastolic arterial pressure and an elevated CVP were found to correlate with a high AKI incidence in septic patients [45–48].

Overzealous fluid treatment may result in interstitial edema which may worsen AKI or hamper renal recovery [49]. This underscores the potential role of venous congestion as one of the factors potentially implicated in the pathogenesis of septic AKI. CVP-directed fluid resuscitation in septic shock might harm the kidney if the target point is not correctly determined. Consequently, conservative fluid management [44] and permissive hypofiltration ("unburdening" the kidney by providing early renal replacement therapy, avoiding new injurious events such as fluid overload, and initiating therapies to improve survival and avoid ongoing loss of kidney function) [50, 51] are emerging treatment options in septic AKI. CVP should play a "limiting" rather than a target role within fluid resuscitation protocols [52]. Chen et al. found that early goal-directed diuretic therapy can improve the prognosis of sepsis [53]. In 105 patients with septic shock, Wang et al. showed that CVP was associated with kidney, liver, and lung function, sequential organ failure assessment scores, and lactate. Patients whose CVP remained below 8 mmHg during 7 days had a higher survival rate [54]. However, hypovolemia and renal hypoperfusion may occur in AKI patients if a too excessive fluid removal is pursued with diuretics or extracorporeal therapy [55].

Taken together, CVP plays an important role in the development of septic AKI by actively sustaining renal venous congestion and enhancing sepsis-related tissue edema.

A high CVP should be avoided

Healthy persons have a low CVP [56]. A high CVP does not always signify fluid overload, yet may impede RBF return to the right atrium and increase the risk of AKI. Ventricular preload is determined by transmural pressure, which is the difference between intracardiac and extracardiac intrathoracic pressure. Changes in right or left ventricular compliance, pulmonary hypertension, pulmonary venous disease, chronic airway disease, positive pressure ventilation, cardiac tamponade, pleural effusion, and increased intra-abdominal pressure all can increase intrathoracic or pericardial pressure [57] and thus augment CVP, decrease venous return, and potentially injure the kidney. Any elevation or significant change in CVP may refer to either presence or severity of a particular disease process and its response to treatment (Fig. 1).

Intra-abdominal hypertension

Intra-abdominal hypertension is defined as an intra-abdominal pressure exceeding 1.6 kPa. Abdominal compartment syndrome is diagnosed when the intra-abdominal pressure persists above 2.7 kPa in association with new organ dysfunction or failure. Various diseases

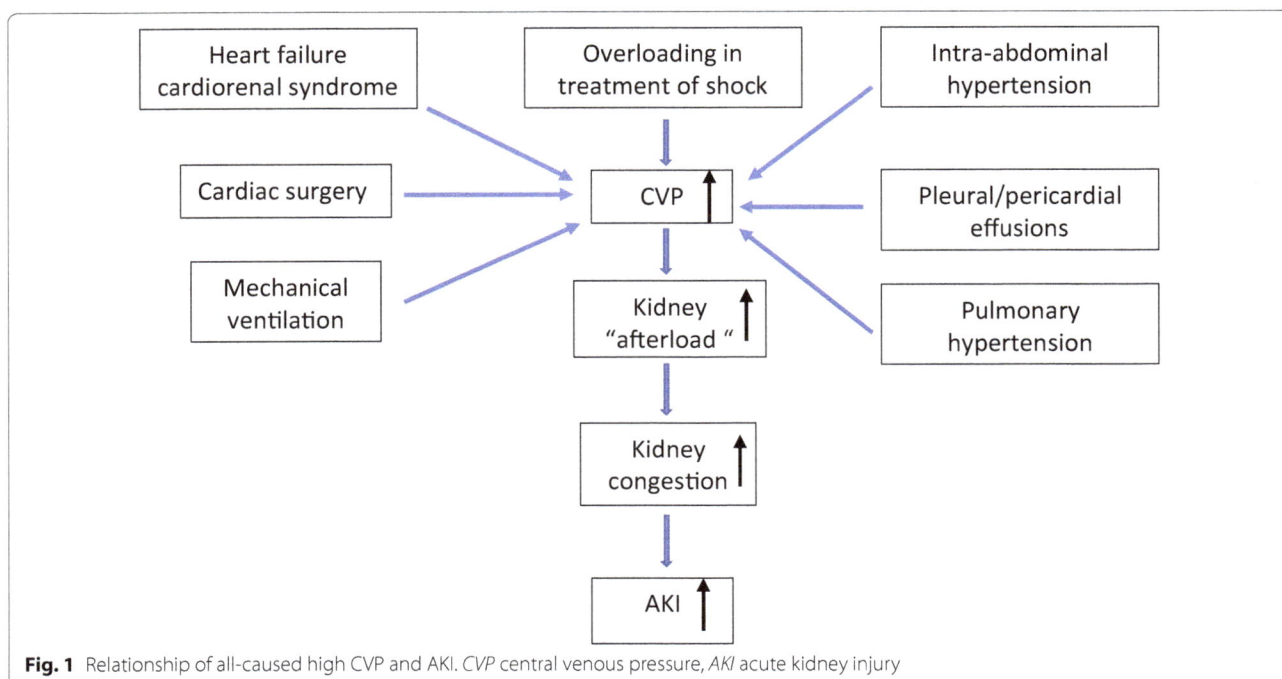

Fig. 1 Relationship of all-caused high CVP and AKI. *CVP* central venous pressure, *AKI* acute kidney injury

or conditions (e.g., pancreatitis, bile peritonitis, intra-abdominal hemorrhage, large abdominal masses, blunt abdominal trauma, recent abdominal surgery, ...) but also ample fluid resuscitation may cause abdominal hypertension and abdominal compartment syndrome [58–61]. Sepsis is an important trigger of AKI in postoperative and trauma patients with intra-abdominal hypertension [62]. AKI related to high intra-abdominal pressure is mainly due to an increase in inferior vena cava and intrathoracic pressure resulting in CVP elevation. A close relationship exists between an increased intra-abdominal pressure and the presence of oliguria and a high serum creatinine. The impact of diuretics on CVP and recovery of renal function is limited. However, lowering intra-abdominal pressure decreased CVP, restored diuresis, and normalized serum creatinine levels [61]. In a swine model, elevated intra-abdominal pressure increased renal venous, pleural, wedge, and pulmonary artery pressures, whereas cardiac index and urine output decreased. Intravascular volume expansion significantly increased urine output [63]. Decreasing intra-abdominal pressure to offer more space for volume expansion may be the best option to lower CVP.

Cardiac surgery

The CVP recorded 6 h after elective or urgent coronary artery bypass grafting was a strong and independent predictor of mortality and AKI [64]. The risk-adjusted OR for AKI was 5.5 (95% CI 1.93, 15.5; $p = 0.001$) with every

5 mmHg rise in CVP for patients with a CVP < 9 mmHg. For patients with a CVP ≥ 9 mmHg at 6 h, risk-adjusted OR was 1.3 (95% CI 1.01, 1.65; $p = 0.045$) with every 5 mmHg rise in CVP [64]. Guinot et al. observed that renal dysfunction in cardiac surgery patients was associated with early postoperative vena cava dilatation and elevated CVP, secondary to an increase in right heart filling pressure due to impaired right ventricular diastolic function [65].

Mechanical ventilation

Mechanical ventilation, especially when combined with high positive end-expiratory pressure (PEEP), prone positioning, and lung recruitment maneuvers, induces a high CVP [57, 66, 67]. Lung recruitment decreased renal arterial blood flow and perfusion of renal cortex and medulla in both healthy pigs and in pigs with endotoxin-induced pulmonary arterial hypertension [66, 67]. A balance must be sought between adequate blood volume, lowest CVP, and lowest intrathoracic pressure by carefully titrating PEEP under hemodynamic monitoring [68].

Specific conditions

Pleural and pericardial effusions are often associated with an increase in CVP. Pleural or pericardial puncture and drainage will reduce CVP. An increased CVP is a hallmark of diseases accompanied by pulmonary hypertension. Specific treatments (e.g., inhaled nitric oxide) can decrease pulmonary pressure and CVP, yet may increase

AKI risk [69]. The intrinsic response of renal vessels must thus always be weighed against the potential benefit of decreasing CVP when treating the primary disease.

The "optimal" CVP should be personalized and kept as low as possible

Currently, no exact definition of "lowest possible CVP" can be given except that it should be a CVP that assures adequate cardiac output and preserves organ perfusion. It becomes evident that a personalized approach is needed to aim at the most optimal CVP. In different patient populations or cohorts of similar patients with different disease stages, this optimal CVP level also will be different. A retrospective analysis of more than 500,000 CVP recordings in more than 9000 patients showed that the highest quartile of mean CVP during the first 3 days [mean (SD); 17.4 (4.1) mmHg] was associated with a 33.6% higher adjusted risk of death as compared with the lowest quartile [7.4 (1.9) mmHg]. Poor secondary outcomes (i.e., prolonged mechanical ventilation or vasopressor use, longer ICU and hospital stay) were also associated with higher quartiles of elevated mean CVP. Prolonged duration of CVP > 10 mmHg was significantly higher in non-survivors [70]. Keeping CVP and fluid in balance is more challenging in patients exhibiting a high CVP but no volume overload. In addition, extracting volume is not always the best way to decrease CVP. Overzealous use of diuretics or excessive ultrafiltration may indeed cause unwarranted volume loss resulting in lower cardiac preload, CO, and RBF. Strict and continuous monitoring of cardiac output, CVP, and kidney perfusion is imperative to avoid under- or over-treatment [71, 72]. Patients with acute heart failure and a CVP < 10 cm H2O were more likely to develop worsening renal function within the first 24 h than those presenting with a CVP > 15 cm H2O [73]. This does not imply that a higher CVP must be targeted in this population but rather that a volume "deficit" due to excessive fluid restriction or elimination should absolutely be avoided. Any decision to lower CVP should be individualized. Improving lung–right heart interactions that sustain an elevated CVP in heart failure and cardiorenal syndrome appears to be more efficacious than reducing intravascular volume [26, 30].

Conclusions

CVP is an innate pressure that is not only affected by manipulation of intravascular volume (fluid administration, restriction, or elimination) but also determined by various disease processes (intra-abdominal hypertension, pulmonary hypertension,...) or treatment (mechanical ventilation). Irrespective of volume status, an elevated CVP may harm the kidney by impeding renal venous return and causing renal interstitial edema. Individualizing CVP measurements and keeping CVP as low as possible should be encouraged to preserve kidney function or to avoid unnecessary renal damage.

Abbreviations
AKI: acute kidney injury; CVP: central venous pressure; MAP: mean arterial pressure; RVP: renal venous pressure; RPP: renal perfusion pressure; CO: cardiac output; RBF: renal blood flow; MSFP: mean system filling pressure; EGDT: early goal-directed therapy; PEEP: positive end-expiratory pressure.

Authors' contributions
XC performed the literature search and wrote the first draft of the paper. XW, PMH, HDS, and DL reviewed and contributed to the manuscript. All authors read and approved the final manuscript.

Author details
[1] Pittsburgh Heart, Lung, Blood and Vascular Medicine Institute, University of Pittsburgh, 200 Lothrop Street, BST E1240, Pittsburgh, PA 15261, USA. [2] Department of Critical Care Medicine, Peking Union Medical College Hospital, Peking Union Medical College, Chinese Academy of Medical Sciences, 1 Shuaifuyuan, Dongcheng District, Beijing 100073, China. [3] Department of Intensive Care, Centre Hospitalier Universitaire Brugmann, Brugmann University Hospital, 4 Place Van Gehuchtenplein, 1020 Brussels, Belgium. [4] Department of Intensive Care, University Hospital, Vrije Universiteit Brussel (VUB), 101, Laarbeeklaan, Jette 1090 Brussels, Belgium.

Acknowledgements
Thanks to Dr. Wenzhao Chai, Hongmin Zhang, Rongli Yang, Qing Zhang, and Suwei Li's help in the formatting of the idea. Thanks to Dr. John A. Kellum's comments. Thanks to Seth Morrisroe for draft editing.

Competing interests
The authors declare that they have no competing interests.

Funding
Not applicable.

References
1. Parmar A, Langenberg C, Wan L, May CN, Bellomo R, Bagshaw SM. Epidemiology of septic acute kidney injury. Curr Drug Targets. 2009;10(12):1169–78.
2. Kellum JA. Why are patients still getting and dying from acute kidney injury? Curr Opin Crit Care. 2016;22(6):513–9.
3. Matejovic M, Ince C, Chawla LS, Blantz R, Molitoris BA, Rosner MH, et al. Renal hemodynamics in AKI. In search of new treatment targets. J Am Soc Nephrol JASN. 2016;27(1):49–58.
4. Zhang H, Liu D, Wang X, Chen X, Zhang Q, Tang B, et al. Variations of renal vascular score and resistive indices in septic shock patients. Zhonghua Yi Xue Za Zhi. 2014;94(27):2102–5.
5. Badin J, Boulain T, Ehrmann S, Skarzynski M, Bretagnol A, Buret J, et al. Relation between mean arterial pressure and renal function in the

early phase of shock: a prospective, explorative cohort study. Crit Care. 2011;15(3):R135.

6. Gambardella I, Gaudino M, Ronco C, Lau C, Ivascu N, Girardi LN. Congestive kidney failure in cardiac surgery: the relationship between central venous pressure and acute kidney injury. Interact Cardiovasc Thorac Surg. 2016;23(5):800–5.

7. Bagshaw SM, Delaney A, Jones D, Ronco C, Bellomo R. Diuretics in the management of acute kidney injury: a multinational survey. Contrib Nephrol. 2007;156:236–49.

8. Chuasuwan A, Kellum JA. Cardio-renal syndrome type 3: epidemiology, pathophysiology, and treatment. Semin Nephrol. 2012;32(1):31–9.

9. Jones SL, Martensson J, Glassford NJ, Eastwood GM, Bellomo R. Loop diuretic therapy in the critically ill: a survey. Crit Care Resusc. 2015;17(3):223–6.

10. Fiaccadori E. Fluid overload in acute kidney injury: an underestimated toxin? G Ital Nefrol. 2011;28(1):11.

11. Marik PE, Baram M, Vahid B. Does central venous pressure predict fluid responsiveness? A systematic review of the literature and the tale of seven mares. Chest. 2008;134(1):172–8.

12. Ho KM. Pitfalls in haemodynamic monitoring in the postoperative and critical care setting. Anaesth Intensive Care. 2016;44(1):14–9.

13. Chen KP, Cavender S, Lee J, Feng M, Mark RG, Celi LA, et al. Peripheral edema, central venous pressure, and risk of AKI in critical illness. Clin J Am Soc Nephrol. 2016;11(4):602–8.

14. Magder S, Bafaqeeh F. The clinical role of central venous pressure measurements. J Intensive Care Med. 2007;22(1):44–51.

15. Gelman S. Venous function and central venous pressure: a physiologic story. Anesthesiology. 2008;108(4):735–48.

16. Magder S. Understanding central venous pressure: not a preload index? Curr Opin Crit Care. 2015;21(5):369–75.

17. Magder S. Volume and its relationship to cardiac output and venous return. Crit Care. 2016;20:271.

18. Honore PM, Jacobs R, Hendrickx I, Bagshaw SM, Joannes-Boyau O, Boer W, et al. Prevention and treatment of sepsis-induced acute kidney injury: an update. Ann Intensive Care. 2015;5(1):51.

19. Winton FR. The influence of venous pressure on the isolated mammalian kidney. J Physiol. 1931;72(1):49–61.

20. Brengelmann GL. A critical analysis of the view that right atrial pressure determines venous return. J Appl Physiol. 2003;94(3):849–59.

21. Beard DA, Feigl EO. Understanding Guyton's venous return curves. Am J Physiol Heart Circ Physiol. 2011;301(3):H629–33.

22. Den Hartog EA, Versprille A, Jansen JR. Systemic filling pressure in intact circulation determined on basis of aortic vs. central venous pressure relationships. Am J Physiol. 1994;267(6 Pt 2):H2255–8.

23. Gupta K, Sondergaard S, Parkin G, Leaning M, Aneman A. Applying mean systemic filling pressure to assess the response to fluid boluses in cardiac post-surgical patients. Intensive Care Med. 2015;41(2):265–72.

24. Hinshaw LB, Brake CM, Iampietro PF, Emerson TE Jr. Effect of increased venous pressure on renal hemodynamics. Am J Physiol. 1963;204:119–23.

25. Burban M, Hamel JF, Tabka M, de La Bourdonnaye MR, Duveau A, Mercat A, et al. Renal macro- and microcirculation autoregulatory capacity during early sepsis and norepinephrine infusion in rats. Crit Care. 2013;17(4):R139.

26. Guazzi M, Gatto P, Giusti G, Pizzamiglio F, Previtali I, Vignati C, et al. Pathophysiology of cardiorenal syndrome in decompensated heart failure: role of lung-right heart-kidney interaction. Int J Cardiol. 2013;169(6):379–84.

27. Toyoda D, Fukuda M, Iwasaki R, Terada T, Sato N, Ochiai R, et al. The comparison between stroke volume variation and filling pressure as an estimate of right ventricular preload in patients undergoing renal transplantation. J Anesth. 2015;29(1):40–6.

28. Cui K, Wang X, Zhang H, Chai W, Liu D. The application of combined central venous pressure and oxygen metabolism parameters monitoring in diagnosing septic shock-induced left ventricular dysfunction. Zhonghua Nei Ke Za Zhi. 2015;54(10):855–9.

29. Zhang HM, Liu DW, Wang XT, Long Y, Shi Y, Chai WZ, et al. Correlation between pressure and volume parameters of septic shock patients with cardiac depression. Zhonghua Wai Ke Za Zhi [Chin J Surg]. 2010;48(3):201–4.

30. McCullough PA, Kellum JA, Haase M, Muller C, Damman K, Murray PT, et al. Pathophysiology of the cardiorenal syndromes: executive summary from the eleventh consensus conference of the acute dialysis quality initiative (ADQI). Contrib Nephrol. 2013;182:82–98.

31. Damman K, van Deursen VM, Navis G, Voors AA, van Veldhuisen DJ, Hillege HL. Increased central venous pressure is associated with impaired renal function and mortality in a broad spectrum of patients with cardiovascular disease. J Am Coll Cardiol. 2009;53(7):582–8.

32. Mullens W, Abrahams Z, Francis GS, Sokos G, Taylor DO, Starling RC, et al. Importance of venous congestion for worsening of renal function in advanced decompensated heart failure. J Am Coll Cardiol. 2009;53(7):589–96.

33. Ohuchi H, Ikado H, Noritake K, Miyazaki A, Yasuda K, Yamada O. Impact of central venous pressure on cardiorenal interactions in adult patients with congenital heart disease after biventricular repair. Congenit Heart Dis. 2013;8(2):103–10.

34. Romagnoli S, Ricci Z, Ronco C. Therapy of acute kidney injury in the perioperative setting. Curr Opin Anaesthesiol. 2017;30(1):92–9.

35. Mebazaa A. Congestion and cardiorenal syndromes. Contrib Nephrol. 2010;165:140–4.

36. Saito S, Uchino S, Takinami M, Uezono S, Bellomo R. Postoperative blood pressure deficit and acute kidney injury progression in vasopressor-dependent cardiovascular surgery patients. Crit Care. 2016;20:74.

37. Rivers E, Nguyen B, Havstad S, Ressler J, Muzzin A, Knoblich B, et al. Early goal-directed therapy in the treatment of severe sepsis and septic shock. N Engl J Med. 2001;345(19):1368–77.

38. Rhodes A, Evans LE, Alhazzani W, Levy MM, Antonelli M, Ferrer R, et al. Surviving sepsis campaign: international guidelines for management of sepsis and septic shock: 2016. Crit Care Med. 2017;45(3):486–552.

39. Pro CI, Yealy DM, Kellum JA, Huang DT, Barnato AE, Weissfeld LA, et al. A randomized trial of protocol-based care for early septic shock. N Engl J Med. 2014;370(18):1683–93.

40. Angus DC, Yealy DM, Kellum JA, Pro CI. Protocol-based care for early septic shock. N Engl J Med. 2014;371(4):386.

41. Investigators A, Group ACT, Peake SL, Delaney A, Bailey M, Bellomo R, et al. Goal-directed resuscitation for patients with early septic shock. N Engl J Med. 2014;371(16):1496–506.

42. Mouncey PR, Osborn TM, Power GS, Harrison DA, Sadique MZ, Grieve RD, et al. Protocolised Management In Sepsis (ProMISe): a multicentre randomised controlled trial of the clinical effectiveness and cost-effectiveness of early, goal-directed, protocolised resuscitation for emerging septic shock. Health Technol Assess. 2015;19(97):i–xxv, 1–150.

43. Ahmed W, Memon JI, Rehmani R, Al Juhaiman A. Outcome of patients with acute kidney injury in severe sepsis and septic shock treated with early goal-directed therapy in an intensive care unit. Saudi J Kidney Dis Transpl. 2014;25(3):544–51.

44. Schrier RW. Fluid administration in critically ill patients with acute kidney injury. Clin J Am Soc Nephrol. 2010;5(4):733–9.

45. Marik PE. Iatrogenic salt water drowning and the hazards of a high central venous pressure. Ann Intensive Care. 2014;4:21.

46. Legrand M, Dupuis C, Simon C, Gayat E, Mateo J, Lukaszewicz AC, et al. Association between systemic hemodynamics and septic acute kidney injury in critically ill patients: a retrospective observational study. Crit Care. 2013;17(6):R278.

47. Wong BT, Chan MJ, Glassford NJ, Martensson J, Bion V, Chai SY, et al. Mean arterial pressure and mean perfusion pressure deficit in septic acute kidney injury. J Crit Care. 2015;30(5):975–81.

48. Chen XK, Li SW, Liu DW, Yang RL, Zhang HM, Zhang H, et al. Effects of central venous pressure on acute kidney injury in septic shock. Zhonghua Yi Xue Za Zhi. 2011;91(19):1323–7.

49. Prowle JR, Bellomo R. Fluid administration and the kidney. Curr Opin Crit Care. 2010;16(4):332–6.

50. Chawla LS, Kellum JA, Ronco C. Permissive hypofiltration. Crit Care. 2012;16(4):317.

51. Chen X, Yang R, Liu D. Permissive hypohemofiltration and blood purification to salvage acute kidney injury. Zhonghua Nei Ke Za Zhi. 2014;53(6):428–30.

52. Pinsky MR, Kellum JA, Bellomo R. Central venous pressure is a stopping rule, not a target of fluid resuscitation. Crit Care Resusc. 2014;16(4):245–6.

53. Chen XK, Ding Q, Liu DW, Li WX, Huang LF, Sui F, et al. Effects of early goal-directed diuresis therapy on the outcomes of critical ill patients. Zhonghua Yi Xue Za Zhi. 2013;93(23):1815–8.

54. Wang XT, Yao B, Liu DW, Zhang HM. Central venous pressure dropped early is associated with organ function and prognosis in septic shock patients: a retrospective observational study. Shock. 2015;44(5):426–30.

55. Prowle JR, Echeverri JE, Ligabo EV, Ronco C, Bellomo R. Fluid balance and acute kidney injury. Nat Rev Nephrol. 2010;6(2):107–15.

56. Pinsky MR, Payen D. Functional hemodynamic monitoring. Crit Care. 2005;9(6):566–72.

57. Berger D, Moller PW, Weber A, Bloch A, Bloechlinger S, Haenggi M, et al. Effect of PEEP, blood volume, and inspiratory hold maneuvers on venous return. Am J Physiol Heart Circ Physiol. 2016;311(3):H794–806.

58. Chen XK, Li WX. Intra-abdominal hypertension induced acute kidney injury: pressure overweigh volume. Zhonghua Yi Xue Za Zhi. 2012;92(15):1009–11.

59. Mohmand H, Goldfarb S. Renal dysfunction associated with intra-abdominal hypertension and the abdominal compartment syndrome. J Am Soc Nephrol. 2011;22(4):615–21.

60. Ross EA. Congestive renal failure: the pathophysiology and treatment of renal venous hypertension. J Card Fail. 2012;18(12):930–8.

61. Wu YF, Zheng YP, Zhang N, Liu H, Zheng QX, Yang FT, et al. Study on the correlation between the changes in intra-abdominal pressure and renal functional in the patients with abdominal compartment syndrome. Eur Rev Med Pharmacol Sci. 2015;19(19):3682–7.

62. Honore PM, Jacobs R, Joannes-Boyau O, De Regt J, Boer W, De Waele E, et al. Septic AKI in ICU patients. diagnosis, pathophysiology, and treatment type, dosing, and timing: a comprehensive review of recent and future developments. Ann Intensive Care. 2011;1(1):32.

63. Bloomfield GL, Blocher CR, Fakhry IF, Sica DA, Sugerman HJ. Elevated intra-abdominal pressure increases plasma renin activity and aldosterone levels. J Trauma. 1997;42(6):997–1004 (**discussion-5**).

64. Williams JB, Peterson ED, Wojdyla D, Harskamp R, Southerland KW, Ferguson TB, et al. Central venous pressure after coronary artery bypass surgery: does it predict postoperative mortality or renal failure? J Crit Care. 2014;29(6):1006–10.

65. Guinot PG, Abou-Arab O, Longrois D, Dupont H. Right ventricular systolic dysfunction and vena cava dilatation precede alteration of renal function in adult patients undergoing cardiac surgery: an observational study. Eur J Anaesthesiol. 2015;32(8):535–42.

66. Daudel F, Gorrasi J, Bracht H, Brandt S, Krejci V, Jakob SM, et al. Effects of lung recruitment maneuvers on splanchnic organ perfusion during endotoxin-induced pulmonary arterial hypertension. Shock. 2010;34(5):488–94.

67. Nunes S, Rothen HU, Brander L, Takala J, Jakob SM. Changes in splanchnic circulation during an alveolar recruitment maneuver in healthy porcine lungs. Anesth Analg. 2004;98(5):1432–8.

68. Vieillard-Baron A, Matthay M, Teboul JL, Bein T, Schultz M, Magder S, et al. Experts' opinion on management of hemodynamics in ARDS patients: focus on the effects of mechanical ventilation. Intensive Care Med. 2016;42(5):739–49.

69. Ruan SY, Huang TM, Wu HY, Wu HD, Yu CJ, Lai MS. Inhaled nitric oxide therapy and risk of renal dysfunction: a systematic review and meta-analysis of randomized trials. Crit Care. 2015;19:137.

70. Li DK, Wang XT, Liu DW. Association between elevated central venous pressure and outcomes in critically ill patients. Ann Intensive Care. 2017;7(1):83.

71. Honore PM, Pierrakos C, Spapen HD. Relationship between central venous pressure and acute kidney injury in critically ill patients. Annu Update Intensive Care Emerg Med. 2019.

72. Legrand M, Soussi S, Depret F. Cardiac output and CVP monitoring… to guide fluid removal. Crit Care. 2018;22(1):89.

73. Uthoff H, Breidthardt T, Klima T, Aschwanden M, Arenja N, Socrates T, et al. Central venous pressure and impaired renal function in patients with acute heart failure. Eur J Heart Fail. 2011;13(4):432–9.

22

Severe metabolic acidosis after out-of-hospital cardiac arrest: risk factors and association with outcome

Matthieu Jamme[1,3], Omar Ben Hadj Salem[1,3], Lucie Guillemet[1,3], Pierre Dupland[1], Wulfran Bougouin[1,3,4], Julien Charpentier[1], Jean-Paul Mira[1,3], Frédéric Pène[1,3], Florence Dumas[2,3,4], Alain Cariou[1,3,4*] and Guillaume Geri[1,3,4]

Abstract

Background: Metabolic acidosis is frequently observed as a consequence of global ischemia–reperfusion after out-of-hospital cardiac arrest (OHCA). We aimed to identify risk factors and assess the impact of metabolic acidosis on outcome after OHCA.

Methods: We included all consecutive OHCA patients admitted between 2007 and 2012. Using admission data, metabolic acidosis was defined by a positive base deficit and was categorized by quartiles. Main outcome was survival at ICU discharge. Factors associated with acidosis severity and with main outcome were evaluated by linear and logistic regressions, respectively.

Results: A total of 826 patients (68.3% male, median age 61 years) were included in the analysis. Median base deficit was 8.8 [5.3, 13.2] mEq/l. Male gender ($p = 0.002$), resuscitation duration ($p < 0.001$), initial shockable rhythm ($p < 0.001$) and post-resuscitation shock ($p < 0.001$) were associated with an increased level of acidosis. ICU mortality rate increased across base deficit quartiles (39.1, 59.2, 76.3 and 88.3%, p for trend < 0.001), and base deficit was independently associated with ICU mortality ($p < 0.001$). The proportion of CPC 1 patients among ICU survivors was similar across base deficit quartiles (72.8, 67.1, 70.5 and 62.5%, $p = 0.21$), and 7.3% of patients with a base deficit higher than 13.2 mEq/l survived to ICU discharge with complete neurological recovery.

Conclusion: Severe metabolic acidosis is frequent in OHCA patients and is associated with poorer outcome, in particular due to refractory shock. However, we observed that about 7% of patients with a very severe metabolic acidosis survived to ICU discharge with complete neurological recovery.

Keywords: Metabolic acidosis, Out-of-hospital cardiac arrest, Post-resuscitation syndrome, Outcome

Background

Among successfully resuscitated out-of-hospital cardiac arrest (OHCA) patients admitted to the intensive care unit (ICU) after return of spontaneous circulation (ROSC), the occurrence of a "post-cardiac arrest syndrome" is the leading cause of early mortality. This syndrome is related to multi-organ ischemic reperfusion injury and may lead to multi-organ failure in the early hours after resuscitation [1].

Acidosis is frequently observed in this context [2] and is often multifactorial, resulting from major metabolic disturbances (increased levels of blood lactate, phosphate, unmeasured anions, acute kidney injury) as well as respiratory disturbances. Metabolic acidosis has well-known deleterious effects including decrease of cardiac contractility [3], arterial vasodilatation [4], impairment of the inflammatory and immune response [5] leading to an increased risk of multi-organ failure. Accordingly, a strong association between the depth of acidosis and

*Correspondence: alain.cariou@aphp.fr
[1] Medical Intensive Care Unit, Cochin University Hospital (APHP), 27 rue du Faubourg Saint Jacques, 75014 Paris, France

poor outcome has been previously demonstrated in critically ill patients [6, 7]. Even though intuitive in OHCA patients, data on the prevalence and the severity of metabolic acidosis at ICU admission are scarce. Moreover, data on the prognostic impact of metabolic acidosis in these patients and on the proportion of patients with severe metabolic acidosis discharged alive from ICU are lacking.

In the present study, we aimed to describe the outcome of successfully resuscitated OHCA patients with metabolic acidosis and to identify factors associated with severe acidosis and survival to ICU discharge.

Methods
Study population
In the present analysis, we screened all consecutive OHCA patients admitted to our cardiac arrest center between January 2007 and December 2012 (IRB number CE-SRLF 12-384). We then selected patients who evidenced a metabolic acidosis at ICU admission, defined by a positive base deficit, as described above. We only excluded patients who did not get ROSC in the prehospital setting and who received CPR at time of ICU admission.

Data collection and definitions
Cardiac arrest characteristics, in-hospital management and outcome data were prospectively collected according to the Utstein style [8]. The following information was recorded prospectively for each patient: demographic data, clinical parameters, cardiac arrest location, time from collapse to basic life support (BLS) and time from BLS to ROSC, initial rhythm, admission blood lactate level, temperature management and ICU mortality. Post-resuscitation shock was defined as the need for vasopressors (epinephrine or norepinephrine) lasting more than 6 h despite adequate fluid loading or the need for mechanical circulatory assistance (intra-aortic balloon pump) [9]. We reviewed patients' charts in order to collect information that could impact ICU admission bicarbonate level, i.e., the use of intravenous bicarbonate during resuscitation, the existence of chronic respiratory condition and chronic kidney disease in the past medical history.

Laboratory values were computed from medical files and extracted from the patient data management system (Clinisoft, GE Healthcare). We specifically collected arterial blood gas (pH, PCO_2 [mmHg], PO_2 [mmHg], bicarbonate [$mmol^{-1}$]), arterial blood lactate, hemoglobin, potassium, phosphorus, blood creatinine and urea levels. We determined the occurrence and the severity of acute kidney injury within the first 48 h using the KDIGO definition [10].

Metabolic acidosis was defined by a positive base deficit (i.e., negative base excess). Base deficit was calculated according to the Van Slyke equation [11, 12] and expressed in mEq/l. We then divided the study population in quartiles of base deficit.

Early management
As previously described [13], our local practices include a strategy of early imaging work-up performed within the first 24 h after an immediate assessment of the feasibility of further investigations by the Emergency Medical Services (EMS) and ICU physicians. According to this strategy, we consider immediate coronary angiography in all patients without obvious extra-cardiac cause of cardiac arrest, regardless of the initial rhythm and ECG changes. In case of suspected extra-cardiac cause and in the absence of an obvious etiology, a CT scan can also be performed at admission (brain CT scan and chest CT pulmonary angiography). After this early imaging procedure, patients are then admitted to ICU. Arterial blood gas is taken as soon as possible, i.e., either at the cath laboratory arrival, or at ICU admission if the patient was directly admitted to the ICU. Renal replacement therapy is initiated at ICU admission in case of severe metabolic acidosis (defined by a pH lower than 7.20 and an admission bicarbonate level lower than 20 mmol/l) and/or in case of life-threatening hyperkalemia (defined by blood potassium level higher than 6 mmol/l with electrocardiographic findings suggestive of hyperkalemia) [2]. Therapeutic hypothermia was performed using surface cooling, using a 33 °C temperature target.

Outcomes
The main outcome was survival at ICU discharge. Neurological outcome and cause of death were our secondary outcomes. The cause of death was defined for each non-survivor as related to post-cardiac arrest shock, when death occurred as a direct consequence of shock (including subsequent multi-organ failure), or related to neurological injury if this led to withdrawal of life-sustaining therapy or brain death [9]. Neurological outcome at ICU discharge was assessed using the Cerebral Performance Categories score [14]. Briefly, CPC score ranges from 1 to 5: 1 is a normal neurological state while 4 means vegetative state and 5 death.

Statistical analysis
Continuous variables were presented as median [interquartile] and categorical variables as counts (percentages). Baseline characteristics were compared according to the presence of acidemia using Mann–Whitney test, and Pearson Chi-square test or the Fisher's exact test, as appropriate, for continuous and categorical variables,

respectively. Characteristics between quartiles of base excess were compared using Cuzick test and trend Pearson Chi-square test for continuous and categorical variables, respectively.

To evaluate prognostic performance of base deficit, admission pH, arterial lactate and bicarbonate level, we picked up thresholds corresponding to a specificity of 100% (i.e., no survivor above the threshold).

Factors associated with base excess were identified using a multivariable linear regression. Normal distribution of residuals was checked as well as heteroscedasticity. Factors associated with ICU mortality were assessed using a multivariable logistic regression. The multivariable model was built using all variables significantly associated with ICU mortality in univariate analysis ($p < 0.05$). The goodness-of-fit of the model was evaluated using the Hosmer–Lemeshow test.

This analysis was repeated in the following subgroups of patients, as sensitivity analyses: patients without prehospital bicarbonate infusion and patients without either chronic respiratory disease or chronic kidney disease. We also performed a sensitivity analysis including arterial blood lactate level in the multivariable model to assess a potential interaction between lactate level and base deficit. We thus included a cross-produced factor, and both lactate level and base deficit were included as continuous variables in the model.

All statistical tests were two-sided using a type I error of 0.05 unless otherwise mentioned. Analyses were performed using Stata 14.1 (Stata Corp, College Station, TX).

Results

A total of 899 resuscitated OHCA patients were admitted to the study hospital during the study period. We excluded 27 patients without ROSC at ICU admission, one patient with DNR order and 2 patients with no available arterial blood gases at ICU admission. Among the 869 remaining patients with acid–base status available, 43 patients did not have metabolic acidosis, and we included 826 patients in the analysis.

Baseline characteristics of the studied population

Most of the included patients were male (68.3%) of median age of 61 [iqr 50–73] years (Table 1). An initial shockable rhythm was observed in 414 (50.1%) cases, and the median time from collapse to ROSC was 20 [iqr 13–30] min. Post-resuscitation shock occurred in 480 (58.1%) cases. Acute kidney injury (AKI) was observed in 548/791 (69.3%) patients (baseline creatinine level was unknown in 35/45 patients with chronic kidney disease). Renal replacement therapy (RRT) was initiated within the first 24 h in 40.6% of cases. Even if indicated, 13 patients

did not receive RRT because of major hemodynamic instability ($n = 10$) or early withdrawal of life-sustaining therapy ($n = 3$).

Factors associated with severity of metabolic acidosis

Arterial acidemia (pH < 7.38) was observed in the majority of patients at ICU admission (n = 743, 90.0%) with a median pH at ICU admission at 7.22 [7.11, 7.31] and a blood bicarbonate level of 17.5 [14.0, 20.4] mmol/l. Median base deficit was 8.8 [iqr 5.3, 13.2] mEq/l (Additional file 1: Figure S1). Median base deficit was 3.3 [iqr 2.5, 5.3] and 9.5 [iqr 5.9, 13.8] in patients without and with acidemia ($p < 0.001$). There were, respectively, 61, 19, 2 and 0 patients without acidemia in base deficit quartiles. The proportion of witnessed cases and of initial shockable rhythm decreased across base deficit quartiles while time interval from collapse to ROSC increased across the quartiles (16, 20, 22 and 29 min, p for trend < 0.001) (Table 1). Left ventricular ejection fraction did not differ in the 4 quartiles of base deficit (median = 40% in the four quartiles). In multivariable linear regression, male gender (beta estimate − 1.51 [95% confidence interval − 2.45, − 0.56]) and initial shockable rhythm (− 2.36 [− 3.41, − 1.31]) were negatively associated with base deficit. Conversely, time interval between collapse to ROSC (+ 0.09 per min [0.06, 0.12]) and the occurrence of post-resuscitation shock (+ 2.45 [1.60, 3.29]) was independently associated with base deficit (Table 2).

Association between base deficit, ICU mortality and cause of death

Overall, 543 (65.7%) patients died in ICU. ICU mortality rate increased across base deficit quartiles (39.1, 59.2, 76.3 and 88.3%, p for trend < 0.001). ICU mortality was 42.2 versus 68.4% in patients without and with acidemia ($p < 0.001$). After adjustment for confounders, we observed an association between base deficit and mortality at ICU discharge (odds ratio 1.76 [1.07, 2.91], 3.82 [2.20, 6.65], 5.13 [2.67, 9.88] for 5–9, 9–13 and > 13 categories with base deficit < 5 as reference category, respectively) (Table 3). Similar results were obtained in patients without prehospital bicarbonate infusion and without either chronic respiratory disease or chronic kidney disease. We observed a strong interaction between base deficit and lactate level (p for interaction = 0.004).

Brain damage was the leading cause of death ($n = 367$, 67.6%), while refractory shock was responsible for 173 (31.9%) deaths. Three patients died in ICU from septic shock without brain anoxic injury. Death related to refractory shock was more frequent in the subgroup of patients with the most severe metabolic acidosis (13.6, 22.1, 28.5 and 49.5% across base deficit quartiles).

Table 1 Baseline characteristics of the 826 patients included in the study according to quartiles of base deficit

Variable	All patients $n=826$	Base deficit quartiles				p value
		[0–5] $n=207$	[5–9] $n=206$	[9–13] $n=207$	>13 $n=206$	
Demographics						
Male gender	564 (68.3)	156 (75.4)	148 (71.8)	139 (67.1)	121 (58.7)	<0.001
Age (year)	61 [50, 73]	60 [51, 71]	64 [51, 77]	60 [49, 72]	62 [51, 74]	0.678
OHCA characteristics						
Public setting	262 (31.8)	79 (38.3)	71 (34.5)	70 (33.8)	42 (20.4)	<0.001
Witnessed CA	698 (87.0)	181 (90.5)	183 (92.0)	177 (88.5)	157 (77.3)	<0.001
Bystander CPR	444 (55.8)	122 (62.2)	122 (60.7)	99 (49.5)	101 (51.0)	0.004
Initial VF/VT	414 (50.1)	129 (62.3)	121 (58.7)	92 (44.4)	72 (35.0)	<0.001
Collapse to ROSC, min	20 [13, 30]	16 [10, 25]	20 [14, 27]	22 [15, 33]	29 [20, 40]	<0.001
Prehosp. infusion of bicar.	113 (13.7)	17 (8.2)	22 (10.7)	28 (13.5)	46 (22.3)	<0.001
Chronic respiratory disease	42 (5.1)	11 (5.3)	14 (6.8)	8 (3.9)	9 (4.4)	0.399
Chronic kidney disease	45 (5.5)	5 (2.4)	12 (5.9)	14 (6.9)	14 (7.0)	0.039
Biological characteristics at ICU admission						
pH	7.22 [7.11, 7.31]	7.33 [7.28, 7.39]	7.27 [7.21, 7.32]	7.18 [7.13, 7.25]	7.03 [6.92, 7.11]	<0.001
PCO_2 (mmHg)	42.8 [36.0, 51.2]	41.5 [36.8, 49.7]	42.3 [36.3, 50.5]	43.5 [35.7, 52.3]	43.5 [35.1, 52.5]	0.554
Bicarbonate level (mmol/l)	17.5 [14.0, 20.4]	21.8 [20.7, 22.9]	19.1 [17.8, 20.0]	16.0 [15.0, 16.9]	10.8 [8.7, 12.7]	<0.001
Urea level (mmol/l)	7.3 [5.7, 10.2]	6.8 [5.3, 8.9]	7.3 [5.8, 9.8]	7.5 [5.8, 10.6]	8.1 [5.7, 13.2]	<0.001
Creatinine level (μmol/l)	106 [78, 146]	87 [69, 111]	102 [77, 130]	114 [86, 148]	136 [101, 190]	<0.001
Phosphorus level (mmol/l)	1.7 [1.1, 2.5]	1.2 [0.9, 1.7]	1.4 [1.0, 1.9]	1.9 [1.3, 2.5]	2.9 [2.1, 3.8]	<0.001
Lactate level (mmol/l)	5.2 [2.5, 9.2]	2.5 [1.6, 4.3]	4.0 [2.3, 5.7]	6.5 [3.5, 8.8]	11.2 [7.6, 15.0]	<0.001
Base deficit (mEq/l)	8.8 [5.3, 13.2]	3.6 [2.8, 4.5]	6.8 [6.0, 7.9]	10.8 [9.7, 11.9]	17.8 [15.2, 21.0]	<0.001
In-hospital characteristics						
Cardiac cause-related CA	436 (56.2)	136 (68.7)	122 (61.3)	103 (54.5)	75 (39.5)	<0.001
Post-resus. shock	480 (58.1)	87 (42.0)	109 (52.9)	119 (57.5)	165 (80.1)	<0.001
Acute kidney injury[a]						<0.001
No AKI	243 (30.7)	104 (51.5)	71 (35.9)	59 (30.3)	9 (4.6)	
KDIGO 1	65 (8.2)	12 (5.9)	27 (13.6)	19 (9.7)	7 (3.6)	
KDIGO 2	45 (5.7)	17 (8.4)	13 (6.6)	10 (5.1)	5 (2.6)	
KDIGO 3	438 (55.4)	69 (34.2)	87 (43.9)	107 (54.9)	175 (89.7)	
Coronary angiography	556 (67.3)	145 (70.0)	150 (72.8)	135 (65.2)	126 (61.2)	0.019
Therapeutic hypothermia	717 (86.8)	186 (89.9)	182 (88.3)	185 (89.4)	164 (79.6)	0.005
RRT at day-1	335 (40.6)	42 (20.4)	56 (27.2)	89 (43.0)	148 (71.8)	<0.001

OHCA out-of-hospital cardiac arrest, *CPR* cardiopulmonary resuscitation, *ROSC* restoration of spontaneous circulation, *AKI* acute kidney injury, *KDIGO* kidney disease improving global outcome, *RRT* renal replacement therapy

p value for trend has been calculated using a Chi-square trend test for binary variables and Cuzick test for ordinal and continuous variables

[a] Missing data are related to the missingness of basal level of creatinine in patients with chronic kidney disease

Overall, the proportion of CPC1 patients decreased across the base deficit quartile while it was similar among patients discharged alive (72.8, 67.1, 70.5 and 62.5%, $p=0.21$) (Fig. 1). Among patients with the most severe acidosis, clinical characteristics except initial rhythm and in-hospital management were similar between patients who died and those who were discharged alive from ICU (Additional file 2: Table S1).

No patient survived with a base deficit higher than 25 mmol/l, a pH lower than 6.72, a blood bicarbonate

level lower than 8.6 mmol/l or an admission arterial blood lactate level higher than 20 mmol/l (Additional file 3: Table S2).

Discussion

In the present study, we found that metabolic acidosis was almost constantly observed at ICU admission in OHCA patients. Metabolic acidosis was related to the initial rhythm and the time interval from collapse to ROSC. Furthermore, we observed that metabolic acidosis

Table 2 Factors associated with base deficit in multivariable linear regression

Variable	Coefficient	95% confidence interval	p value
Age, per year	− 0.01	− 0.03, 0.02	0.670
Male gender	− 1.51	− 2.45, − 0.56	0.002
Public setting	− 0.85	− 1.76, 0.06	0.067
Witnessed CA	− 1.35	− 2.91, 0.22	0.091
Bystander CPR	0.69	− 0.17, 1.56	0.117
Collapse to ROSC, per min	0.09	0.06, 0.12	< 0.001
Initial VF/VT	− 2.36	− 3.41, − 1.31	< 0.001
Post-resus. shock	2.45	1.60, 3.29	< 0.001
Cardiac cause-related CA	− 0.16	− 1.21, 0.89	0.761

CA cardiac arrest, CPR cardiopulmonary resuscitation, ROSC restoration of spontaneous circulation

Table 3 Factors associated with ICU mortality in multivariable logistic regression

Variable	Odds ratio	95% confidence interval	p value
Age (year)	1.03	1.02, 1.05	< 0.001
Male gender	1.39	0.87, 2.22	0.164
Public setting	0.63	0.41, 0.97	0.034
Witnessed CA	0.96	0.39, 2.35	0.931
Bystander CPR	0.76	0.50, 1.16	0.200
Initial VF/VT	0.43	0.26, 0.71	0.001
Collapse to ROSC, per min	1.05	1.03, 1.07	< 0.001
Cardiac cause-related CA	0.48	0.29, 0.80	0.005
Post-resus. shock	1.31	0.89, 1.96	0.181
Base deficit quartiles (mEq/l)			
< 5	1.00	1.00, 1.00	
5–9	1.76	1.07, 2.91	0.026
9–13	3.82	2.20, 6.65	< 0.001
> 13	5.13	2.67, 9.88	< 0.001

CA cardiac arrest; CPR cardiopulmonary resuscitation; ROSC restoration of spontaneous circulation

was associated with ICU mortality in a severity-dependent manner and was also associated with refractory shock. However, we also found that about 10% of patients with a very severe metabolic acidosis (median base deficit > 13.2 mEq/l) survived to ICU discharge with good neurological recovery.

In the present study, metabolic acidosis was severe and strongly determined by the initial cardiac rhythm and the time interval from collapse to ROSC. While several studies have already reported the occurrence of acidosis after cardiac arrest, the present study reports findings from a large cohort of OHCA patients using a reproducible and reliable definition of metabolic acidosis [15–18]. To the best of our knowledge, the present study is the largest study focusing on the prevalence and the prognostic impact of metabolic acidosis in successfully resuscitated OHCA patients. Moreover, several studies reported metabolic acidosis using either pH and/or blood lactate level [19, 20]. This probably includes some patients with exclusive respiratory acidosis, especially in countries where there is no use of advanced airway in the field, and simultaneously misses some patients with compensated metabolic acidosis. This is the reason why we used the base deficit calculation without using pH. Furthermore, the association we observed between severity of metabolic acidosis and both resuscitation duration and initial rhythm may reflect the goodness-of-fit of such a measure with the degree and the duration of inadequate perfusion [21]. Thus, we showed that lactate level was an important contributor of metabolic acidosis but not sufficient to exhaustively describe it [22, 23]. In the present study, acidosis strongly correlated with both lactate level and phosphorus level, highlighting the fact that metabolic acidosis after OHCA is not only related to increase of lactate level but also to accumulation of unmeasured anions partially because of frequent acute kidney injury. This additional finding may explain the association we observed between severity of metabolic acidosis and ICU mortality as acute kidney injury has been demonstrated as an independent marker of ICU mortality after out-of-hospital cardiac arrest [2, 24].

Our findings support a strong association between severity of metabolic acidosis at ICU admission after OHCA and ICU mortality. Interestingly, we were able to provide cause of death and observed that ICU mortality in the most severe patients included in the present study was mostly related to refractory multi-organ failure. The association between metabolic acidosis and ICU mortality has been reported in different subgroups of critically ill patients: trauma [25], sepsis [26] as well as cardiac arrest [27–29]. Nolan et al. [27] reported a significant increase of 45% of in-hospital mortality per 0.1 point of pH decrease below 7.25. In the same manner, Chien et al. [29] reported an odds ratio of survival to hospital discharge of 10 for patients with a pH higher than 7.07 [95% confidence interval 2.1, 47.7]. Although pH is a simple measure to obtain at ICU admission, it does not distinguish metabolic and respiratory acidosis. Indeed, PCO_2 increase after ROSC may largely contribute to acidemia [30, 31]. Thus, we chose to consider base deficit, more likely to reflect metabolic acidosis and ischemia. We evidenced a severity-manner relationship between base

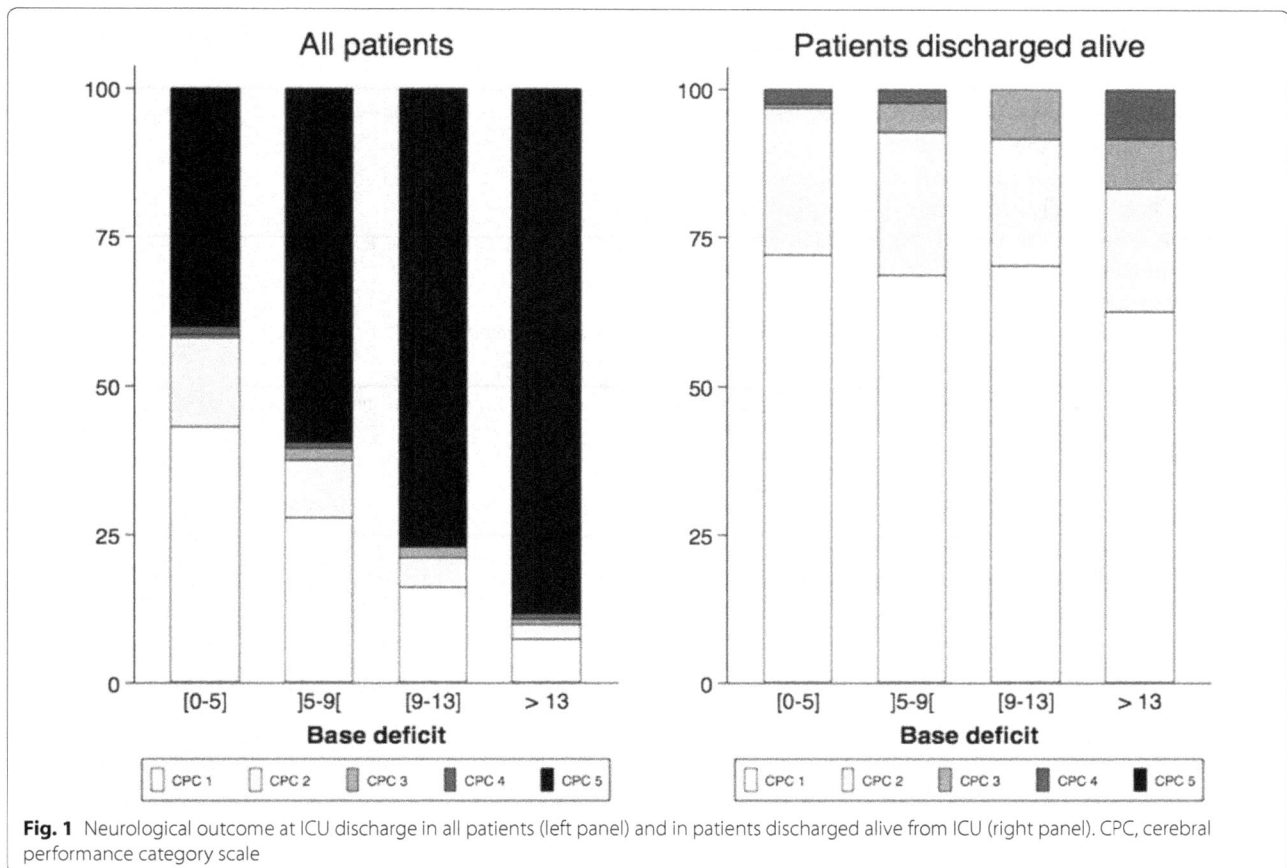

Fig. 1 Neurological outcome at ICU discharge in all patients (left panel) and in patients discharged alive from ICU (right panel). CPC, cerebral performance category scale

deficit and survival to hospital discharge. Physicians may be aware that pH may add information to base deficit, as we observed that patients with acidemia had worse prognosis than those without. These findings are fully consistent with those previously published in some smaller cohorts [17, 28, 32, 33]. Besides the correlation between base deficit and duration of resuscitation efforts, metabolic acidosis may be associated with mortality by its hemodynamic effects, as depression of ventricular function, catecholamine release and reduction of ventricular responsiveness to catecholamines [4]. Interestingly, we did not evidence any relationship between metabolic acidosis and myocardial function, assessed by the left ventricle ejection function. This might suggest that in our cohort, metabolic acidosis may worsen vasoplegia in a more intensive manner and explain the increase of deaths related to refractory shock we observed across the base deficit quartiles.

We observed a survival rate of about 10% in the fourth quartile of base deficit, i.e., in patients with the most severe metabolic acidosis. In 1985, Weil et al. did not observe any survivor with a pH below 7.25 and an arterial lactate level higher than 7 mmol/l. However, this study was published 30 years ago and in-hospital management of successfully resuscitated OHCA patients has greatly improved since this publication [34]. In the study reported by Chien et al., the lowest pH associated with survival was 6.86 while Nolan et al. reported a survival rate of less than 1% below 6.70, about 3% between 6.70 and 6.80 and about 7% between 6.80 and 6.90 [27, 29]. Recently, Ilicki et al. [35] described 6 OHCA survivors with an initial pH lower than 6.90. However, among these cases, 3 had another underlying cause of acidemia (either ketoacidosis or metformin intoxication), and 2 had hemorrhagic shock. The comparison according to vital status at ICU discharge in this subgroup of patients did not evidence any in-hospital factors that could be associated with survival. We were particularly interested in the similar rate of renal replacement therapy in these patients regardless of the vital status at ICU discharge. Despite acidosis severity (almost three quarters of patients received renal replacement therapy within the first 24 h), several patients survived without aggressive treatment of metabolic acidosis and we did not find any additional factor that could differentiate these patients. Moreover, prehospital infusion of bicarbonate appeared to be strongly correlated with ICU mortality and seemed to be a surrogate marker of the severity assessed by the prehospital team.

We acknowledge several limitations in the present study. First, due to the retrospective design, we are not able to confirm the causality of the association we observed. Despite adjustment for prehospital and in-hospital confounders, we cannot be sure that metabolic acidosis might only be a mediator rather than an independent predictor of ICU mortality. Second, we specifically collected information about acidosis of OHCA patients included in analysis previously performed that focused on the prognostic impact of acute kidney injury in this setting [3]. Thus, we were not able to extend the study period beyond 2012. However, we do believe the results we observed would be similar in a more recent cohort. Third, we were not able to collect additional information on the pathogenesis of the metabolic acidosis. We did not collect chloremia, albumin or magnesium level, which could have allowed us to explore more deeply metabolic acidosis mechanisms. Fourth, we did not collect repeated measurements of base deficit, which prevented us to evaluate the prognostic impact of metabolic acidosis correction or acidosis duration. Last, we did not collect renal replacement therapy details, which could partly explain the differences between survivors and patients who died in the fourth quartile of base deficit.

Conclusion

Metabolic acidosis was observed in 95% of OHCA patients admitted to the ICU. Initial rhythm and time interval from collapse to ROSC were independently associated with base deficit. Base deficit was strongly associated with ICU mortality especially from refractory shock but seems to have no impact on neurological recovery in patients who were discharged alive. A substantial proportion of patients admitted with a very severe metabolic acidosis were discharged alive with a good neurological performance.

Abbreviations

OHCA: out-of-hospital cardiac arrest; ICU: intensive care unit; ROSC: return of spontaneous circulation; BLS: basic life support; PCO_2: partial pressure

in carbon dioxide; PO_2: partial pressure in oxygen; KDIGO: kidney disease: improving renal outcome; EMS: emergency medical service; ECG: electrocardiogram; CPC: cerebral performance category score; RRT: renal replacement therapy.

Authors' contributions

MJ, AC and GG designed the study. MJ, OBHS, LG, PD, WB, JC, JPM, FP, AC and GG collected the data. MJ and GG performed the statistical analysis and wrote the manuscript. OBHS, LG, PD, WB, JC, JPM, FP, FD and AC reviewed the manuscript. MJ, AC and GG take responsibility for the integrity of the work. All authors read and approved the final manuscript.

Author details

[1] Medical Intensive Care Unit, Cochin University Hospital (APHP), 27 rue du Faubourg Saint Jacques, 75014 Paris, France. [2] Emergency Department, Cochin University Hospital (APHP), Paris, France. [3] Paris Descartes University, Paris, France. [4] INSERM U970, Sudden Death Expertise Centre, Paris Cardiovascular Research Centre, Paris, France.

Acknowledgements

We thank Nancy Kentish-Barnes for her help in preparing the manuscript.

Competing interests

GG was granted by the French Intensive Care Society, the Assistance Publique Hôpitaux de Paris and by the Schueller-Bettencourt Foundation. The remaining authors have disclosed that they do not have any potential competing interests.

Funding

Not applicable.

References

1.   Neumar RW, Nolan JP, Adrie C, Aibiki M, Berg RA, Böttiger BW, et al. Post-cardiac arrest syndrome: epidemiology, pathophysiology, treatment, and prognostication. A consensus statement from the International Liaison Committee on Resuscitation (American Heart Association, Australian and New Zealand Council on Resuscitation, European Resuscitation Council, Heart and Stroke Foundation of Canada, InterAmerican Heart Foundation, Resuscitation Council of Asia, and the Resuscitation Council of Southern Africa); the American Heart Association Emergency Cardiovascular Care Committee; the Council on Cardiovascular Surgery and Anesthesia; the Council on Cardiopulmonary, Perioperative, and Critical Care; the Council on Clinical Cardiology; and the Stroke Council. Circulation. 2008;118(23):2452–83.
2.   Geri G, Guillemet L, Dumas F, Charpentier J, Antona M, Lemiale V, et al. Acute kidney injury after out-of-hospital cardiac arrest: risk factors and prognosis in a large cohort. Intensive Care Med. 2015;41(7):1273–80.
3.   Wildenthal K, Mierzwiak DS, Myers RW, Mitchell JH. Effects of acute lactic acidosis on left ventricular performance. Am J Physiol. 1968;214(6):1352–9.
4.   Kellum JA, Song M, Venkataraman R. Effects of hyperchloremic acidosis on arterial pressure and circulating inflammatory molecules in experimental sepsis. Chest. 2004;125(1):243–8.
5.   Kellum JA, Song M, Li J. Science review: extracellular acidosis and the immune response: clinical and physiologic implications. Crit Care Lond Engl. 2004;8(5):331–6.
6.   Gunnerson KJ, Saul M, He S, Kellum JA. Lactate versus non-lactate metabolic acidosis: a retrospective outcome evaluation of critically ill patients. Crit Care. 2006;10(1):R22.
7.   Jung B, Rimmele T, Le Goff C, Chanques G, Corne P, Jonquet O, et al. Severe metabolic or mixed acidemia on intensive care unit admission: incidence, prognosis and administration of buffer therapy. A prospective, multiple-center study. Crit Care Lond Engl. 2011;15(5):R238.
8.   Perkins GD, Jacobs IG, Nadkarni VM, Berg RA, Bhanji F, Biarent D, et al. Cardiac arrest and cardiopulmonary resuscitation outcome reports: update of the Utstein Resuscitation Registry Templates for Out-of-Hospital Cardiac Arrest: a statement for healthcare professionals from a task force of the International Liaison Committee on Resuscitation (American Heart Association, European Resuscitation Council, Australian and New Zealand Council on Resuscitation, Heart and Stroke Foundation of Canada, InterAmerican Heart Foundation, Resuscitation Council of Southern Africa, Resuscitation Council of Asia); and the American Heart Association Emergency Cardiovascular Care Committee and the Council on Cardiopulmonary, Critical Care, Perioperative and Resuscitation. Circulation. 2015;132(13):1286–300.

9. Lemiale V, Dumas F, Mongardon N, Giovanetti O, Charpentier J, Chiche J-D, et al. Intensive care unit mortality after cardiac arrest: the relative contribution of shock and brain injury in a large cohort. Intensive Care Med. 2013;39(11):1972–80.

10. Kdigo AKI. Workgorup. KDIGO clinical practice guideline for acute kidney injury. Kidney Int Suppl. 2012;2(1):1.

11. Siggaard-Andersen O. The van Slyke equation. Scand J Clin Lab Investig Suppl. 1977;146:15–20.

12. Morgan TJ, Clark C, Endre ZH. Accuracy of base excess—an in vitro evaluation of the Van Slyke equation. Crit Care Med. 2000;28(8):2932–6.

13. Chelly J, Mongardon N, Dumas F, Varenne O, Spaulding C, Vignaux O, et al. Benefit of an early and systematic imaging procedure after cardiac arrest: insights from the PROCAT (Parisian Region Out of Hospital Cardiac Arrest) registry. Resuscitation. 2012;83(12):1444–50.

14. Jennett B, Bond M. Assessment of outcome after severe brain damage. Lancet Lond Engl. 1975;1(7905):480–4.

15. Spindelboeck W, Gemes G, Strasser C, Toescher K, Kores B, Metnitz P, et al. Arterial blood gases during and their dynamic changes after cardiopulmonary resuscitation: a prospective clinical study. Resuscitation. 2016;106:24–9.

16. Edmonds-Seal J. Acid-base studies after cardiac arrest. A report on 64 cases. Acta Anaesthesiol Scand Suppl. 1966;23:235–41.

17. Langhelle A, Tyvold SS, Lexow K, Hapnes SA, Sunde K, Steen PA. In-hospital factors associated with improved outcome after out-of-hospital cardiac arrest. A comparison between four regions in Norway. Resuscitation. 2003;56(3):247–63.

18. Prause G, Ratzenhofer-Comenda B, Smolle-Jüttner F, Heydar-Fadai J, Wildner G, Spernbauer P, et al. Comparison of lactate or BE during out-of-hospital cardiac arrest to determine metabolic acidosis. Resuscitation. 2001;51(3):297–300.

19. Momiyama Y, Yamada W, Miyata K, Miura K, Fukuda T, Fuse J, et al. Prognostic values of blood pH and lactate levels in patients resuscitated from out-of-hospital cardiac arrest. Acute Med Surg. 2017;4(1):25–30.

20. Chien D-K, Lin M-R, Tsai S-H, Sun F-J, Liu T-C, Chang W-H. Survival prediction of initial blood pH for nontraumatic out-of-hospital cardiac arrest patients in the emergency department. Int J Gerontol. 2010;4(4):171–5.

21. Takasu A, Sakamoto T, Okada Y. Arterial base excess after CPR: The relationship to CPR duration and the characteristics related to outcome. Resuscitation. 2007;73(3):394–9.

22. Makino J, Uchino S, Morimatsu H, Bellomo R. A quantitative analysis of the acidosis of cardiac arrest: a prospective observational study. Crit Care

Lond Engl. 2005;9(4):R357–62.

23. Funk G-C, Doberer D, Sterz F, Richling N, Kneidinger N, Lindner G, et al. The strong ion gap and outcome after cardiac arrest in patients treated with therapeutic hypothermia: a retrospective study. Intensive Care Med. 2009;35(2):232–9.

24. Sandroni C, Dell'anna AM, Tujjar O, Geri G, Cariou A, Taccone FS. Acute kidney injury after cardiac arrest: a systematic review and meta-analysis of clinical studies. Minerva Anestesiol. 2016;82(9):989–99.

25. Rutherford EJ, Morris JA, Reed GW, Hall KS. Base deficit stratifies mortality and determines therapy. J Trauma. 1992;33(3):417–23.

26. Noritomi DT, Soriano FG, Kellum JA, Cappi SB, Biselli PJC, Libório AB, et al. Metabolic acidosis in patients with severe sepsis and septic shock: a longitudinal quantitative study. Crit Care Med. 2009;37(10):2733–9.

27. Nolan JP, Laver SR, Welch CA, Harrison DA, Gupta V, Rowan K. Outcome following admission to UK intensive care units after cardiac arrest: a secondary analysis of the ICNARC Case Mix Programme Database. Anaesthesia. 2007;62(12):1207–16.

28. Grubb NR, Elton RA, Fox KA. In-hospital mortality after out-of-hospital cardiac arrest. Lancet Lond Engl. 1995;346(8972):417–21.

29. Chien D-K, Chang W-H, Tsai S-H, Chang K-S, Chen C-C, Su Y-J. Outcome on non-traumatic out-of-hospital cardiac arrest in the elderly. Int J Gerontol. 2008;2(2):60–6.

30. Kim Y-J, Lee YJ, Ryoo SM, Sohn CH, Ahn S, Seo D-W, et al. Role of blood gas analysis during cardiopulmonary resuscitation in out-of-hospital cardiac arrest patients. Medicine (Baltimore). 2016;95(25):e3960.

31. Yannopoulos D, Matsuura T, McKnite S, Goodman N, Idris A, Tang W, et al. No assisted ventilation cardiopulmonary resuscitation and 24-hour neurological outcomes in a porcine model of cardiac arrest. Crit Care Med. 2010;38(1):254–60.

32. Maupain C, Bougouin W, Lamhaut L, Deye N, Diehl J-L, Geri G, et al. The CAHP (Cardiac Arrest Hospital Prognosis) score: a tool for risk stratification after out-of-hospital cardiac arrest. Eur Heart J. 2016;37(42):3222–8.

33. Martinell L, Nielsen N, Herlitz J, Karlsson T, Horn J, Wise MP, et al. Early predictors of poor outcome after out-of-hospital cardiac arrest. Crit Care Lond Engl. 2017;21(1):96.

34. Weil MH, Grundler W, Yamaguchi M, Michaels S, Rackow EC. Arterial blood gases fail to reflect acid–base status during cardiopulmonary resuscitation: a preliminary report. Crit Care Med. 1985;13(11):884–5.

35. Ilicki J, Djärv T. Reply to Letter: Survival in extremely acidotic cardiac arrest patients depends on etiology of acidosis. Resuscitation. 2017;113:e25.

Permissions

List of Contributors

Constantine J. Karvellas
Division of Gastroenterology (Liver Unit), Department of Critical Care Medicine, University of Alberta, 1-40 Zeidler Ledcor Building, Edmonton, AB T6G-2X8, Canada

Jaime L. Speiser
Department of Public Health Sciences, Medical University of South Carolina, Charleston, SC, USA

Mélanie Tremblay and Christopher F. Rose
Hepato-Neuro Laboratory, CRCHUM, Université de Montréal, Montreal, Canada

William M. Lee
Division of Digestive and Liver Diseases, Department of Internal Medicine, University of Texas Southwestern Medical Center, Dallas, TX, USA

Gretchen L. Sacha, Simon W. Lam, Heather Torbic, Stephanie N. Bass, Sarah C. Welch and Seth R. Bauer
Department of Pharmacy, Cleveland Clinic, 9500 Euclid Avenue (Hb-105), Cleveland, OH 44195, USA

Abhijit Duggal
Respiratory Institute, Cleveland Clinic, Cleveland, OH, USA

Robert S. Butler
Department of Quantitative Health Sciences, Cleveland Clinic, Cleveland, OH, USA

Hui-Bin Huang, Jin-Min Peng, Li Weng, Chun-Yao Wang, Wei Jiang and Bin Du
Medical ICU, Peking Union Medical College Hospital, Peking Union Medical College and Chinese Academy of Medical Sciences, 1 Shuai Fu Yuan, Beijing 100730, People's Republic of China

Hui-Bin Huang
Department of Critical Care Medicine, The First Affiliated Hospital of Fujian Medical University, Fuzhou, China

Maryse A. Wiewel, Brendon P. Scicluna, Lonneke A. van Vught, Arie J. Hoogendijk and Tom van der Poll
Center for Experimental and Molecular Medicine, Academic Medical Center, University of Amsterdam, Meibergdreef 9, Room G2-130, 1105 AZ Amsterdam, The Netherlands
The Center for Infection and Immunity Amsterdam, Academic Medical Center, University of Amsterdam, Meibergdreef 9, 1105 AZ Amsterdam, The Netherlands

Brendon P. Scicluna and H. Zwinderman
Department of Clinical Epidemiology, Bioinformatics, and Biostatistics, Academic Medical Center, University of Amsterdam, Meibergdreef 9, 1105 AZ Amsterdam, The Netherlands

René Lutter
Department of Respiratory Medicine and Experimental Immunology, Academic Medical Center, University of Amsterdam, Meibergdreef 9, 1105 AZ Amsterdam, The Netherlands

Janneke Horn and Marcus J. Schultz
Department of Intensive Care, Academic Medical Center, University of Amsterdam, Meibergdreef 9, 1105 AZ Amsterdam, The Netherlands

Olaf L. Cremer
Department of Intensive Care Medicine, University Medical Center Utrecht, Heidelberglaan 100, 3584 CX Utrecht, The Netherlands

Marc J. Bonten
Julius Center for Health Sciences and Primary Care, University Medical Center Utrecht, Heidelberglaan 100, 3584 CX Utrecht, The Netherlands
Department of Medical Microbiology, University Medical Center Utrecht, Heidelberglaan 100, 3584 CX Utrecht, The Netherlands

Tom van der Poll
Division of Infectious Diseases, Academic Medical Center, University of Amsterdam, Meibergdreef 9, 1105 AZ Amsterdam, The Netherlands

Thibault Duburcq, Arthur Durand, Mercedes Jourdain, Sebastien Préau, Erika Parmentier-Decrucq, Daniel Mathieu, Julien Poissy and Raphaël Favory
Centre de Réanimation - Rue Emile Laine, CHU de Lille – Hôpital R Salengro, 59037 Lille Cedex, France

Valery Gmyr, François Pattou and Mercedes Jourdain
INSERM U1190 Translational Research for Diabetes, Univ Lille, 59000 Lille, France
European Genomic Institute for Diabetes, 59000 Lille, France

Antoine Tournoys and Viviane Gnemmi
Centre de Biologie Pathologie, CHU Lille, 59000 Lille, France

Fabienne Tamion and Emmanuel Besnier
Medical Intensive Care Unit, Rouen University Hospital, Rouen, France

Arthur Durand and Raphaël Favory
LIRIC Inserm U995 Glycation: From Inflammation to Aging, 59000 Lille, France

Luigi Pisani, Jan-Paul Roozeman, Fabienne D. Simonis, Antonio Giangregorio, Sophia M. van der Hoeven, Laura R. Schouten, Janneke Horn, Ary Serpa Neto, Arjen M. Dondorp, Lieuwe D. Bos and Marcus J. Schultz
Department of Intensive Care, Academic Medical Center, Meibergdreef 9, 1105 AZ Amsterdam, The Netherlands

Fabienne D. Simonis, Sophia M. van der Hoeven, Lieuwe D. Bos and Marcus J. Schultz
Laboratory of Experimental Intensive Care and Anesthesiology (LEICA), Academic Medical Center, Amsterdam, The Netherlands

Salvatore Grasso
Anesthesia and Intensive Care Unit, Department of Emergency and Organ Transplantation, University of Bari Aldo Moro, Bari, Italy

Laura R. Schouten
Department of Pediatrics, Academic Medical Center, Amsterdam, The Netherlands

Lieuwe D. Bos
Department of Pulmonology, Academic Medical Center, Amsterdam, The Netherlands

Ary Serpa Neto
Department of Critical Care Medicine, Hospital Israelita Albert Einstein, São Paulo, Brazil

Emir Festic
Pulmonary and Critical Care Medicine, Mayo Clinic, Jacksonville, FL, USA

Luigi Pisani, Arjen M. Dondorp and Marcus J. Schultz
Mahidol–Oxford Research Unit (MORU), Faculty of Tropical Medicine, Mahidol University, Bangkok, Thailand

Jean Louis Trouillet
Service de Réanimation, Groupe Hospitalier Pitié-Salpêtrière, Assistance Publique-Hôpitaux de Paris, Paris, France

Olivier Collange
Hôpitaux Universitaires de Strasbourg, Nouvel Hôpital Civil, Pôle d'Anesthésie-Réanimation Chirurgicale, SAMU, SMUR, NHC, 1 Place de l'Hôpital, 67000 Strasbourg, France
EA 3072, FMTS, Université de Strasbourg, Strasbourg, France

Fouad Belafia
Intensive Care Unit and Department of Anesthesiology, Research Unit INSERM U1046, University of Montpellier Saint Eloi Hospital and Montpellier School of Medicine, Montpellier, France

François Blot
Medical-Surgical Intensive Care Unit, Gustave Roussy Cancer Campus, Villejuif, France

Franck Jegoux
Service ORL et Chirurgie Cervico-maxillo-Faciale, CHU PONTCHAILLOU, Rue H. Le Guilloux, 35033 Rennes Cedex 9, France

Erwan L'Her
LaTIM INSERM UMR 1101, Université de Bretagne Occidentale, Rue Camille Desmoulins, 29200 Brest Cedex, France
Médecine Intensive et Réanimation, CHRU de Brest, Boulevard Tanguy Prigent, 29200 Brest Cedex, France

Sebastien Vergez
ORL Chirurgie Cervicofaciale, CHU Toulouse Rangueil-Larrey, 24 chemin de Pouvourville, 31059 Toulouse Cedex 9, France

Julien Amour
Département d'Anesthésie et de Réanimation Chirurgicale, Institut de Cardiologie, Groupe Hospitalier Pitié-Salpêtrière, 47-83 Boulevard de l'Hôpital, 75013 Paris, France

Max Guillot
EA 3072,FMTS, Université de Strasbourg, Strasbourg, France
Hôpitaux Universitaires de Strasbourg, Hôpital de Hautepierre, Réanimation Médicale, Avenue Molière, 67200 Strasbourg, France

Renato Carneiro de Freitas Chaves, Thiago Domingos Corrêa, Ary Serpa Neto, Bruno de Arruda Bravim, Ricardo Luiz Cordioli, Fabio Tanzillo Moreira, Karina Tavares Timenetsky and Murillo Santucci Cesar de Assunção
Intensive Care Unit, Hospital Israelita Albert Einstein, Av. Albert Einstein, 627/701, 5th Floor, São Paulo, SP 05651-901, Brazil

Thiago Domingos Corrêa
Intensive Care Unit, Hospital Municipal Dr. Moysés Deutsch - M'Boi Mirim, São Paulo, SP, Brazil

Ary Serpa Neto
Department of Intensive Care, Academic Medical Center, University of Amsterdam, Amsterdam, The Netherlands

Christos Filis
3rd Department of Internal Medicine, "Sotiria" Hospital, National and Kapodistrian University of Athens, 152 Mesogion Av., 115 27 Athens, Greece

Ioannis Vasileiadis and Antonia Koutsoukou
Intensive Care Unit, 1st Department of Respiratory Medicine, "Sotiria" Hospital, National and Kapodistrian University of Athens, 152 Mesogion Av., 115 27 Athens, Greece

Guo-guang Ma, Guang-wei Hao, Xiao-mei Yang, Du-ming Zhu, Lan Liu, Hua Liu, Guo-wei Tu and Zhe Luo
Department of Critical Care Medicine, Zhongshan Hospital, Fudan University, No. 180 Fenglin Road, Shanghai 200032, Xuhui District, People's Republic of China

Maria Giuseppina Annetta, Davide Silvestri, Domenico Luca Grieco, Alessio Maccaglia, Giovanna Mercurio, Anselmo Caricato and Massimo Antonelli
Department of Anesthesia and Intensive Care, Fondazione Policlinico Universitario 'A.Gemelli', Largo A.Gemelli, 8, 00168 Rome, Italy

Mauro Pittiruti
Department of Surgery, Fondazione Policlinico Universitario 'A.Gemelli', Rome, Italy

Michele Fabio La Torre and Nicola Magarelli
Department of Radiology, Fondazione Policlinico Universitario 'A.Gemelli', Rome, Italy

Andreas Drolz, Thomas Horvatits, Kevin Roedl, Karoline Rutter, Richard Brunner, Christian Zauner, Michael Trauner, Bruno Schneeweiss and Valentin Fuhrmann
Division of Gastroenterology and Hepatology, Department of Internal Medicine III, Medical University of Vienna, Vienna, Austria

Andreas Drolz, Thomas Horvatits, Kevin Roedl, Karoline Rutter and Valentin Fuhrmann
Department of Intensive Care Medicine, University Medical Center, Hamburg-Eppendorf, Martinistraße 52, 20246 Hamburg, Germany

Peter Schellongowski
Division of Oncology and Infectious Diseases, Department of Internal Medicine I, Medical University of Vienna, Vienna, Austria

Gottfried Heinz
Division of Cardiology, Department of Internal Medicine II, Medical University of Vienna, Vienna, Austria

Georg-Christian Funk
Department of Respiratory and Critical Care Medicine, and Ludwig Boltzmann Institute for COPD, Otto-Wagner Hospital, Vienna, Austria

Ferran Roche-Campo, Alexandre Bedet, Emmanuel Vivier, Laurent Brochard and Armand Mekontso Dessap
Service de Réanimation Médicale, DHU A-TVB, Hôpitaux Universitaires Henri Mondor, Assistance Publique – Hôpitaux de Paris, 51 Avenue du Maréchal de Lattre de Tassigny, 94010 Créteil Cedex, France

Ferran Roche-Campo
Servei de Medicina Intensiva, Hospital Verge de la Cinta, Tortosa, Tarragona, Spain

Alexandre Bedet and Armand Mekontso Dessap
Groupe de Recherche Clinique CARMAS, Institut Mondor de Recherche Biomédicale, Faculté de Médecine de Créteil, Université Paris Est Créteil, 94010 Créteil, France

Emmanuel Vivier
Service de Réanimation Polyvalente, Centre hospitalier Saint-Joseph Saint-Luc, Lyon, France

Laurent Brochard
Keenan Research Centre and Critical Care Department, St Michael's Hospital, Toronto, Canada
Interdepartmental Division of Critical Care Medicine, University of Toronto, Toronto, Canada

Jordi Vallés, Susana Millán, Emili Díaz, Ignacio Martín-Loeches, Paula Saludes, Jorge Lema, Montse Batlle, Néstor Bacelar and Antoni Artigas
Critical Care Department, Hospital-Sabadell, Corporació Sanitària Universitària Parc Taulí, ParcTauli s/n, 08208 Sabadell, Spain

Jordi Vallés, Antoni Artigas and Antoni Artigas
Universitat Autonoma Barcelona, Sabadell, Spain

Jordi Vallés, Emili Díaz, Ignacio Martín-Loeches, Antoni Artigas and Antoni Artigas
CIBERES Enfermedades Respiratorias, Valladolid, Spain

Eva Castanyer, Xavier Gallardo, Marta Andreu and Mario Prenafeta
UDIAT, Hospital Universitari Parc Taulí, Sabadell, Spain

Christine K. Federspiel
Division of Nephrology, Department of Medicine, University of California, San Francisco, San Francisco, CA 94143-0532, USA

Christine K. Federspiel, Theis S. Itenov and Morten H. Bestle
Department of Anesthesiology, Nordsjællands Hospital, University of Copenhagen, Copenhagen, Denmark

Kala Mehta
Department of Epidemiology and Biostatistics, University of California, San Francisco, San Francisco, USA

Raymond K. Hsu
Division of Nephrology, Department of Medicine, University of California, San Francisco, San Francisco, USA

Kathleen D. Liu
Divisions of Nephrology and Critical Care Medicine, Departments of Medicine and Anesthesia, University of California, San Francisco, San Francisco, CA 94143-0532, USA

Benoit Pilmis
Service de maladies infectieuses et tropicales, Hôpital Necker Enfants malades, Service de maladies infectieuses et tropicales, Université Paris Descartes, Paris, France
Equipe mobile de microbiologie clinique, Groupe Hospitalier Paris Saint-Joseph, Paris, France

Vincent Jullien
Service de Pharmacologie, Hôpital Européen Georges Pompidou, Université Paris Descartes, Paris, France
INSERM U1129, Paris, France

Alexis Tabah
Intensive Care Unit, The Redcliffe Hospital, Brisbane, Australia
Burns, Trauma and Critical Care Research Centre, The University of Queensland, Brisbane, Australia

Jean-Ralph Zahar
Département de Microbiologie Clinique, Unité de Contrôle et de Prévention du risque Infectieux, Groupe Hospitalier Paris Seine Saint-Denis, AP-HP, CHU Avicenne, 125 rue de Stalingrad, 9300 Bobigny, France
Infection Control Unit, IAME, UMR 1137, Université Paris 13, Sorbonne Paris Cité, Paris, France

Christian Brun-Buisson
Réanimation médicale, Hôpital Henri Mondor, Université Paris Est Créteil (UPEC), Créteil, France

Karim Jaffal, Julien Poissy, Anahita Rouze, Sébastien Preau, Boualem Sendid, Marjorie Cornu and Saad Nseir
Critical Care Center, CHU Lille, 59000 Lille, France

Julien Poissy, Anahita Rouze, Sébastien Preau, Boualem Sendid, Marjorie Cornu and Saad Nseir
U995-LIRIC-Lille Inflammation Research International Center, Univ. Lille, 59000 Lille, France

Julien Poissy, Anahita Rouze, Sébastien Preau, Boualem Sendid, Marjorie Cornu and Saad Nseir
Inserm, U995, 59000 Lille, France

Boualem Sendid and Marjorie Cornu
Laboratory of Mycology and Parasitology, CHU Lille, 59000 Lille, France

Keyvan Razazi, Faten May, Nicolas de Prost, Christian Brun-Buisson and Guillaume Carteaux
AP-HP, DHU A-TVB, Service de Réanimation Médicale, Hôpitaux Universitaires Henri Mondor, 94010 Créteil, France

Keyvan Razazi, Sébastien Jochmans, Faten May, Nicolas de Prost, Christian Brun-Buisson, Guillaume Carteaux and Armand Mekontso Dessap
Faculté de Médecine de Créteil, IMRB, GRC CARMAS, Université Paris Est Créteil, 94010 Créteil, France

Keyvan Razazi, Keyvan Razazi and Armand Mekontso Dessap
Unité U955 (Institut Mondor de Recherche Biomédicale), INSERM, Créteil, France

Florence Boissier
Service de Réanimation Médicale, Centre Hospitalier Universitaire de Poitiers, Poitiers 86021, France
AP-HP, Service de Réanimation Médicale, Hôpital Européen Georges Pompidou, 75015 Paris, France

Mathilde Neuville
AP-HP, Réanimation Médicale et des Maladies Infectieuses, Hôpital Bichat Claude Bernard, Paris, France

Sébastien Jochmans
Département de Médecine Intensive, Groupe Hospitalier Sud Ile-de-France, Hôpital de Melun, 77011 Melun, France

Martial Tchir
Service de Réanimation, Centre Hospitalier de Villeneuve-Saint-Georges, 94190 Villeneuve-Saint-Georges, France

Claudia Scorcella, Elisa Damiani, Roberta Domizi, Silvia Pierantozzi, Stefania Tondi, Andrea Carsetti, Silvia Ciucani, Valentina Monaldi, Mara Rogani, Benedetto Marini, Erica Adrario, Rocco Romano and and Abele Donati
Anaesthesia and Intensive Care, Department of Biomedical Sciences and Public Health, Università Politecnica delle Marche, via Tronto 10/a, 60126 Ancona, Italy

Can Ince
Department of Translational Physiology, Academic Medical Centre, University of Amsterdam, Meibergdreef 9, 1105 AZ Amsterdam, The Netherlands

E. Christiaan Boerma
Department of Intensive Care, Medical Centre Leeuwarden, Henri Dunantweg 2, 8934 AD Leeuwarden, The Netherlands

Sylvain Jean-Baptiste, Jonathan Messika, Stéphane Gaudry, Didier Dreyfuss and Jean-Damien Ricard
Medico-Surgical Intensive Care Unit, AP-HP, Hôpital Louis Mourier, 178 rue des Renouillers, 92700 Colombes, France

Jonathan Messika, Didier Dreyfuss and Jean-Damien Ricard
IAME, UMR 1137, INSERM, 75018 Paris, France
IAME, UMR 1137, Univ Paris Diderot, Sorbonne Paris Cité, 75018 Paris, France

David Hajage
Département de Biostatistiques, Santé Publique et Information Médicale, AP-HP, Hôpital Pitié-Salpêtrière, 75013 Paris, France
Univ Pierre et Marie Curie, Sorbonne Universités, 75013 Paris, France

David Hajage and Stéphane Gaudry
ECEVE, U1123, CIC-EC 1425, INSERM, 75010 Paris, France
ECEVE, UMRS 1123, Univ Paris Diderot, Sorbonne Paris Cité, 75010 Paris, France

Julie Barbieri and Benoit Coffin
Gastroenterology Unit, AP-HP, Hôpital Louis Mourier, 178 rue des Renouillers, 92700 Colombes, France

Henri Duboc and Benoit Coffin
Univ Paris Diderot, Sorbonne Paris Cité, 75018 Paris, France

Xiukai Chen
Pittsburgh Heart, Lung, Blood and Vascular Medicine Institute, University of Pittsburgh, 200 Lothrop Street, BST E1240, Pittsburgh, PA 15261, USA

Xiaoting Wang and Dawei Liu
Department of Critical Care Medicine, Peking Union Medical College Hospital, Peking Union Medical College, Chinese Academy of Medical Sciences, 1 Shuaifuyuan, Dongcheng District, Beijing 100073, China

Patrick M. Honore
Department of Intensive Care, Centre Hospitalier Universitaire Brugmann, Brugmann University Hospital, 4 Place Van Gehuchtenplein, 1020 Brussels, Belgium

Herbert D. Spapen
Department of Intensive Care, University Hospital, Vrije Universiteit Brussel (VUB), 101, Laarbeeklaan, Jette 1090 Brussels, Belgium

Matthieu Jamme, Omar Ben Hadj Salem, Lucie Guillemet, Pierre Dupland, Wulfran Bougouin, Julien Charpentier, Jean-Paul Mira, Frédéric Pène, Alain Cariou and Guillaume Geri
Medical Intensive Care Unit, Cochin University Hospital (APHP), 27 rue du Faubourg Saint Jacques, 75014 Paris, France

Florence Dumas
Emergency Department, Cochin University Hospital (APHP), Paris, France

Matthieu Jamme, Omar Ben Hadj Salem, Lucie Guillemet,Florence Dumas, Alain Cariou and Guillaume Geri
Paris Descartes University, Paris, France

Wulfran Bougouin, Florence Dumas, Alain Cariou and Guillaume Geri
INSERM U970, Sudden Death Expertise Centre, Paris Cardiovascular Research Centre, Paris, France

Index

www.ingramcontent.com/pod-product-compliance
Lightning Source LLC
Chambersburg PA
CBHW061243190326
41458CB00011B/3563